Student Workbook for

Modern Dental Assisting

Fourteenth Edition

Debbie S. Robinson, CDA, MS
Former Research Assistant Professor,
Department of Nutrition,
Gilling's School of Global Public Health
Former Research Assistant, and Project Coordinator, UNC-CH Adams School of Dentistry,
Former Director, Dental Assisting and Dental Assisting Specialty Program,
UNC-CH Adams, School of Dentistry

ELSEVIER

Elsevier
3251 Riverport Lane
St. Louis, Missouri 63043

STUDENT WORKBOOK FOR MODERN DENTAL ASSISTING,
FOURTEENTH EDITION

Notice

Practitioners and researchers must always rely on their own experience and knowledge in evaluating
and using any information, methods, compounds or experiments described herein. Because of rapid
advances in the medical sciences, in particular, independent verification of diagnoses and drug dosages
should be made. To the fullest extent of the law, no responsibility is assumed by Elsevier, authors, editors
or contributors for any injury and/or damage to persons or property as a matter of products liability,
negligence or otherwise, or from any use or operation of any methods, products, instructions, or ideas
contained in the material herein.

Previous editions copyrighted 2021, 2018, 2015, 2012, 2009, 2005, 2002, 1999, 1995, 1990, 1985, 1980, and 1976.

Senior Content Strategist: Kelly Skelton
Senior Content Development Specialist: Rebecca M. Leenhouts
Publishing Services Manager: Deepthi Unni
Project Manager: Sheik Mohideen K
Design Direction: Amy Buxton

Printed in India

Last digit is the print number: 9 8 7 6 5 4 3 2 1

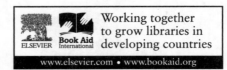

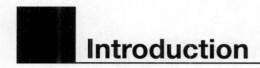

Introduction

The student workbook is designed to prepare you for the preclinical, clinical, and administrative procedures presented in *Modern Dental Assisting,* Fourteenth Edition (MDA 14). The pages can be easily removed for assignment submission and placed in your notebook with corresponding lecture notes. Workbook chapters relate directly to the chapters in the textbook, with each containing questions and exercises to help you practice, comprehend, and master the chapter content.

CHAPTER EXERCISES

Chapters include a variety of exercises: short answer questions derived from the learning outcomes; fill-in-the-blank statements from the key terms; multiple-choice questions that parallel the recall questions; and case studies and activities that draw from additional chapter topics to draw knowledge from other chapters and the *Interactive Dental Office,* which is located on the companion Evolve website. Answers to the workbook exercises are available from your instructor.

In addition to the exercises, you will also find cordinated video clips noted at the back of a chapter under "Electronic Resources" to view on the companion Evolve site. We have also incorporated Dentrix software into the office practice management exercises in the following chapters (26, 28, 62, and 63). You will be introduced to both the business and clinical areas of dentistry by providing practice exercises on how to use the system, in addition to exercises that incorporate the patients from the *Interactive Dental Office.*

COMPETENCY SHEETS

Competency is a method used to evaluate mastery of preclinical, clinical, administrative, and advanced skills. The competency sheets are designed to give you the opportunity to practice a skill until mastered. A space on the form allows for three different evaluations: self, peer, and instructor and/or dentist. The evaluation system provides an objective grading scale, which reflects a step-by-step competency for each procedure at all levels. A space for reviewer comments is available, along with an area for documentation of evaluation, date, and grade. Each procedure from the textbook has a corresponding competency sheet which appears individually so that it can be submitted to your instructor or supervisor as completed.

CLINICAL EXTERNSHIP GUIDE

A clinical externship is an integral part of your education. We are excited to include this in MDA 14 Workbook, the "Dental Assisting Clinical Externship Guide." The content in this section observes the CODA Accreditation Standards that are required for a student to gain competence by having a minimum of 300 hours of clinical experience in two or more offices with fifty percent in a general practice setting.

The material includes an organized method to document assigned externship sites; required time sheets to be maintained; a record of clinical activities and business office skills; a student journal of clinical activity; and seminar content for discussion.

FLASHCARDS

Flashcards included with the workbook are made up of key terms and information from the textbook. They include knowledge on the sciences, medical emergencies, infection control, radiography, dental materials, instruments, and general and specialty dental procedures. You can use the flashcards as a bonus study tool.

We wish you much success in your studies and your chosen profession of dental assisting!

Debbie S. Robinson

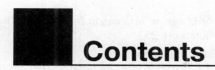

Contents

1 History of Dentistry

SHORT-ANSWER QUESTIONS

1. Describe the role of Hippocrates in history.

2. State the basic principle of the Hippocratic Oath.

3. Name the first woman to graduate from a college of dentistry.

4. Name the first woman to practice dentistry in the United States.

5. Name the first African American woman to receive a dental degree in the United States.

6. Name the first African American to receive the DMD degree from Harvard University.

7. Discuss the contributions of Horace H. Hayden and Chapin A. Harris.

8. Describe two major contributions of G. V. Black.

9. Name the first dentist to employ a dental assistant.

10. Name the first Native American Indian dentist.

11. Name the scientist who discovered x-rays.

12. Name the physician who first used inhalation sedation for tooth extractions.

13. Discuss the purpose and activities of the National Museum of Dentistry.

FILL-IN-THE-BLANK STATEMENTS

Select the best term from the list below and complete the following statements.

forensic dentistry
Ida Gray-Rollins
Saint Apollonia
Paul Revere
preceptorship
Wilhelm Conrad Roentgen

1. _____ was the first dental assistant.

2. Studying under the guidance of one already in the profession is referred to as a _____.

3. _____ known as the 'Patroness of Dentistry' for those suffering a dental problem.

4. _____ was an American silversmith by trade, and amateur dentist because of his skills.

5. _____ discovered radiographs.

6. _____ was the first African-American woman in the United States to earn a formal DDS degree.

MULTIPLE-CHOICE QUESTIONS

Complete each question by circling the best answer.

1. Hesi-Re was _____.
   a. the first female dentist
   b. the earliest recorded dentist
   c. the first dental assistant
   d. the first dental hygienist

2. Dental disease dates back to the _____
   a. nineteenth century
   b. eighteenth century
   c. ancient betinnings
   d. renaissance

3. Who is considered "The Father of Medicine"?
   a. Hippocrates
   b. G. V. Black
   c. Pierre Fauchard
   d. Paul Revere

4. What does the Hippocratic Oath promise?
   a. To heal all
   b. To treat dental problems in patients of all ages
   c. To act ethically and refrain from doing harm
   d. To include dentistry in medicine

5. What type of dental procedures did the Romans practice?
   a. Oral hygiene
   b. Gold crowns
   c. Tooth extraction
   d. All of the above

6. Which artist first distinguished different types of teeth in the mouth?
   a. Claude Monet
   b. Leonardo da Vinci
   c. Vincent van Gogh
   d. Peter Max

2

Chapter **1 History of Dentistry**

7. Who is referred to as the *father of surgery?*
   a. Ambroise Paré
   b. Hippocrates
   c. G. V. Black
   d. Pierre Fauchard

8. Who is referred to as the *father of modern dentistry?*
   a. Ambroise Paré
   b. Hippocrates
   c. G. V. Black
   d. Pierre Fauchard

9. Who was John Greenwood's famous patient?
   a. Paul Revere
   b. George Washington
   c. Leonardo da Vinci
   d. Hippocrates

10. Which famous colonial patriot first used forensic evidence?
    a. Paul Revere
    b. George Washington
    c. Abraham Lincoln
    d. Betsy Ross

11. The nineteeth century is credited as _____ in dentistry?
    a. A guild of Barbers
    b. Age of Reason
    c. Industrial Growth
    d. The Birth of a profession

12. Who is credited with establishing the first dental school in America?
    a. Chapin Harris
    b. Horace Wells
    c. G. V. Black
    d. Edmund Kells

13. Who discovered x-rays*?*
    a. Chapin Harris
    b. Horace Wells
    c. Wilhelm Conrad Roentgen
    d. Edmund Kells

14. Who is credited with employing the first dental assistant?
    a. Chapin Harris
    b. Horace Wells
    c. G. V. Black
    d. Edmund Kells

15. The first dentist to use inhalation anesthesia in dentistry was _____.
    a. Chapin Harris
    b. Horace Wells
    c. G. V. Black
    d. Edmund Kells

16. Who was the first female dentist in the United States?
    a. Emeline Roberts-Jones
    b. Lucy B. Hobbs-Taylor
    c. G. V. Black
    d. W. B. Saunders

17. Who was the first woman to graduate from dental school?
    a. Emmeline Roberts-Jones
    b. Lucy B.Hobbs-Taylor
    c. G. V. Black
    d. W. B. Saunders

18. Where is the National Museum of Dentistry located?
    a. New Orleans, Louisiana
    b. San Francisco, California
    c. Baltimore, Maryland
    d. Seattle, Washington

19. In what year was the first edition of *Modern Dental Assisting* published?
    a. 1982
    b. 1973
    c. 1976
    d. 1981

20. In what year was Robert Tanner Freeman accepted at Harvard Dental school?
    a. 1867
    b. 1900
    c. 1928
    d. 1865

ACTIVITY

The practice of dentistry has changed dramatically over the past 50 years. To compare the dental experiences of various generations, ask the following questions of one or two people in each of the following age groups: 15 to 25, 26 to 40, and 55 years and older. Compare and analyze their answers to see how dentistry and people's perceptions about dentistry have changed.

Questions to Ask

1. How do you feel about going to the dentist?

2. Do you expect to keep all of your teeth throughout your life? Why or why not?

3. What is the biggest change you have noticed in receiving dental care during your life?

4. What are your feelings about the profession of dentistry?

2 | The Dental Healthcare Team

SHORT-ANSWER QUESTIONS

1. List the members of the dental healthcare team and explain the role of each in a dental practice.

2. Describe the minimal educational requirements for each dental healthcare team member.

3. Name and describe each recognized dental specialty.

FILL-IN-THE-BLANK STATEMENTS

Select the best term from the list below and complete the following statements.

dental assistant
dental hygienist
dental laboratory technician
dental public health
dentist
endodontist
oral and maxillofacial radiology

oral and maxillofacial surgery
oral pathology
orthodontics
pediatric dentistry
periodontics
prosthodontics

1. An auxilary who is qualified to provide chairside support to the dentist is a(n) _____.

2. The specialty concerned with the diagnosis and treatment of the supporting structures of the tooth is _____.

3. The specialty concerned with the use of advanced imaging to detect tumors and disease of the jaws, head, and neck is _____.

4. A(n) _____ is a practioner qualified in the prevention, diagnosis and treatment of teeth.

5. A profession that fabricates replacements of teeth specified by a written prescription from the dentist is a(n) _____.

6. A(n) _____ is a licensed auxiliary who provides preventive, therapeutic, and educational care.

7. The specialty of promoting dental health through organized community efforts is _____.

8. _____ is the specialty that is concerned with diseases of the oral structures.

9. A(n) _____ is one who specializes in diseases of the pulp.

10. _____ is the diagnosis and surgical treatment of diseases, injuries and defects of the head and neck regions.

11. _____ is the specialty that is concerned with the correction of malocclusions.

12. _____ is the specialty that is concerned with the restoration and replacement of natural teeth.

13. _____ is the area of dentistry that specializes in children from birth through adolescence.

MULTIPLE-CHOICE QUESTIONS

Complete each question by circling the best answer.

1. Who would not be considered a member of the dental healthcare team?
   a. Dental hygienist
   b. Dental supply company
   c. Dental laboratory technician
   d. Dental assistant

2. What is the minimal length of education for dental hygiene licensure?
   a. 1 academic year
   b. 2 academic years
   c. 3 academic years
   d. 4 academic years

3. What is the minimal length of education for an ADA-accredited dental assisting program?
   a. 1 academic year
   b. 2 academic years
   c. 3 academic years
   d. 4 academic years

4. What is the minimal length for an ADA-accredited dental laboratory technician program?
   a. 1 academic year
   b. 2 academic years
   c. 3 academic years
   d. 4 academic years

5. What must a dental laboratory technician receive from the dentist before fabricating and delivering an indirect restoration or prosthesis?
   a. The patient record
   b. A text from the dentist
   c. A prescription from the dentist
   d. A drawing of the indirect restoration or prosthesis

ACTIVITY

As a dental assisting student, you are embarking on an exciting career with many opportunities awaiting you after graduation. It is not too early to think about the career choices you will make. After reading Chapter 2, answer the following questions to help you formulate long-term career goals.

1. What attracted you to select dental assisting as a career choice?

2. Are you interested in continuing your education to become a dental hygienist, dentist or dental specialist? Which specialty and why?

3 The Professional Dental Assistant

SHORT-ANSWER QUESTIONS

1. Describe the difference between being a professional and being an employee.

2. Describe the characteristics of a professional dental assistant.

3. Describe the personal qualities of a dental assistant.

4. Describe how your personal characteristics meet the qualities of a good dental assistant.

5. Identify career opportunities for the educationally qualified dental assistant.

6. Describe the role of the Dental Assisting National Board.

7. Describe the purpose of the American Dental Assistants Association.

8. Describe the benefits of membership in the American Dental Assistants Association.

FILL-IN-THE-BLANK STATEMENTS

Select the best term from the list below and complete the following statements.

American Dental Assistants Association
Certified Dental Assistant
Dental Assisting National Board
Professional

1. The professional organization that represents the profession of dental assisting is the _____.

2. The national agency that is responsible for administering the certification examination and issuing certification is the

_____.

7

3. The credential earned who has passed the certification examination and remains current through continuing education is a _____.

4. A _____ is a person who does a job that requires special training, education and skill.

MULTIPLE-CHOICE QUESTIONS

Complete each question by circling the best answer.

1. The essentials of professional appearance include _____.
   a. good health
   b. good grooming
   c. appropriate dress
   d. all of the above

2. How does a professional demonstrate responsibility?
   a. Arriving on time
   b. Volunteering to help
   c. Being cooperative
   d. All of the above

3. What is the purpose of the ADAA?
   a. To advance the careers of dental assistants
   b. To promote the dental assisting profession
   c. To enhance the delivery of high-quality dental healthcare
   d. All of the above

4. What credential is issued by the DANB?
   a. Registered dental assistant
   b. Certified dental assistant
   c. Licensed dental assistant
   d. Bachelor's degree

5. What pathway of certification is available for an international DDS?
   a. Pathway I
   b. Pathwayy II
   c. Pathway III
   d. All of the above

6. The position of the dental assistant that can legally provide intraoral functions is the _____.
   a. Administrative assistant
   b. Circulating assistant
   c. Expanded function assistant
   d. Sterilization assistant

ACTIVITIES

1. Go to https://www.danb.org/About-DANB/News-and-Events/Press-Releases and review the topics of the most recent postings. Which of the topics interest you and why.

2. Engage your classmates in a discussion of the personal and professional characteristics they think would be desirable and nondesirable in a dental assistant. Explain why each of the desirable characteristics is important.

3. As the patient of your personal dental practice, what characteristics of the dental assistant impress you the most?

4 Ethics and Code of Conduct in Dentistry

SHORT-ANSWER QUESTIONS

1. Explain the basic principles of ethics.

2. State the Code of Ethics of the American Dental Assistants Association.

3. Explain the difference between being "legal" and being "ethical."

4. Identify sources of early learning of ethics.

5. Describe the model for ethical decision making.

FILL-IN-THE-BLANK STATEMENTS

Select the best term from the list below and complete the following statements.

autonomy
code of ethics
ethics
veracity
nonmaleficence

1. _____ equates to truthfulness.

2. Voluntary standards of behavior established by a profession are a(n) _____.

3. _____ is self-determination.

4. _____ are moral standards of conduct and rules or principles that govern proper conduct.

5. _____ is to do no harm to the patient.

MULTIPLE-CHOICE QUESTIONS

Complete each question by circling the best answer.

1. A basic principle of ethics is _____.
   a. autonomy
   b. justice
   c. non-maleficence
   d. all of the above

2. What is established as a guide to professional behavior?
   a. Code of conduct
   b. Code of ethics
   c. Code of honor
   d. Code of medicine

3. Ethics are _____.
   a. required by law
   b. open to individual interpretation
   c. settled by court decisions
   d. clear and direct

4. What does the ethical principle of non-maleficence mean?
   a. The right of privacy
   b. To help others
   c. To treat people fairly
   d. To do no harm

5. Confidentiality refers to a person's
   a. Beneficence
   b. Autonomy
   c. Justtice
   d. Veracity

ACTIVITIES

1. Aside from the examples in your textbook, provide an example for each of the following ethical principles and describe how each example could relate to a situation in your dental assisting class.
   - Principle of justice

   - Principle of autonomy

   - Principle of beneficence

   - Principle of nonmaleficence

2. In small groups, each group develop a specific Code of Ethics for your dental assisting class. Present these to each group to discuss and agree to abide by. How do you think these specific codes will affect the class dynamics for the coming year?

5 Dentistry and the Law

SHORT-ANSWER QUESTIONS

1. What is the purpose of the Dental Practice Act?

2. Describe the types of supervision for the certified dental assistant.

3. Give an example that could be considered patient abandonment.

4. Give an example of contributory negligence in the dental practice.

5. Give examples of civil law and criminal law in the dental profession.

6. What is the difference between written and implied consent?

7. Describe the procedure for documenting informed consent.

8. Explain when it is necessary to obtain an informed refusal.

9. Describe the exceptions for disclosure.

10. What is the role of the dental team regarding child abuse and neglect.

FILL-IN-THE-BLANK STATEMENTS

Select the best term from the list below and complete the following statements.

abandonment	**implied contract**
Board of Dentistry	**licensure**
civil law	**malpractice**
contract law	**mandated reporter**
criminal law	**patient of record**
dental auxiliary	**reciprocity**
direct supervision	*res gestae*
due care	*res ipsa loquitur*
expanded function	*respondeat superior*
expressed contract	**state Dental Practice Act**
general supervision	**written consent**
implied consent	

1. A(n) _____ is a term to describe the dental assistant, a dental hygienist, or a dental laboratory technician.

2. A(n) _____ is an individual who has been examined, diagnosed, and treatment planned by the dentist.

3. _____ is a level of supervision in which the dentist is physically present.

4. A(n) _____ is an intraoral function delegated to an auxiliary that requires the additional skill and training before performing it.

5. _____ is a legal doctrine that holds the employer liable for the acts of the employee.

6. The _____ protects the public from incompetent dental health care providers.

7. _____ is each state's agency that adopts rules and regulations and implements the state Dental Practice Act.

8. _____ gives a person the legal right to practice in a specific state.

9. _____ is the category of law that deals with the relations of individuals or corporations.

10. _____ is a system that allows individuals in one state to obtain a license in another state without retesting.

11. Terminating the dentist–patient relationship without a reasonable notice to the patient is _____.

12. _____ is just, proper, and sufficient care or the absence of negligence.

13. _____ category of law that involves violations against the state or government.

14. _____ is a level of supervision in which the dentist has given instructions but does not need not be physically present.

15. _____ is professional negligence.

16. _____ is the patient's action indicating agreement to undergo treatment.

17. Binding agreements involve _____.

18. A contract that is verbal or written is a(n) _____.

19. A contract that is established by actions and not words is a(n) _____.

20. _____ includes a written explanation of the diagnostic findings, the prescribed treatment, and the reasonable expectations regarding the results of treatment.

21. _____ is a statement that is made at the time of an alleged negligent act and is admissible as evidence in a court of law.

22. A(n) _____ is a professional who is required by state law to report known or suspected child abuse.

23. _____ means that the act speaks for itself.

MULTIPLE-CHOICE QUESTIONS

Complete each question by circling the best answer.

1. The purpose of being licensed is _____.
   a. to make more money
   b. to protect the public from incompetent practitioners
   c. to keep count of the number of professionals in the field
   d. to have laws to follow

2. Who interprets the state Dental Practice Act?
   a. The governor of the state
   b. The American Dental Association
   c. The state legislature
   d. The state dental board

3. Reciprocity allows a licensed practitioner to _____.
   a. treat patients from another practice
   b. prescribe drugs
   c. practice in another state
   d. specialize in another field of dentistry

4. *Respondeat superior* states that _____.
   a. a patient can be seen by another dentist without records
   b. an employer is responsible for the actions of his or her employees
   c. a dentist can treat patients in another state
   d. a dentist can specialize and practice that specialty

5. If a dentist is physically present when a dental auxiliary is performing an expanded function, the dentist is providing _____.
   a. direct supervision
   b. physical supervision
   c. general supervision
   d. legal supervision

6. When a dentist discontinues treatment after it has begun, the dentist has implemented _____.
   a. a felony
   b. abuse
   c. abandonment
   d. a disservice

7. When can a dentist refuse to treat a patient with HIV infection?
   a. When the staff does not want to treat patients with HIV infection
   b. Under no conditions
   c. When the patient has a dental condition that would be better treated by a specialist
   d. All of the above

8. When a patient receives proper sufficient care, he or she is receiving _____.
   a. poor care
   b. due care
   c. professional care
   d. dental care

9. A category of law can include _____.
   a. civil
   b. professional
   c. contract
   d. a and c

10. Which is a type of contract?
    a. Professional
    b. Expressed
    c. Implied
    d. b and c

11. How would a professional prevent a malpractice suit?
    a. Have the patient be seen by another dentist
    b. Practice prevention and communication with the patient
    c. Have a lawyer meet with the patient
    d. Schedule appointments further apart

12. Which of the following components is/are necessary for a malpractice suit to occurr?
    a. Duty of care
    b. Dereliction in treatment
    c. Direct cause
    d. All of the above

13. What term describes an alleged negligent act and is admissible as evidence in a court of law?
    a. *Res ipsa loquitur*
    b. *Res gestae*
    c. Pro bono
    d. Due care

14. A patient that enters a dental office is demonstrating

    _____.
    a. implied consent
    b. verbal consent
    c. written consent
    d. legal consent

15. To provide evidence, where would a broken appointment be recorded?
    a. daily schedule
    b. ledger
    c. patient record
    d. recall list

16. What is the objective of reporting a suspected case of child abuse?
    a. To start legal proceedings
    b. To have documentation
    c. To protect the child from further abuse
    d. To punish the abuser

17. Who are considered "mandated reporters" in reporting abuse or neglect?
    a. Professionals required by state law to report known or suspected cases of child abuse
    b. Reporters from a newspaper following a story
    c. Individuals elected to give advice
    d. Written documents on known or suspected cases of child abuse

ACTIVITIES

1. Obtain a copy of your state Dental Practice Act and review the regulations that are critical for dental assistants.

2. Obtain a list of the expanded functions delegated in your state and identify the types of supervision necessary for each function.

3. Describe the practice limitations for a dental assistant in your state.

6 | General Anatomy

SHORT-ANSWER QUESTIONS

1. Explain the difference between anatomy and physiology.

2. Describe the imaginary planes and associated body directions used to divide the body into sections.

3. The body is organized at different units. Name the four units.

4. Identify and describe the components of a cell.

5. Identify and describe the four types of tissues in the human body.

6. Name and give location of the two major body cavities.

FILL-IN-THE-BLANK STATEMENTS

Select the best term from the list below and complete the following statements.

anatomic position	distal	parietal
anatomy	epithelial	physiology
anterior	horizontal plane	proximal
appendicular	medial	stem cells
axial	midsagittal plane	superior
cranial cavity	nucleus	visceral
cytoplasm	organelle	

1. _____ is the study of the shape and structure of the human body.

2. _____ is the study of the functions of the human body.

3. The body is in the _____ when it is erect and facing forward with arms at the sides and the palms facing up.

4. The _____ is a vertical plane that divides the body into equal left and right halves.

5. The _____ divides the body into superior (upper) and inferior (lower) portions.

6. The gel-like fluid inside the cell is _____.

7. A specialized part of the cell that performs a definite function is an _____.

8. The _____ is the control center of a cell.

9. The _____ is a cavity that houses the brain.

10. _____ is a type of tissue that forms the covering for all body surfaces.

11. _____ is a part that is above another portion, or closer to the head.

12. _____ means toward the front.

13. _____ means toward, or nearer to, the midline of the body.

14. _____ means the part is closer to the trunk of the body.

15. _____ is the opposite of proximal, the part that is farther away from the trunk of the body.

16. _____ pertains to internal organs or the covering of organs.

17. Closer to point of attachment, or to trunk of body _____.

18. The region of the body that consists of the arms and legs is the _____.

19. _____ are immature, unspecialized cells capable of replication and differentiation into other types of cells or tissues.

20. _____ pertains to the walls of a body cavity.

MULTIPLE-CHOICE QUESTIONS

Complete each question by circling the best answer.

1. Anatomy is the study of _____.
   a. function
   b. form and structure
   c. internal organs
   d. veins and arteries

2. Physiology is the study of _____.
   a. function
   b. form and structure
   c. internal organs
   d. veins and arteries

3. The imaginary line that divides the body into upper and lower portions is the _____.
   a. frontal
   b. midsagittal
   c. horizontal
   d. lateral

4. The imaginary line that divides the body into equal right and left halves is the _____.
   a. frontal
   b. midsagittal
   c. horizontal
   d. lateral

5. _____ is the portion of the cell that carries genetic information.
   a. Cytoplasm
   b. Cell wall
   c. Mitochondria
   d. Nucleus

6. Body tissues that bind and support other tissues are _____.
   a. epithelial
   b. muscle
   c. connective
   d. nerve

7. The organizational levels of the body are cells, tissues, organs, and _____.
   a. bones
   b. systems
   c. brain
   d. reproductive

8. The two major cavities in the body are _____.
   a. sagittal and ventral
   b. dorsal and median
   c. cranial and thoracic
   d. dorsal and ventral

9. The axial portion of the body consists of the _____.
   a. head
   b. neck
   c. trunk
   d. all of the above

10. The appendicular portion of the body consists of the _____.
    a. head
    b. arms
    c. legs
    d. b and c

11. What is the simplest organizational level of the human body?
    a. Tissues
    b. Organs
    c. Body systems
    d. Cells

12. The federal government's lead agency for scientific research on oral, dental, and craniofacial disease is the _____.
    a. FDA
    b. EPA
    c. NIDCR
    d. OSHA

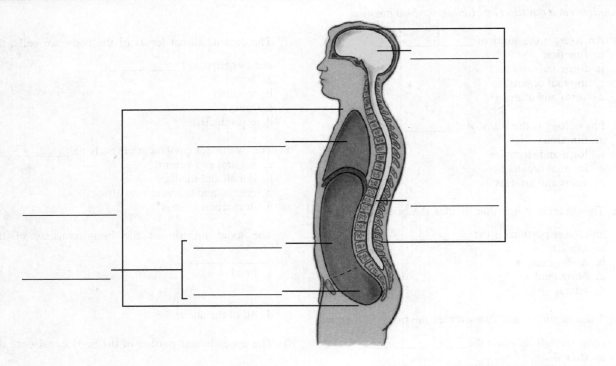

(From Applegate EJ: The anatomy and physiology learning system, ed 4, St Louis, Saunders, 2011.)

1. Label the illustration of the body cavities.
   a. Cranial cavity

   b. Ventral cavity

   c. Dorsal cavity

   d. Pelvic cavity

   e. Thoracic cavity

   f. Spinal cavity

   g. Abdominal cavity

   h. Abdominopelvic cavity

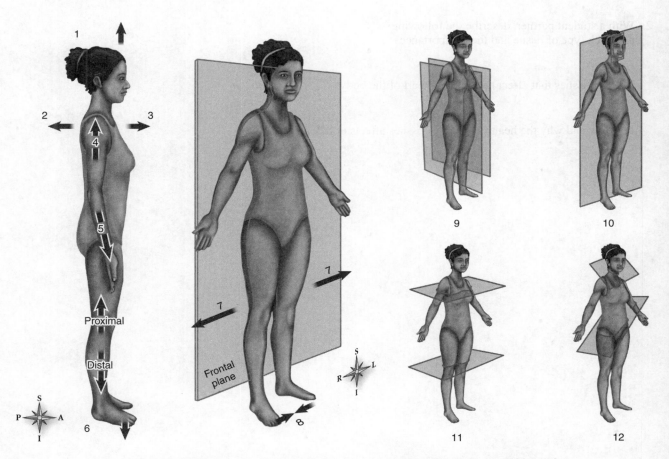

(From Patton KT, Thibodeau GA: Structure & function of the body, ed 16, St. Louis, 2020, Mosby)

2. Label the body in anatomical position.

   a. Transverse plane (transverse)
   b. Lateral view
   c. Superior
   d. Frontal plane (coronal)
   e. Medial view

   f. Inferior
   g. Proximal
   h. Anterior
   i. Sagittal planes
   j. Posterior

ACTIVITIES

1. With a student partner, discuss why the study of general anatomy is important for a dental assistant. Try to think of at least five reasons.

2. With a student partner, describe the following:
   a. Each type of tissue and their importance

   b. The tissues that affect the orofacial part of the body

   c. How and why the health of various tissues affects oral health

7 General Physiology

SHORT-ANSWER QUESTIONS

1. Name each body system.

2. Give the purpose of each body system.

3. Describe the components of each body system.

4. Explain how each body system functions.

5. Describe the signs and symptoms of common disorders related to each body system.

6. Give examples of conditions that require the interaction of body systems.

FILL-IN-THE-BLANK STATEMENTS

Select the best term from the list below and complete the following statements.

appendicular skeleton	**muscle insertion**
arteries	**muscle origin**
suture	**neurons**
axial skeleton	**osteoblasts**
cancellous bone	**pericardium**
cartilage	**periosteum**
central nervous system	**peripheral nervous system**
compact bone	**peristalsis**
integumentary system	**Sharpey fibers**
involuntary muscles	**veins**
joints	

1. The portion of the skeleton that consists of the skull, spinal column, ribs, and sternum is the _____.

2. The portion of the skeleton that consists of the upper extremities, the shoulder girdle plus the lower extremities and pelvic girdle is the _____.

3. _____ is a specialized connective tissue that covers all bones of the body.

4. Cells that are associated with bone formation are _____.

5. _____ anchors the periosteum to the bone.

6. _____ forms the outer layer of bones, where it is needed for strength.

7. The _____ is the lighter bone found in the interior of bones.

8. _____ is a tough connective, nonvascular, elastic tissue.

9. Structural areas where two or more bones come together are _____.

10. _____ is a term used when bones articulate and form a joint.

11. _____ are muscles that function automatically, without conscious control.

12. The location where the muscle begins is the _____.

13. The location where the muscle ends is the _____.

14. The _____ is a double-walled sac that encloses the heart.

15. Blood vessels that carry blood away from the heart are _____.

16. Blood vessels that carry blood to the heart are _____.

17. The _____ is composed of the brain and spinal cord.

18. The _____ is composed of the cranial nerves and spinal nerves.

19. _____ direct nerve impulses.

20. A rhythmic action that moves food through the digestive tract is _____.

21. The _____ involves the skin.

MULTIPLE-CHOICE QUESTIONS

Complete each question by circling the best answer.

1. The skeleton is divided into axial and _____ sections.
   a. peripheral
   b. appendicular
   c. frontal
   d. parietal

2. The connective tissue that covers all bones is the _____.
   a. nervous
   b. muscle
   c. epithelial
   d. periosteum

3. The two types of bone are compact and _____.
   a. cortical
   b. trabeculae
   c. cancellous
   d. periosteum

4. Cartilage is found _____
   a. outside of bones
   b. where bones join
   c. inside of bones
   d. in the teeth

5. Another term for the articulation of bones that form a jagged line is a _____
   a. cartilage
   b. bone
   c. bone marrow
   d. suture

6. Which of the following is/are type(s) of muscle tissue?
   a. Smooth
   b. Skeletal
   c. Cardiac
   d. All of the above

7. Which muscle is striated in appearance but resembles smooth muscle in action?
   a. Smooth
   b. Striated
   c. Cardiac
   d. Skeletal

8. Which of the following is a muscular disorder?
   a. Contusion
   b. Endocarditis
   c. Multiple sclerosis
   d. Gout

9. A function of the circulatory system is _____.
   a. to transport nutrients and oxygen to body cells
   b. to transport carbon dioxide to body cells
   c. to regulate body temperature and chemical stability
   d. a and c

10. The heart chambers consist of the atria and _____.
   a. pulmonic
   b. aortic
   c. mitral
   d. ventricles

11. Which of the following is/are function(s) of a blood vessel?
   a. To carry blood away from the heart
   b. To connect the arterial and venous system
   c. To carry blood toward the heart
   d. All of the above

12. The primary function of the lymph system is to _____.
   a. carry blood away from the heart
   b. provide the body with nutrients
   c. regulate body temperature and chemical stability
   d. rid body of toxins, waste, and and harmful microorganisms

13. What make(s) up the lymph system?
   a. Lymph vessels
   b. Lymph nodes
   c. Lymph fluid
   d. All of the above

14. What system(s) is considered the cummunication system of the body
   a. Central nervous system
   b. Autonomic nervous system
   c. Peripheral nervous system
   d. a and c

15. The peripheral nervous system is divided into the autonomic and _____ nervous systems.
   a. somatic
   b. autonomic
   c. peripheral
   d. central

16. The type of neuron that carries impulses toward the brain and spinal cord is _____.
   a. associative
   b. motor
   c. sensory
   d. synapse

17. The main function of the respiratory system is _____.
   a. to carry blood throughout the body
   b. to deliver oxygen to the body
   c. to give the body the ability to move
   d. to contribute to the immune system

18. What is the role of the digestive system?
   a. It breaks down the food you eat for energy
   b. To deliver oxygen to the body
   c. To give the body the ability to move
   d. To contribute to the immune system

19. Which is not an action of the digestive system?
   a. Ingestion
   b. Sensory function
   c. Movement
   d. Absorption

20. The primary function of the endocrine system is to:
   a. Control growth
   b. Deliver oxygen to the body
   c. Form and eliminate urine
   d. Regulate the body's activities with hormones

21. The primary function of the urinary system is to;
   a. Transport oxygen to cells
   b. Defend against disease
   c. Eliminate waste from the body
   d. Regulate body temperature

22. Which body system includes the skin?
   a. Skeletal
   b. Integumentary
   c. Nervous
   d. Muscular

23. Which of the following is an example of an appendage?
   a. Hair
   b. Nails
   c. Glands
   d. All of the above

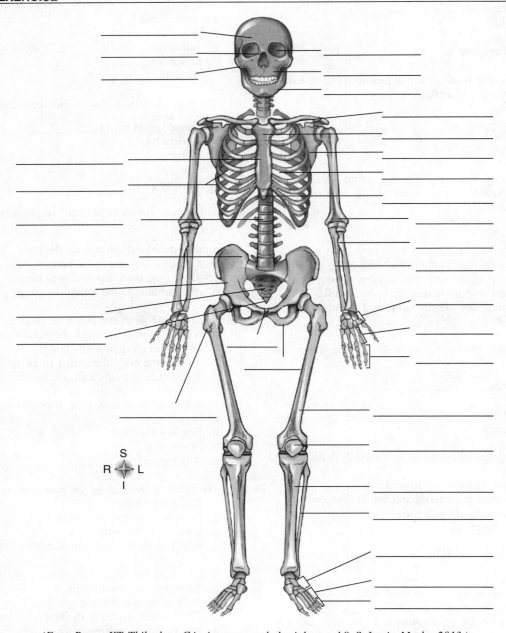

(From Patton KT, Thibodeau GA: Anatomy and physiology, ed 8, St Louis, Mosby, 2013.)

1. Label the bones in the skeletal system.

a. Greater trochanter	l. Ribs	w. Radius
b. Metatarsals	m. Costal cartilage	x. Ilium
c. Manubrium	n. Xiphoid process	y. Sacrum
d. Nasal bone	o. Femur	z. Carpals
e. Zygomatic bone	p. Orbit	aa. Metacarpals
f. Ulna	q. Vertebral column	bb. Pubis
g. Mandible	r. Phalanges	cc. Ischium
h. Tarsals	s. Fibula	dd. Sternum
i. Frontal bone	t. Coccyx	ee. Patella
j. Clavicle	u. Humerus	ff. Tibia
k. Scapula	v. Coxal (hip) bone	gg. Maxilla

ACTIVITY

Exercise is an important factor in good health. Aerobic exercise is a good way to stay healthy, and increase the efficiency of the body's intake of oxygen. It is recommended that everyone exercise 20 minutes a day, three to five times a week.

To find your optimum level of exertion, subtract your age from the number 220 and then multiply the result by 85%. This gives you the maximum heart rate for your age. To see whether you are achieving the maximum level of exertion, take your pulse for 15 seconds immediately after exercising.

8 Oral Embryology and Histology

1. Define *embryology* and *histology*.

2. Describe the three periods of prenatal development.

3. Describe the steps in the formation of the palate.

4. List the stages in the development of a tooth.

5. What genetic and environmental factors can affect dental development?

6. Explain the difference between the clinical and the anatomic crown.

7. Name and describe the types of tissues within a tooth.

8. Name and describe the three types of dentin.

9. Describe the structure and location of the dental pulp.

10. Name and describe the components of the periodontium.

11. Describe the functions of the periodontal ligaments.

12. Describe the types of oral mucosa and give an example of each.

FILL-IN-THE-BLANK STATEMENTS

Select the best term from the list below and complete the following statements.

ameloblasts	masticatory mucosa
cementoblasts	odontoblasts
cementoclasts	osteoclasts
conception	periodontium
embryology	prenatal development
embryonic period	stratified squamous epithelium
exfoliation	succedaneous
histology	

1. _____ is the study of prenatal development.

2. _____ is the study of the structure and function of tissues on a microscopic level.

3. _____ begins at the start of pregnancy and continues until birth.

4. The _____ extends from the beginning of the second week to the end of the eighth week.

5. The union of the male sperm and the ovum of the female is _____.

6. _____ teeth are permanent teeth with primary predecessors; examples are the anterior teeth and premolars.

7. The tissues that support the teeth in the alveolar bone are _____.

8. Enamel-forming cells are _____.

9. _____ are dentin-forming cells.

10. _____ are cementum-forming cells.

11. Cells that resorb cementum are _____.

12. _____ are cells that resorb bone.

13. The normal process of shedding primary teeth is _____.

14. Oral mucosa is made up of _____.

15. Oral mucosa that covers the hard palate, dorsum of the tongue, and gingiva is _____.

MULTIPLE-CHOICE QUESTIONS

Complete each question by circling the best answer.

1. Name the first period of prenatal development.
   a. Embryonic period
   b. Fetal period
   c. Preimplantation period
   d. Embryo

2. Which period of prenatal development is the most critical?
   a. Embryonic period
   b. Fetal period
   c. Preimplantation period
   d. Embryo

3. The embryonic layer that differentiates into cartilage, bones, and muscles is _____.
   a. endoderm
   b. ectoderm
   c. mesoderm
   d. phisoderm

4. Which branchial arch forms the bones, muscles, and nerves of the face and the lower lip?
   a. First
   b. Second
   c. Third
   d. Fourth

5. Which branchial arch forms the sides and front of the neck?
   a. First
   b. Second
   c. Third
   d. Fourth

6. The hard and soft palates are formed by the union of the primary and secondary _____.
   a. maxillary processes
   b. premaxilla
   c. palates
   d. palatine processes

7. When does the development of the human face occur in prenatal period?
   a. Second and third week
   b. Third and fourth week
   c. Fifth to eighth week
   d. Ninth to twelfth week

8. Which of the following environmental influences during pregnancy may cause anomalies?
   a. Infections
   b. Drugs
   c. Exposure to radiation
   d. All of the above

9. What factor(s) can have a prenatal influence on dental development?
   a. Genetics
   b. Environment
   c. Physical causes
   d. a and b

10. Name the process for the laying down or adding of bone.
    a. Deposition
    b. Discharge
    c. Resorption
    d. Drift

11. Name the process of bone loss or removal.
    a. Deposition
    b. Discharge
    c. Resorption
    d. Drift

12. Growth, calcification, and _____ are the three primary periods in tooth formation.
    a. bud
    b. eruption
    c. cap
    d. bell

13. The final stage in the growth period is the _____.
    a. bud
    b. cap
    c. bell
    d. calcification

14. Dentin that forms before eruption and makes up the bulk of the tooth is _____?
    a. Secondary dentin
    b. Primary dentin
    c. Tertiary dentin
    d. Prenatal dentin

15. What is the name of the process by which teeth move into a functional position in the oral cavity?
    a. Eruption
    b. Exfoliation
    c. Development
    d. Resorption

16. The portion of a tooth that is visible in the mouth is the _____.
    a. anatomic crown
    b. enamel crown
    c. facial crown
    d. clinical crown

17. The cementoenamel junction is located _____.
    a. on the occlusal surface
    b. between the dentin and the enamel
    c. between the pulp and the cementum
    d. between the cementum and the enamel

18. _____ is the hardest substance in the human body.
    a. bone
    b. enamel
    c. dentin
    d. cartilage

19. What is the the largest mineral component in enamel?
    a. Calcium
    b. Magnesium
    c. Iron
    d. Palladium

20. Pain is transmitted through dentin by way of _____.
    a. dentinal tubules
    b. dentinal fibers
    c. odontoblasts
    d. nerves

21. The type of dentin that is also known as *reparative dentin* is _____.
    a. primary dentin
    b. secondary dentin
    c. tertiary dentin
    d. odontoblasts

22. The pulp is made up of _____.
    a. blood vessels
    b. bone
    c. nerves
    d. a and c

23. What types of cells form the intercellular substance of the pulp?
    a. Odontoblasts
    b. Fibroblasts
    c. Cementoblasts
    d. Dentinoblasts

24. The primary function of the periodontium is _____.
    a. to support the tooth
    b. to maintain the tooth
    c. to retain the tooth
    d. all of the above

25. Which type of oral mucosa forms the inside of the cheeks, lips, and soft palate?
    a. Masticatory mucosa
    b. Specialized mucosa
    c. Lining mucosa
    d. Gingival mucosa

LABELING EXERCISES

1. Label the illustration of a dental pulp.

    a. Coronal pulp
    b. Pulp horns
    c. Accessory canal
    d. Apical foramen
    e. Radicular pulp

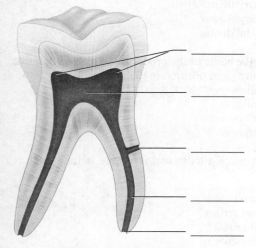

(© Elsevier Collection.)

30

2. Label the illustration of the periodontium.

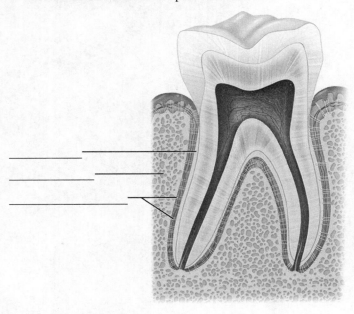

(© Elsevier Collection.)

    a. Cementum
    b. Alveolar bone
    c. Periodontal ligament

TOPICS FOR DISCUSSION

Expectant parents wonder whether their child will be male or female, will be tall or short, or will have brown eyes or blue. Many expectant parents do not realize that all of these attributes are determined at the instant of conception. All expectant parents want a healthy baby to be born. Ask your friends or relatives who have children the following questions. If they cannot answer them, perhaps you can answer for them.

Questions to Ask

1. Which trimester is the most critical for the development of the baby?

2. By which week of pregnancy are all of the primary teeth developed?

3. Is it safe to take drugs or drink alcohol during pregnancy?

4. What does the baby look like 1 month after conception?

5. What is the rule of thumb in determining a delivery date?

Chapter **8 Oral Embryology and Histology**

9 Head and Neck Anatomy

SHORT-ANSWER QUESTIONS

1. List the regions of the head.

2. List the bones of the cranium and face.

3. List the muscles of the head and neck.

4. Give the circulatory routes of the blood vessels in the head and neck.

5. List the components of the temporomandibular joint.

6. Describe the action of the temporomandibular joint.

7. Give the locations of the major and minor salivary glands and associated ducts.

8. Describe and locate the divisions of the trigeminal nerve.

9. Give the location of the major lymph node sites of the body.

10. Give the location of the paranasal sinuses of the skull.

11. Describe how your knowledge of head and neck anatomy can enlighten your clinical practice.

FILL-IN-THE-BLANK STATEMENTS

Select the best term from the list below and complete the following statements.

abducens nerve
articular space
buccal
circumvallate lingual papillae
cranium
greater palatine nerve
infraorbital region
lacrimal bones

masseter muscle
occipital region
parotid duct
salivary glands
sternocleidomastoid
temporomandibular disorder
temporomandibular joint
trapezius

1. The eight bones that cover and protect the brain are the _____.

2. The _____ nerve serves the posterior hard palate and the posterior lingual gingiva.

3. _____ surface pertains to structures closest to the inner cheek.

4. Large tissue projections on the tongue are _____.

5. The region of the head that is located below the orbital region is the _____.

6. Paired facial bones that help form the medial wall of the orbit are the _____.

7. The _____ is the strongest and most obvious muscle of mastication.

8. The _____ is the region of the head overlying the occipital bone and covered by the scalp.

9. The _____ produce saliva.

10. One of the cervical muscles that divides the neck region into anterior and posterior cervical triangles is the _____.

11. The space between the capsular ligament and the surfaces of the glenoid fossa and the condyle is the _____.

12. The _____ is the sixth cranial nerve, which serves the eye muscle.

13. A joint on each side of the head that allows for movement of the mandible is the _____.

14. _____ is a disease process associated with the TMJ.

15. The _____ is one of the cervical muscles that lifts the clavicle and scapula to shrug the shoulder.

16. The _____ is associated with the parotid salivary gland, which opens into the oral cavity at the parotid papilla.

MULTIPLE-CHOICE QUESTIONS

Complete each question by circling the best answer.

1. The regions of the head include the frontal, parietal, occipital, temporal, orbital, nasal, infraorbital, buccal, oral, mental, and _____.
   a. mandible
   b. maxilla
   c. zygomatic
   d. lacrimal

2. What bone forms the forehead?
   a. Occipital
   b. Frontal
   c. Parietal
   d. Zygomatic

3. What bone forms the back and base of the cranium?
   a. Parietal
   b. Temporal
   c. Occipital
   d. Frontal

4. Which bone forms the cheek?
   a. Sphenoid
   b. Zygomatic
   c. Temporal
   d. Nasal

5. Which bones form the upper jaw and hard palate?
   a. Zygomatic
   b. Sphenoid
   c. Mandible
   d. Maxilla

6. Name the only movable bone of the skull.
   a. Coronoid process
   b. Temporal
   c. Mandible
   d. Maxilla

7. Where is the mental foramen located?
   a. Maxilla
   b. Coronoid process
   c. Mandible
   d. Glenoid process

8. What are the basic types of movement of the temporo-mandibular joint?
   a. Up and down
   b. Hinge and glide
   c. Side to side
   d. Back and forth

9. What type of sign or symptom may a patient who is experiencing temporomandibular disorder exhibit?
   a. Migraine
   b. Nausea
   c. Fever
   d. Pain

10. Which cranial nerve innervates all muscles of mastication?
    a. Third
    b. Fourth
    c. Fifth
    d. Sixth

11. What is the name of the horseshoe-shaped bone where the muscles of the tongue and the floor of the mouth attach?
    a. Hyoid
    b. Sphenoid
    c. Mandible
    d. Vomer

12. Which of the major salivary glands is the largest?
    a. Submandibular
    b. Sublingual
    c. Parotid
    d. Submaxillary

13. What is another name for the parotid duct?
    a. Duct of Rivinus
    b. von Ebner's salivary gland
    c. Wharton's duct
    d. Stensen's duct

14. Which artery is behind the ramus and has five branches?
    a. Infraorbital artery
    b. Facial artery
    c. Inferior alveolar artery
    d. Lingual artery

15. Which artery supplies the maxillary molars, premolar teeth, and gingiva?
    a. Inferior alveolar artery
    b. Posterior superior alveolar artery
    c. Facial artery
    d. Lingual artery

16. How many pairs of cranial nerves are connected to the brain?
    a. 4 pairs
    b. 6 pairs
    c. 10 pairs
    d. 12 pairs

17. Which division of the trigeminal nerve subdivides into the buccal, lingual, and inferior alveolar nerves?
    a. Mandibular division
    b. Facial division
    c. Lingual division
    d. Maxillary division

18. In which type of dental examination would lymph nodes be palpated?
    a. Physical examination
    b. Intraoral examination
    c. Extraoral examination
    d. Radiographic examination

19. What is the term for enlarged or palpable lymph nodes?
    a. Lymphadenopathy
    b. Xerostomia
    c. Parkinson's disease
    d. Lymphitis

LABELING EXERCISES

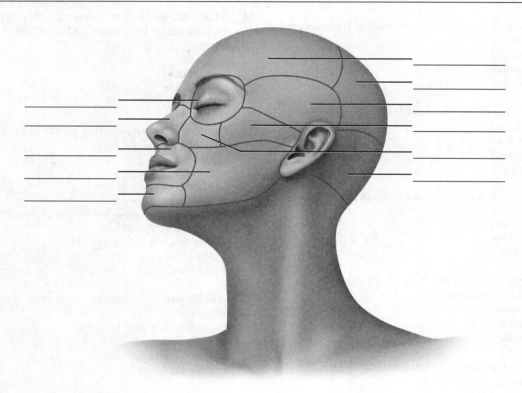

(© Elsevier Collection.)

1. Label the regions of the head.
    a. Zygomatic
    b. Frontal
    c. Oral
    d. Mental
    e. Occipital
    f. Parietal
    g. Nasal
    h. Buccal
    i. Infraorbital
    j. Temporal
    k. Orbital

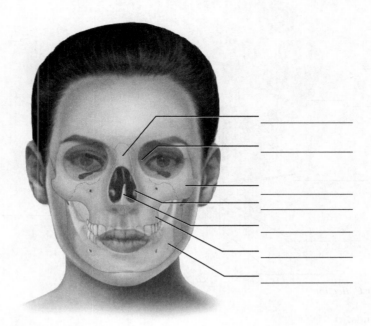

(© Elsevier Collection.)

2. Label the facial bones and overlying facial tissue.
   a. Maxilla
   b. Nasal bone
   c. Inferior nasal concha
   d. Mandible

   e. Vomer
   f. Lacrimal bone
   g. Zygomatic bone

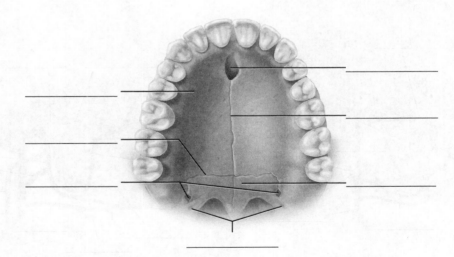

(© Elsevier Collection.)

3. Label the bones and landmarks of the hard palate.
   a. Incisive foramen
   b. Transverse palatine suture
   c. Greater palatine foramina
   d. Horizontal plate of the palatine bone

   e. Lesser palatine foramina
   f. Medial palatine suture
   g. Palatine process of the maxilla

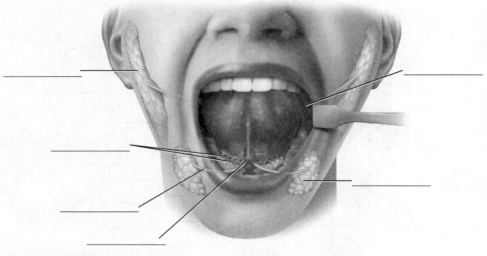

(© Elsevier Collection.)

4. Label the salivary glands.
   a. Sublingual ducts
   b. Parotid papilla
   c. Submandibular duct

   d. Parotid salivary gland
   e. Sublingual caruncle
   f. Submandibular salivary gland

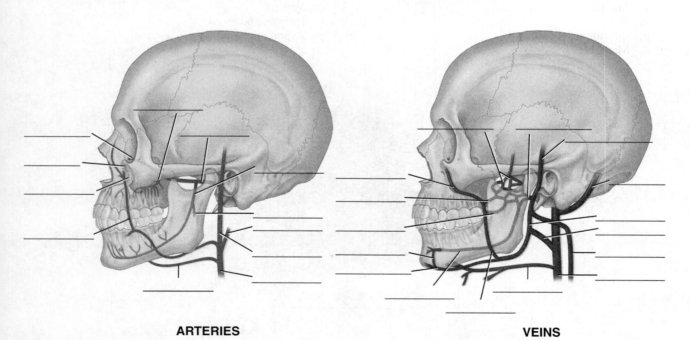

ARTERIES   **VEINS**

(© Elsevier Collection.)

5. Label the major arteries and veins of the face and oral cavity.
   a. Pterygoid plexus
   b. Superficial temporal
   c. Maxillary
   d. Lingual
   e. Buccal
   f. Deep facial
   g. Inferior alveolar
   h. Middle superior alveolar
   i. Facial
   j. Internal jugular
   k. Posterior auricular
   l. Mylohyoid
   m. Common carotid
   n. Anterior facial
   o. Infraorbital
   p. Retromandibular
   q. Mental
   r. External jugular
   s. Internal carotid
   t. Anterior superior alveolar
   u. Submental
   v. External carotid
   w. Common facial

TOPICS FOR DISCUSSION

One of the most important responsibilities of the clinical assistant is to control moisture during a dental procedure. Moisture can contaminate the operative site, prevent a dental material from setting, and cause a dental sealant to fail, or be a reason to restart a procedure.

1. What type of moisture could interfere with a dental procedure?

2. How is saliva produced?

3. Locate where in the mouth saliva would be produced.

4. Describe ways to control moisture during a dental procedure.

10 Landmarks of the Face and Oral Cavity

SHORT-ANSWER QUESTIONS

1. Name the landmarks of the face.

2. Name the landmarks of the oral cavity.

3. Describe the structures found in the vestibular region of the oral cavity.

4. Describe the area of the oral cavity proper.

5. Describe the characteristics of normal gingival tissue.

6. Describe the functions of the taste buds.

FILL-IN-THE-BLANK STATEMENTS

Select the best term from the list below and complete the following statements.

ala of the nose
anterior naris
canthus
Fordyce's spots
gingiva
glabella
labial commissure
labial frenum

mental protuberance
nasion
philtrum
septum
tragus
vermilion border
vestibule

1. The _____ is the fold of tissue at the corner of the eyelid.

2. The wing-like tip of the outer side of each nostril is the _____.

3. The _____ is the rectangular area from under the nose to the midline of the upper lip.

4. The _____ is the cartilage projection anterior to the external opening of the ear.

5. The _____ is the midpoint between the eyes, just below the eyebrows.

6. The _____ is the smooth surface of the frontal bone, also directly above the root of the nose.

7. The tissue that divides the nasal cavity into two nasal fossae is the _____.

8. The _____ is also referred to as the *nostril*.

9. The part of the mandible that forms the chin is the _____.

10. The _____ is the darker-colored border around the lips.

11. The _____ is the angle at the corner of the mouth where the upper and lower lips join.

12. The space between the teeth and the inner mucosa lining of the lips and cheeks is the _____.

13. _____ are normal variations that sometimes appear on the buccal mucosa.

14. The _____ is a band of tissue that passes from the facial oral mucosa at the midline of the arch to the midline of the inner surface of the lip.

15. The masticatory mucosa that covers the alveolar processes of the jaws and surrounds the necks of the teeth is the _____.

MULTIPLE-CHOICE QUESTIONS

Complete each question by circling the best answer.

1. What region of the face extends from the eyebrows to the hairline?
   a. Temple
   b. Zygomatic malar
   c. Forehead
   d. Nose

2. The line that marks a color change from your face to your lips is referred to as the _____.
   a. commissure
   b. vermilion border
   c. Fordyce
   d. labial frenum

3. What type of tissue covers the oral cavity?
   a. Mucous membrane
   b. Epithelial
   c. Squamous
   d. Stratified

4. Besides the oral cavity proper, name the other region of the oral cavity.
   a. Gingiva
   b. Tongue
   c. Lips
   d. Vestibule

5. The structure that passes from the oral mucosa to the facial midline of the mandibular arch is the _____.
   a. tongue
   b. frenum
   c. uvula
   d. incisive papilla

6. What is the proper term for "gums"?
   a. Epithelia
   b. Incisive
   c. Skin
   d. Gingiva

7. What is another term for unattached gingiva?
   a. Interdental gingiva
   b. Gingival groove
   c. Free gingiva
   d. Attached gingiva

8. What is another term for interdental gingiva?
   a. Interdental papilla
   b. Gingival groove
   c. Free gingiva
   d. Attached gingiva

9. What is the name of the pear-shaped pad of tissue behind the maxillary incisors?
   a. Palatine rugae
   b. Incisive papilla
   c. Palatine raphe
   d. Uvula

10. What is the name of the hanging pear-shaped projection of tissue at the border of the soft palate?
   a. Palatine rugae
   b. Free gingiva
   c. Uvula
   d. Incisive papilla

11. What is the correct term for the upper surface of the tongue?
   a. Frontal
   b. Dorsum
   c. Ventral
   d. Apex

12. The thin fold of the mucous membrane that extends from the floor of the mouth to the underside of the tongue is the _____.
   a. sublingual fold
   b. sublingual caruncle
   c. lingual frenum
   d. incisive frenum

LABELING EXERCISE

1. Label the features of the face.

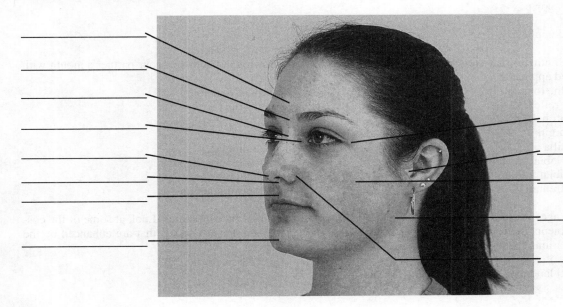

   a. Canthus
   b. Inner canthus
   c. Ala
   d. Philtrum
   e. Tragus
   f. Nasion
   g. Glabella
   h. Root
   i. Septum
   j. Anterior naris
   k. Mental protuberance
   l. Angle of the mandible
   m. Zygomatic arch

1. Identify the features of the face. To do this activity, you will need the following:
   - Student partner
   - Cotton-tipped applicator
   - Mask and gloves
   - Dental light / flashlight

   Using the cotton-tipped applicator, point to each of the following structures on your partner's face:
a. Ala of the nose	h. Bridge of the nose
b. Inner canthus and outer canthus of the eye	i. Vermilion border
c. Commissure of the lips	j. Zygomatic arch
d. Tragus	k. Septum
e. Nasion	l. Anterior naris
f. Glabella	m. Mental protuberance
g. Philtrum	n. Angle of the mandible

2. Identify the major landmarks, structures, and normal tissues of the mouth. To do this activity, you will need the following:
   - Student partner
   - Mask, gloves, gown
   - Mouth mirror
   - Cotton-tipped applicator

   Using the mouth mirror for vision and retraction, point to each of following structures in your partner's mouth with the cotton-tipped applicator:
a. Dorsum of the tongue	i. Vestibule of the mouth
b. Area of gag reflex	j. Wharton's duct
c. Hard and soft palates	k. Uvula
d. Gingival margin	l. Palatal rugae
e. Incisive papilla	m. Attached gingivae
f. Mandibular labial frenum	n. Ventral surface of the tongue
g. Maxillary labial frenum	o. Interdental gingivae
h. Sublingual frenum	p. Mucogingival junction

3. Throughout the ages, women have applied makeup to enhance their natural facial features. Look at some of the cosmetic advertisements in current magazines or newspapers, and identify the facial features that are enhanced by the application of various shades of foundation, lipstick, eyeliner, and blush.

   a. What natural landmark is enhanced using lip liner?

   b. Blush is applied over which structure of the face?

   c. How can the use of eyeliner change the appearance of the eyes?

11 Overview of the Dentitions

SHORT-ANSWER QUESTIONS

1. Explain how the size and shape of a tooth determines its function.

2. Describe the function of the molar, premolar, canine, lateral and central teeth.

3. What is unique about the primary, mixed, and permanent dentition?

4. Define occlusion, centric occlusion, and malocclusion.

5. Give the three classes of Angle's classification.

6. Name and describe the three primary systems of tooth numbering.

FILL-IN-THE-BLANK STATEMENTS

Select the best term from the list below and complete the following statements.

anterior
centric occlusion
curve of Spee
deciduous
dentition
distal surface
embrasure
functional occlusion
interproximal space

malocclusion
mandible
masticatory surface
maxilla
mesial surface
occlusion
quadrant
sextant
succedaneous teeth

1. Natural teeth in the dental arch are called _____.

2. Baby or primary teeth are called _____.

3. _____ is the natural contact of the maxillary teeth to the mandibular teeth.

4. Permanent teeth that replace primary teeth are _____.

5. The teeth in the front of the mouth are referred to as _____ teeth.

6. The upper jaw is the _____.

7. The lower jaw is the _____.

8. A _____ is one fourth of the dentition.

9. A _____ is one sixth of the dentition.

10. The _____ is the surface of the tooth toward the midline.

11. The _____ is the surface of the tooth away from the midline.

12. The chewing surface of the teeth is the _____.

13. The _____ is the area between adjacent tooth surfaces.

14. A(n) _____ is a triangular space in the gingival direction between the proximal surfaces of two adjoining teeth in contact.

15. Teeth are in _____ when there is maximum contact between the occluding surfaces of the maxillary and mandibular teeth.

16. Teeth are in _____ when all teeth make contact during biting and chewing movements.

17. _____ is an abnormal or malpositioned relationship of the maxillary teeth to the mandibular teeth when they are in centric occlusion.

18. The _____ is the bend formed by the maxillary and mandibular arches in occlusion.

MULTIPLE-CHOICE QUESTIONS

Complete each question by circling the best answer.

1. The type(s) of dentition individuals have in their lifetime are
   a. Mixed
   b. Primary
   c. Permanent
   d. b and c

2. How many teeth are in the primary dentition?
   a. 10
   b. 20
   c. 28
   d. 32

3. What is the term to describe the four divisions of the dental arches?
   a. Sextant
   b. Maxillary
   c. Mandibular
   d. Quadrant

4. What term is used for the front teeth?
   a. Mesial
   b. Anterior
   c. Occlusal
   d. Posterior

5. What are the most posterior teeth in the mouth?
   a. Centrals
   b. Laterals
   c. Premolars
   d. Molars

6. Which tooth is referred to as the "cornerstone" of the dental arch?
   a. Lateral
   b. Central
   c. Canine
   d. Molar

7. Name the surface of the tooth that faces the tongue.
   a. Lingual
   b. Facial
   c. Mesial
   d. Distal

8. What is the name for the space between two adjacent teeth?
   a. Occlussal space
   b. Bite space
   c. Interproximal space
   d. Facial space

9. The name of the area where adjacent teeth physically touch is the _____.
   a. embrasure
   b. contact area
   c. occlusion
   d. interproximal

10. The name of the triangular space between two adjacent teeth is the _____.
    a. embrasure
    b. contact area
    c. occlusion
    d. interproximal

11. The junction of two tooth surfaces of a tooth is the _____.
    a. margin
    b. proximal surface
    c. line angle
    d. pit

12. Which portion of a tooth is positioned toward the end of the root?
    a. Occlusal one third
    b. Middle one third
    c. Apical one third
    d. Proximal one third

13. The term for how teeth are positioned during chewing is _____.
    a. functional occlusion
    b. malocclusion
    c. mastication
    d. distoclusion

14. An individual who has an incorrect bite has a diagnosis of _____.
    a. functional occlusion
    b. malocclusion
    c. mastication
    d. neutroclusion

15. What term dscribes a class III malocclusion?
    a. Normal occlusion
    b. Distoclusion
    c. Malocclusion
    d. Mesioclusion

16. What classification is neutroclusion?
    a. Class I
    b. Class II
    c. Class III
    d. Class IV

17. What is the name for the arc of the occlusal plane?
    a. Curve of occlusion
    b. Curve of Spee
    c. Curve of molars
    d. Curve of Otho

LABELING EXERCISES

1. Label the surfaces of the teeth.

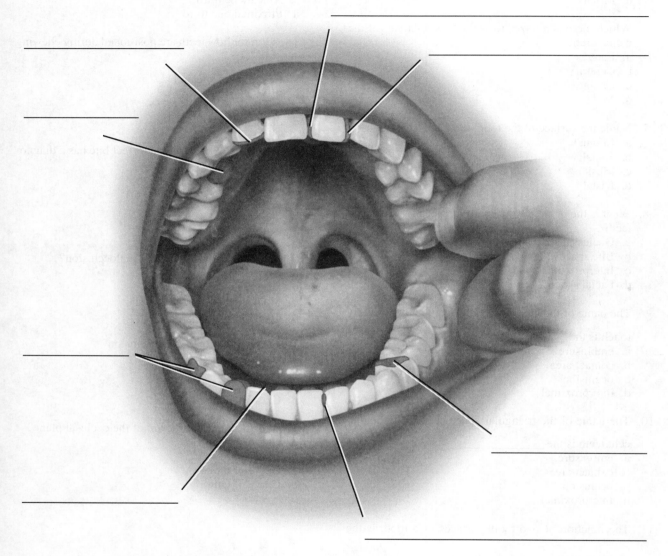

(© Elsevier Collection.)

a. Mesial surface
b. Distal surface
c. Palatal surface
d. Occlusal surface

e. Proximal surface with contact area
f. Incisal surface
g. Lingual surface
h. Facial surfaces (buccal/labial)

2. Place the corresponding tooth number using the universal system chart.

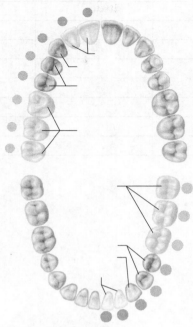

(© Elsevier Collection.)

a. Maxillary central / lateral incisors
b. Maxillary canines
c. Maxillary premolars
d. Maxillary molars

e. Mandibular central / lateral incisors
f. Mandibular canines
g. Mandibular premolars
h. Mandibular molars

ACTIVITY

In the table below, fill in the number of each tooth according to the Universal, Palmer Notation, and ISO/FDI numbering systems. You may wish to refer to a typodont or a study model of the adult and primary dentitions.

	UNIVERSAL	PALMER NOTATION	ISO/FDI
Maxillary right second molar			
Maxillary right first molar			
Maxillary right first premolar			
Maxillary right canine			
Maxillary right lateral			
Maxillary right central			
Maxillary left central			
Maxillary left canine			
Maxillary left second premolar			
Maxillary left first molar			
Maxillary left third molar			
Mandibular left second molar			

	UNIVERSAL	PALMER NOTATION	ISO/FDI
Mandibular left first molar			
Mandibular left canine			
Mandibular left lateral			
Mandibular left central			
Mandibular right central			
Mandibular right canine			
Mandibular right second premolar			
Mandibular right second molar			

12 Tooth Morphology

SHORT-ANSWER QUESTIONS

1. Using the Univerisal numbering system, give the name of the following teeth, (3, 5, 7, 13, 19, 23, 30)

2. What type of dentition is considered posterior teeth? What types of dentition is considered anterior teeth?

3. What surface of teeth are you able to detect a pit?

4. What types of teeth are you able to detect a cusp?

5. What unique features are different of the primary and permanent dentitions?

6. How many posterior teeth are included in the primary dentition?

FILL-IN-THE-BLANK STATEMENTS

Select the best term from the list below and complete the following statements.

canine eminence
central groove
cingulum
cusp
fossa
furcation
imbrication lines

incisal edge
inclined cuspal planes
mamelon
marginal ridge
morphology
non-succedaneous

1. The _____ is an elevation on the occlusal surface of posterior teeth.

2. A wide, shallow depression on the lingual surface of anterior teeth is the _____.

3. _____ is an area between two or more root branches.

4. _____ is the external vertical ridge on the labial surface of the canines.

5. The most prominent developmental groove on occlusal surface of posterior teeth is the _____.

6. The _____ is a raised, rounded area on the cervical third of the lingual surface.

7. Slight ridges that run mesiodistally in the cervical third of anterior teeth are _____.

8. The rounded enamel extension on the incisal edge of incisors is the _____.

9. The rounded, raised border located on the mesial and distal portions of the lingual surface of anterior teeth and the occlusal surface of posterior teeth is the _____.

10. A ridge on each permanent incisor that becomes flattened after wear is the _____.

11. _____ are the sloping areas between cusp ridges.

12. _____ refers to a tooth that does not replace a primary tooth.

13. _____ is the study of the form and shape of teeth.

MULTIPLE-CHOICE QUESTIONS

Complete each question by circling the best answer.

1. How many anterior teeth are in the permanent dentition?
   a. 10
   b. 12
   c. 28
   d. 32

2. What term is given to a permanent tooth that replaces a primary tooth of the same type?
   a. Implant
   b. Crown
   c. Succedaneous
   d. Molar

3. What is the rounded, raised area on the cervical thirds of the lingual surfaces of anterior teeth?
   a. Cingulum
   b. Mamelon
   c. Ridge
   d. Edge

4. What feature do newly erupted central and lateral incisors have on their incisal ridges?
   a. Cingulum
   b. Mamelon
   c. Ridge
   d. Cusp

5. Which teeth are the longest ones in the permanent dentition?
   a. Molars
   b. Central incisors
   c. Premolars
   d. Canines

6. Which teeth are the smallest ones in the permanent dentition?
   a. Maxillary molars
   b. Maxillary laterals
   c. Mandibular premolars
   d. Mandibular incisors

7. What is the name for the developmental horizontal lines on anterior teeth?
   a. Imbrication lines
   b. Marginal lines
   c. Oblique lines
   d. Incisal lines

8. What features border the occlusal surface of a posterior tooth?
   a. Oblique ridges
   b. Triangular ridges
   c. Marginal ridges
   d. Incisal ridges

9. What is the pinpoint depression where two or more grooves meet?
   a. Fossa
   b. Sulcus
   c. Ridge
   d. Pit

10. What occlusal design does the mandibular second premolar have?
    a. Incisal edge
    b. Two cusps
    c. Three cusps
    d. b and c

11. Which term is given to the area where the three roots divide?
    a. Furcation
    b. Bifurcation
    c. Trifurcation
    d. Quadrifurcation

12. What term is given to a tooth that does not replace a primary tooth?
    a. Succedaneous
    b. Non-succedaneous
    c. Supernumerary
    d. Developmental

13. _____is the name of the fifth cusp on a maxillary first molar.
    a. Cingulum
    b. Fossa
    c. Mamelon
    d. Cusp of Carabelli

14. How many roots do mandibular molars have?
    a. One
    b. Two
    c. Three
    d. b or c

15. Which teeth are referred to as the "wisdom" teeth?
    a. Central incisors
    b. Canines
    c. First molars
    d. Third molars

16. The thickness of the enamel covering on a primary tooth is considered _____.
    a. Thin
    b. Medium
    c. Thick
    d. Twice as thick as the enamel on a permanent tooth

17. What method of identification is used in the Universal/National System for the primary dentition?
    a. Numeric
    b. Italicized
    c. Alphabetic
    d. Pictorial

18. Which primary tooth has an H-shaped groove pattern on its occlusal surface?
    a. Maxillary premolar
    b. Mandibular molar
    c. Mandibular premolar
    d. Maxillary molar

19. Which primary tooth is the largest?
    a. Incisor
    b. Canine
    c. Premolar
    d. Molar

LABELING EXERCISES

1. Label the features on the occlusal surface of a permanent posterior tooth.

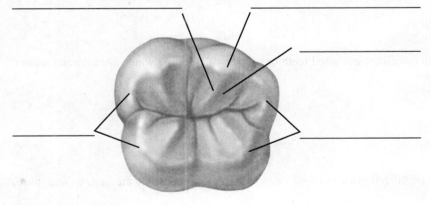

(© Elsevier Collection.)

    a. Cusp ridge
    b. Cusp tip
    c. Inclined cuspal plane
    d. Marginal ridge
    e. Marginal ridge

2. Label the features of a lingual view of a permanent maxillary canine.

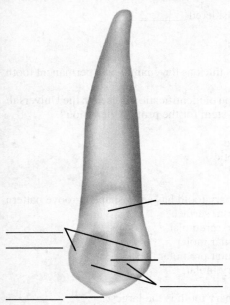

(© Elsevier Collection.)

   a. Cingulum
   b. Lingual ridge
   c. Lingual fossae
   d. Cusp tip
   e. Marginal ridges

ACTIVITIES

1. Look in your mouth and determine whether your mandibular second premolar is a three-cusp or a two-cusp type.

2. From a selection of all permanent teeth (sterilized extracted teeth or models), determine which are first and second premolars.

3. From a selection of all permanent teeth (sterilized extracted teeth or models), determine which are first, second, third, maxillary, and mandibular molars.

4. Examine the teeth of your classmates and note the variations in the cusp of Carabelli.

5. Identify the surfaces and landmarks of the anterior and posterior permanent teeth. To do this activity, you will need the following materials:
   - Typodonts or study models of the permanent dentition
   - Cotton-tipped applicator or explorer

6. Use your cotton-tipped applicator or explorer to point to each of the following surfaces and landmarks of the permanent dentition:

   a. Incisal surface of the maxillary left canine
   b. Labial surface of the mandibular right lateral incisor
   c. Lingual surface of the mandibular left central incisor
   d. Mesial surface of the maxillary right central incisor
   e. Distal surface of the mandibular left lateral incisor
   f. Occlusal surface of the mandibular left first premolar
   g. Lingual surface of the maxillary left first molar
   h. Buccal surface of the mandibular left second molar
   i. Mesial surface of the maxillary right first premolar
   j. Distal surface of the mandibular right second molar
   k. Buccal cusp on the mandibular right second premolar
   l. Occlusal pit on the maxillary right second molar
   m. Marginal ridge on the mandibular left first molar
   n. Cingulum on the maxillary right canine
   o. Lingual fossa on the mandibular left canine
   p. Cusp tip on the maxillary right canine

13 Impact of Oral Public Health

SHORT-ANSWER QUESTIONS

1. What is the objective of dental public health?

2. Give the components of dental public health.

3. Identify sources of systemic fluoride.

4. Describe what is included in a comprehenisve preventive program.

5. What are the three methods of administering fluoride therapy?

6. Describe the effects of excessive amounts of fluoride.

7. What is the purpose of a fluoride needs assessment?

8. Discuss the method of choice of toothbrushing.

FILL-IN-THE-BLANK STATEMENTS

Select the best term from the list below and complete the following statements.

dental public health   systemic fluoride
disclosing agent   topical fluoride
preventive dentistry

1. _____ comprises of education in proper nutrition and a plaque control program.

2. A _____ is applied to teeth to make plaque visible for patient education.

3. Assessment, assurance, development and implementation are functions of _____.

4. Fluoride that is ingested and circulated throughout the body is _____.

5. _____ is fluoride that is applied directly to the teeth.

Complete each question by circling the best answer.

1. What is the goal of preventive dentistry?
   a. To save money
   b. To limit visits to the dentist
   c. To have a healthy mouth
   d. To eliminate the need for dental insurance

2. One of the most common dental diseases is
   _____.
   a. crooked teeth
   b. dental caries
   c. missing teeth
   d. Impacted teeth

3. The goal of a patient education program is to
   _____.
   a. Teach patients how to take care of their teeth and develop sound dental habits
   b. Eliminate visits to the dentist
   c. Teach patients how to educate family members
   d. Save money on dental bills

4. What is the first step in a patient education program?
   a. Insurance approval
   b. Intraoral examination
   c. Listening to the patient
   d. Radiographs

5. Fluoride combats decay by _____.
   a. slowing demineralization
   b. sealing the teeth
   c. enhancing remineralization
   d. both a and c

6. What technique is used in the dental office to deliver fluoride treatment?
   a. Ingestion
   b. Topical
   c. Systemic
   d. Intravenous

7. What dental condition is the result of too much fluoride?
   a. Caries
   b. Gingivitis
   c. Fluorosis
   d. Periodontitis

8. What precaution should be instructed to the child when using fluoridated toothpaste?
   a. Making sure not to swallow the toothpaste
   b. Drink water after brushing
   c. Use the toothpaste only before bedtime
   d. Use the toothpaste only twice a day

9. What is an oral change observed in the older population?
   a. Enamel becomes darker
   b. Pulpal blood decreases
   c. Attrition
   d. All of the above

10. What should patients be instructed to perform daily to remove plaque?
    a. Brush
    b. Rinse with water
    c. Floss
    d. a and c

11. Which type of toothbrush bristles is recommended?
    a. Soft
    b. Medium
    c. Hard
    d. Natural

12. Which method of toothbrushing is generally recommended?
    a. Stillman
    b. Bass
    c. Circular
    d. Back and forth

13. Dental tape is _____.
    a. An oral irrigation dental aid
    b. A flat-type interproximal dental aid
    c. A rounded-type interproximal dental aid
    d. Used for removal of calculus

14. What type(s) of dental floss is most effective for the removal of plaque?
    a. Flavored
    b. Waxed
    c. Unwaxed
    d. b and c

15. Which of the following is recommended after meals and snacks when toothbrushing and flossing are not possible?
    a. Rinse with mouthwash.
    b. Eat an apple.
    c. Rinse with water.
    d. Run the tongue around the teeth.

16. Fluoride varnish is used with which group of patients?
    a. Children
    b. Patients of any age
    c. Adults
    d. Elderly patients

TOPICS FOR DISCUSSION

When you are working in a dental practice, you will see a wide variety of patients with varying ages, personalities, habits, and oral health issues. You want to provide good preventive oral healthcare. How would you handle the following situations?

1. A 10-year-old boy does not think he should give up eating sweets.

2. A 62-year-old woman says she cannot floss because of her arthritis.

3. A mother is afraid to allow her children to have a fluoride treatment because she heard that fluoride is poison.

4. A 50-year-old man with poor oral hygiene is also a heavy smoker.

5. A 32-year-old woman who is 3 months pregnant, and what to be aware of during pregnancy.

MULTIMEDIA PROCEDURES RECOMMENDED REVIEW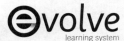

- Applying Topical Fluoride Gel or Foam
- Flossing Techniques
- Toothbrushing Methods

COMPETENCY 13.1: APPLYING TOPICAL FLUORIDE GEL OR FOAM (EXPANDED FUNCTION)

Performance Objective

By following a routine procedure that meets stated protocols, the student will demonstrate the proper technique for applying a topical fluoride gel or foam.

Evaluation and Grading Criteria

3	Student competently met the stated criteria without assistance.
2	Student required assistance in order to meet the stated criteria.
1	Student showed uncertainty when performing the stated criteria.
0	Student was not prepared and needs to repeat the step.
N/A	No evaluation of this step.

Instructor shall define grades for each point range earned on completion of each performance-evaluated task.

Performance Standards

The minimum number of satisfactory performances required before final evaluation is _____.

Instructor shall identify by * those steps considered critical. If a step is missed or minimum competency is not met, the evaluated procedure fails and must be repeated.

PERFORMANCE CRITERIA	*	SELF	PEER	INSTRUCTOR	COMMENTS
1. Selected the appropriate tray and other materials.					
2. Placed personal protective equipment according to the procedure.					
3. Checked to see whether calculus was present and if so, requested the hygienist or dentist remove it.					
4. Positioned the patient and provided patient instructions.					
5. Dispensed the appropriate amount of fluoride material into the tray.					
6. Dried the teeth.					
7. Inserted the tray and placed cotton rolls between the arches.					
8. Promptly placed the saliva ejector and tilted the patient's head forward.					
9. Removed the tray without allowing the patient to rinse or swallow.					

Continued

10. Used the saliva ejector or HVE tip to remove excess saliva and solution.				
11. Instructed the patient not to rinse, eat, drink, or brush the teeth for at least 30 minutes.				
12. Accurately documented the procedure in the patient record.				

ADDITIONAL COMMENTS

Total number of points earned _____

Grade _____ Instructor's initials _____

COMPETENCY 13.2: APPLYING FLUORIDE VARNISH (EXPANDED FUNCTION)

Performance Objective

By following a routine procedure that meets stated protocols, the student will competently and effectively apply fluoride varnish on a patient.

Evaluation and Grading Criteria

 3   Student competently met the stated criteria without assistance.

 2   Student required assistance in order to meet the stated criteria.

 1   Student showed uncertainty when performing the stated criteria.

 0   Student was not prepared and needs to repeat the step.

 N/A   No evaluation of this step.

Instructor shall define grades for each point range earned on completion of each performance-evaluated task.

Performance Standards

The minimum number of satisfactory performances required before final evaluation is _____.

Instructor shall identify by * those steps considered critical. If step is missed or minimum competency is not met, the evaluated procedure fails and must be repeated.

PERFORMANCE CRITERIA	*	SELF	PEER	INSTRUCTOR	COMMENTS
1. Obtained informed consent from the patient or the parent or legal guardian for a minor patient.					
2. Gathered supplies and single-unit dose for application.					
3. Placed personal protective equipment according to the procedure.					
4. Reclined the patient in the ergonomically correct position.					
5. Wiped the teeth to be varnished with the gauze or cotton roll, and inserted the saliva ejector.					
6. Used a cotton-tipped applicator, brush, or syringe-style applicator to apply 0.3 to 0.5 mL of varnish (unit dose) to the clinical crown of teeth.					
7. Used dental floss as needed to draw the varnish interproximally.					
8. Allowed the patient to rinse after the procedure was completed.					
9. Reminded the patient to avoid eating hard foods, drinking hot or alcoholic beverages, brushing, and flossing for at least 4 to 6 hours, or preferably until the day after the application.					

Continued

10. Reminded the patient to drink through a straw for the first few hours after the application.				
11. Accurately documented the procedure in the patient record.				
ADDITIONAL COMMENTS				

Total number of points earned: _____

Grade _____ Instructor's initials _____

COMPETENCY 13.3: ASSISTING THE PATIENT WITH DENTAL FLOSS (EXPANDED FUNCTION)

Performance Objective

By following a routine procedure that meets stated protocols, the student will demonstrate the proper technique for assisting a patient in learning how to use dental floss.

Evaluation and Grading Criteria

3	Student competently met the stated criteria without assistance.
2	Student required assistance in order to meet the stated criteria.
1	Student showed uncertainty when performing the stated criteria.
0	Student was not prepared and needs to repeat the step.
N/A	No evaluation of this step.

Instructor shall define grades for each point range earned on completion of each performance-evaluated task.

Performance Standards

The minimum number of satisfactory performances required before final evaluation is _____.

Instructor shall identify by * those steps considered critical. If step is missed or minimum competency is not met, the evaluated procedure fails and must be repeated.

PERFORMANCE CRITERIA	*	SELF	PEER	INSTRUCTOR	COMMENTS
1. Dispensed the appropriate amount of dental floss; wrapped the excess around the middle or index finger.					
2. Stretched the floss tightly between the fingers, and used the thumb and index finger to guide the floss into place.					
3. Held the floss tightly between the thumb and forefinger of each hand.					
4. Passed the floss gently between the teeth using a sawing motion. Guided the floss to the gumline.					
5. Curved the floss into a C-shape against each tooth, and wiped up and down against tooth surfaces.					
6. Repeated these steps on each side of all teeth in both arches.					
7. Moved a fresh piece of floss into the working position as the floss became frayed or soiled.					

Continued

8. Used a bridge threader to floss under any fixed bridges.					
9. Accurately documented the procedure in the patient record.					

ADDITIONAL COMMENTS

Total number of points earned _____

Grade _____ Instructor's initials _____

14 Nutrition

SHORT-ANSWER QUESTIONS

1. What are the goals of the *Healthy People 2020* report, and why are they important?

2. How do diet and nutrition affect the health of your teeth and gums?

3. Why is the study of nutrition important to the dental team?

4. List the five areas of the MyPlate food guide.

5. Describe the difference between vitamins and minerals.

6. Describe the role and sources of carbohydrates in the daily diet.

7. Explain the need for minerals in a diet.

8. Describe the types of eating disorders.

9. Explain how to interpret food labels.

10. Discuss the requirement for labeling food products.

11. Explain the criteria that must be met for a food to be considered "organic."

12. What foods are considered to be cariogenic?

FILL-IN-THE-BLANK STATEMENTS

Select the best term from the list below and complete the following statements.

amino acids	**nutrients**
anorexia nervosa	**organic**
bulimia	**MyPlate**

1. The current nutrition guide published by the United States Department of Agriculture is the _____.

2. _____ are organic and inorganic chemicals in food that supply energy.

3. Compounds in proteins used by the body to build and repair tissue are _____.

4. _____ is an eating disorder that is caused by an altered self-image.

5. Food products that have been grown without the use of any chemical pesticides, herbicides, or fertilizers are labeled as _____.

6. An eating disorder characterized by binge eating and self-induced vomiting is _____.

MULTIPLE-CHOICE QUESTIONS

Complete each question by circling the best answer.

1. Nutrition is the study of how the body uses food for _____.
   a. growth
   b. repair
   c. maintenance
   d. all of the above

2. The three types of carbohydrates are simple carbohydrates, complex carbohydrates, and _____.
   a. fats
   b. proteins
   c. dietary fiber
   d. water

3. The term used for a food that is capable of causing tooth decay is _____.
   a. nutrient
   b. cariogenic
   c. vitamin
   d. sugar

4. What key nutrients help build and repair the human body?
   a. Fats
   b. Vitamins
   c. Minerals
   d. Proteins

5. How many of the amino acids are essential?
   a. 2
   b. 4
   c. 9
   d. 12

6. A sources of a complete protein is _____.
   a. grains
   b. eggs
   c. pasta
   d. apples

7. Which systemic disease is related to having too much fat in the diet?
   a. Cardiovascular disease
   b. Allergies
   c. Multiple sclerosis
   d. Parkinson's disease

8. Which cholesterol is a "good cholesterol"?
   a. HDL
   b. LDL
   c. DDS
   d. ADA

9. Which vitamins are not destroyed by cooking and are stored in the body?
   a. Organic vitamins
   b. Water-soluble vitamins
   c. Fat-soluble vitamins
   d. Inorganic vitamins

10. Which vitamins are referred to as the "B-complex vitamins"?
    a. Organic vitamins
    b. Water-soluble vitamins
    c. Fat-soluble vitamins
    d. Inorganic vitamins

11. Which vitamin is fat soluble?
    a. Calcium
    b. Riboflavin
    c. Vitamin D
    d. Magnesium

12. Which vitamin is water soluble?
    a. Vitamin A
    b. Vitamin C
    c. Vitamin D
    d. Vitamin K

13. Which nutrient is often called "the forgotten nutrient"?
    a. Calcium
    b. Vitamin C
    c. Iron
    d. Water

14. Which governmental agency regulates the labeling of food products?
    a. FDA
    b. USDA
    c. ADA
    d. OSHA

15. What criteria is used to determine whether a product is "organic"?
    a. Grown without the use of chemical pesticides
    b. Grown without the use of herbicides
    c. Grown without the use of fertilizers
    d. All of the above

16. What eating disorder is characterized as self-starvation?
    a. Anorexia nervosa
    b. Fasting
    c. Bulimia
    d. Dieting

TOPICS FOR DISCUSSION

As a healthcare provider, you are involved in educating your patients about many health issues. Nutrition is one area that cannot be ignored. Not only will lack of proper nutrition contribute to poor health, but it can also contribute to dental disease. Obesity in children has become an epidemic in today's society.

1. What do you think are the main factors that contribute to children being overweight?

2. Describe a commercial that contributes to children's wanting to eat more.

3. Is there one eating habit that contributes to children's being overweight?

4. What should be the role of the dental team in educating families and their children?

5. How can poor nutrition habits affect a person's oral health?

CASE STUDY

Mrs. Diane Hernandez is an active 76-year-old woman. Because she is on a fixed income, her diet is lacking in dairy products, fruits, and vegetables. She tends to eat a lot of premade frozen meals for dinner. She also enjoys between-meal snacks that are high in carbohydrates.

1. What types of between-meal snacks would be healthy alternatives?

2. How could she increase her intake of dairy products, fruits, and vegetables, and stay within her budget?

15 Dental Caries

1. Why is dental caries considered an infectious disease?

2. Describe the process of dental caries.

3. What are the risk factors for dental caries?

4. What is the purpose of using a caries activity test?

5. What are the methods of transmission of oral bacteria?

6. Name the infective agents in the caries process.

7. Describe the role of saliva in oral health.

8. Explain the causes and effects of diet on dental caries.

9. Explain the remineralization process.

10. Distinguish the difference between root caries and smooth surface caries.

11. Describe the methods of detecting dental caries.

12. Name the most common chronic disease in children.

13. What is the difference from CAMBRA and ADA CCS?

14. Describe the technique of a caries detection device.

FILL-IN-THE-BLANK STATEMENTS

Select the best term from the list below and complete the following statements.

CAMBRA   mutans streptococci
caries   pellicle
cavitation   plaque
demineralization   rampant caries
fermentable carbohydrates   remineralization
incipient caries   xerostomia
lactobacillus

1. Another name for tooth decay is _____.

2. _____ is the loss of minerals from the tooth.

3. _____ is the replacement of minerals in the tooth.

4. A type of bacteria primarily responsible for caries is _____.

5. _____ is a type of bacteria that produces lactic acid from carbohydrates.

6. _____ is a colorless, sticky mass of microorganisms that adheres to the tooth surfaces.

7. _____ is the formation of a cavity or hole.

8. _____ is detectable tooth decay that is beginning to form.

9. Decay that develops rapidly and is widespread throughout the mouth is termed _____.

10. _____ is dryness of the mouth caused by abnormal reduction in the amount of saliva.

11. The thin coating of salivary materials that are deposited on tooth surfaces is the _____.

12. Simple carbohydrates such as sucrose, fructose, lactose, and glucose are _____.

13. A system that manages dental caries by risk assessment is _____.

MULTIPLE-CHOICE QUESTIONS

Complete each question by circling the best answer.

1. What type of bacteria is the cause of dental caries?
   a. Spirochetes
   b. Mutans streptococci
   c. Staphylococci
   d. Monocytes

2. What is the soft, sticky, bacterial mass that adheres to teeth?
   a. Decay
   b. Lactobacillus
   c. Plaque
   d. Carbohydrates

3. What mineral in enamel makes the tooth structure easier to dissolve?
   a. Carbonated apatite
   b. Iron
   c. Calcium
   d. Magnesium

4. The three factors necessary for the formation of dental caries are oral biofilm, fermentable carbohydrates, and _____.
   a. saliva
   b. poor toothbrushing habits
   c. a susceptible tooth
   d. non-fluoridated water

5. What is the term for the dissolving of calcium and phosphate from a tooth?
   a. Demineralization
   b. Resorption
   c. Remineralization
   d. Absorption

6. A patient with rapid and extensive formation of caries is given a diagnosis of _____.
   a. malocclusion
   b. xerostomia
   c. rampant caries
   d. temporomandibular disorder

7. Dental caries that occurs under or adjacent to existing dental restorations is termed _____.
   a. gingivitis
   b. periodontitis
   c. rampant caries
   d. recurrent caries

8. How does saliva protect the teeth from dental caries?
   a. Physical actions
   b. Chemical actions
   c. Antibacterial actions
   d. All of the above

CASE STUDY

Jeremy Allen is a 13-year-old patient of the practice. To date, he has received nine restorations and is scheduled to come back for another one. In reviewing his patient record, you notice that most of his restorations are on the chewing surfaces of his teeth.

1. Do you think it is common for a 13-year-old to have this many restorations?

2. What might be the cause for Jeremy's high rate of caries?

3. What term is used to describe the surfaces of the teeth mentioned with restorations?

4. What dental procedures could be indicated to help lower Jeremy's caries rate?

5. How would you educate Jeremy to help reduce his rate of caries?

COMPETENCY 15.1: PERFORMING CARIES DETECTION USING THE KAVO DIAGNODENT CARIES DETECTION DEVICE (EXPANDED FUNCTION)

Performance Objective

By following a routine procedure that meets stated protocols, the student will perform a caries detection procedure using an electronic caries detection device.

Evaluation and Grading Criteria

 3   Student competently met the stated criteria without assistance.

 2   Student required assistance in order to meet the stated criteria.

 1   Student showed uncertainty when performing the stated criteria.

 0   Student was not prepared and needs to repeat the step.

 N/A   No evaluation of this step.

Instructor shall define grades for each point range earned on completion of each performance-evaluated task.

Performance Standards

The minimum number of satisfactory performances required before final evaluation is _____.

Instructor shall identify by * those steps considered critical. If a step is missed or minimum competency is not met, the evaluated procedure fails and must be repeated.

PERFORMANCE CRITERIA	*	SELF	PEER	INSTRUCTOR	COMMENTS
1. Personal protective equipment placed according to procedure.					
Establish Zero Baseline					
2. Before scanning, selected an anatomic reference point on a healthy nonrestored tooth.					
3. Held the probe tip against the tooth at right angles to the surface.					
4. Gently squeezed the gray ring switch of the handpiece.					
5. Successfully established the zero baseline. (Display shows "Set 0," also confirmed by an audible beep.)					
6. Recorded the anatomic location where the zero baseline was established in the patient's dental record for future reference.					
Scanning Procedure					
7. Cleaned and dried the teeth using a prophy brush or other acceptable means.					
8. Identified surfaces of the tooth to be tested.					
9. During examination of suspicious sites, used light contact when touching the tip of the handpiece to the surface of the tooth.					

Continued

10. Placed the probe tip directly on the pits and fissures, making sure the tip was in contact with the long axis of the tooth.				
11. Slowly rotated or rocked the handpiece in a pendulum-like manner when the tip was in contact with the fissure.				
12. Recorded the readings.				
13. After the scan was completed, held the tip in the air and held the gray ring switch until "Set 0" appeared on the display.				
14. Accurately documented procedure in patient record.				

ADDITIONAL COMMENTS

Total number of points earned _____

Grade _____ Instructor's initials _____

COMPETENCY 15.2: PERFORMING CARIES RISK ASSESSMENT (EXPANDED FUNCTION)

Performance Objective

By following a routine procedure that meets stated protocols, the student will perform a caries risk assessment using a caries risk test and comparing the density of mutans streptococci (MS) and lactobacilli (LB) colonies with the corresponding evaluation pictures.

Evaluation and Grading Criteria

<u>3</u>   Student competently met the stated criteria without assistance.

<u>2</u>   Student required assistance in order to meet the stated criteria.

<u>1</u>   Student showed uncertainty when performing the stated criteria.

<u>0</u>   Student was not prepared and needs to repeat the step.

<u>N/A</u>   No evaluation of this step.

Instructor shall define grades for each point range earned on completion of each performance-evaluated task.

Performance Standards

The minimum number of satisfactory performances required before final evaluation is _____.

Instructor shall identify by * those steps considered critical. If a step is missed or minimum competency is not met, the evaluated procedure fails and must be repeated.

PERFORMANCE CRITERIA	*	SELF	PEER	INSTRUCTOR	COMMENTS
1. Personal protective equipment placed according to procedure.					
2. Explained the procedure to the patient.					
3. Instructed the patient to chew the paraffin wax pellet.					
4. Instructed the patient to expectorate into the paper cup.					
5. Removed the agar carrier from the test vial, and placed an $NaHCO_3$ tablet at the bottom of the vial.					
6. Carefully removed the protective foils from the two agar surfaces without touching the agar.					
7. Thoroughly wet both agar surfaces using a pipette. Avoided scratching the agar surface. Held the carrier at an angle while wetting.					
8. Slid the agar carrier back into the vial, and closed the vial tightly.					

Continued

9. Used a waterproof pen to note the name of the patient and the date on the lid of the vial.				
10. Placed the test vial upright in the incubator and incubated at 37° C (99° F) for 49 hours.				
11. Removed the vial from the incubator.				
12. Compared the density of MS and LB colonies with the corresponding evaluation pictures on a chart. *Tip: Hold the agar carrier at a slight angle under a light source to see the colonies clearly.*				
13. Accurately documented procedure in patient record.				

ADDITIONAL COMMENTS

Total number of points earned _____

Grade _____ Instructor's initials _____

16 Periodontal Disease

SHORT-ANSWER QUESTIONS

1. Name the tissues of the periodontium.

2. Describe the prevalence of periodontal disease.

3. Name the structures that make up the periodontium.

4. What systemic factors influence periodontal disease?

5. Give the two main forms of periodontal diseases.

6. Explain the significance of plaque and calculus in periodontal disease.

7. Identify the risk factors that contribute to periodontal disease.

8. Describe the systemic conditions that are linked to periodontal disease.

9. Describe the clinical characteristics of gingivitis.

10. Describe the progression of periodontitis.

FILL-IN-THE-BLANK STATEMENTS

Select the best term from the list below and complete the following statements.

calculus
gingivitis
periodontal diseases
periodontitis

periodontium
plaque
subgingival
supragingival

79

1. A soft deposit on teeth that consists of bacteria and bacterial by-products is _____.

2. _____ is made up of calcium and phosphate salts in the saliva that become mineralized and adhere to the tooth surface.

3. The _____ are structures that surround, support, and are attached to the teeth.

4. Diseases of the periodontium are referred to as _____.

5. _____ refers to the area above the gingiva.

6. _____ refers to the area below the gingiva.

7. Inflammation of the gingival tissue is _____.

8. _____ is an inflammatory disease of the supporting tissues of the teeth.

MULTIPLE-CHOICE QUESTIONS

Complete each question by circling the best answer.

1. Gingivitis is defined as _____.
   a. inflammation of the periodontium
   b. inflammation of the alveolar process
   c. inflammation of the gingival tissue
   d. inflammation of the oral mucosa

2. Which of the following is a clinical sign of gingivitis?
   a. Caries
   b. Redness
   c. Fever
   d. Ulcers

3. Which of the following can be used to reverse gingivitis?
   a. Improve brushing and flossing techniques.
   b. Take antibiotics.
   c. Undergo root planing.
   d. Nothing can reverse gingivitis.

4. Periodontitis is defined as _____.
   a. inflammation of the supporting tissues of the teeth
   b. inflammation of the alveolar process
   c. inflammation of the gingiva
   d. inflammation of the oral mucosa

5. Which of the following systemic diseases is related to periodontal disease?
   a. Cardiovascular disease
   b. Preterm low birth weight
   c. Respiratory disease
   d. All of the above

LABELING EXERCISE

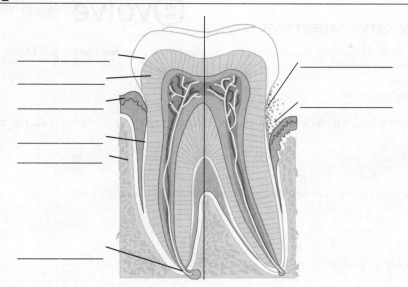

1. Label the cross-section of a tooth and its associated anatomic structures.
   a. Dentin
   b. Calculus
   c. Apical foramen
   d. Periodontal pocket
   e. Cementum
   f. Alveolar bone
   g. Gingiva
   h. Enamel

CASE STUDY

You are working for an orthodontist. Sally Hunter is a 14-year-old patient of the practice. Sally is wearing braces on her teeth and has returned to your office for her 6-week checkup. While removing elastics from her appliances, you note that her gingiva is red and slightly inflamed. You look at her patient record, and there is no indication of this condition at her last checkup.

1. What do you think could cause the redness and inflammation of Sally's gingival tissue?

2. Could there be any other reason for this gingival appearance?

3. Why should there be a note in the patient's chart regarding the oral tissues?

4. What would likely be the orthodontist's diagnosis for Sally's gingiva?

5. How can this problem be alleviated?

Access the Interactive Dental Office on Evolve and click on the patient case for Louisa Van Doren.

- Review Mrs. Van Doren's record.
- Mount her radiographs.
- Answer the following questions.

1. Does Mrs. Van Doren's health history contain any information regarding a condition that could lead to periodontal complications?

2. While viewing Mrs. Van Doren's radiographs, what did you notice about the level of bone?

Chapter **16** **Periodontal Disease**

17 Oral Pathology

SHORT-ANSWER QUESTIONS

1. Explain why a dental assistant should be knowledgeable about oral pathology.

2. List and describe the categories of diagnostic information.

3. Describe the warning signs of oral cancer.

4. Describe the types of oral lesions.

5. Name the five lesions associated with HIV/AIDS.

6. Describe the appearance of lesions associated with the use of smokeless tobacco.

7. Differentiate between chronic and acute inflammation.

8. Identify two oral conditions related to nutritional factors.

9. Describe the oral conditions of a patient with bulimia.

10. Explain the oral conditions with the use of methamphetamine.

FILL-IN-THE-BLANK STATEMENTS

Select the best term from the list below and complete the following statements.

abscess
biopsy
candidiasis
carcinoma
cellulitis
cyst
ecchymosis
erosion
glossitis
granuloma

hematoma
lesion
leukemia
leukoplakia
lichen planus
metastasize
meth mouth
pathology
sarcoma
xerostomia

1. _____ is the study of disease.

2. A pathologic site is considered a(n) _____.

3. _____ is the wearing away of tissue or tooth structure.

4. A(n) _____ is a non-cancerous growth filled with a liquid or semi-solid material with a definite wall.

5. A(n) _____ is a localized collection of pus from a bacterial infection.

6. A swelling or mass of blood collected in one area or organ is a(n) _____.

7. _____ is the medical term for bruising.

8. A cluster or nodule of non-cancerous cells is a _____.

9. _____ is the formation of white spots or patches on the mucosa.

10. A benign, chronic disease that affects the skin and oral mucosa is _____.

11. _____ is a superficial infection that is caused by a yeast-like fungus.

12. _____ is the inflammation of cellular or connective tissue.

13. _____ is a general term used to describe inflammation of the tongue.

14. _____ is a malignant cancer that begins in epithelial tissue.

15. _____ is a malignant cancer found in connective tissue such as muscle or bone.

16. A type of cancer that affects the blood and lymphatic system _____.

17. _____ is dryness of the mouth caused by reduction of saliva.

18. A(n) _____ is the removal of tissue for diagnostic examination.

19. _____ is the spread of disease from one part of the body to another.

20. _____ is the term for the advanced tooth decay caused by the heavy use of methamphetamine.

MULTIPLE-CHOICE QUESTIONS

Complete each question by circling the best answer.

1. What types of lesions are below the surface?
   a. Ulcers
   b. Plaque
   c. Blisters
   d. Bruises

2. What types of lesions are above the surface?
   a. Ulcers
   b. Cysts
   c. Blisters
   d. Bruises

3. What types of lesions are even with the surface?
   a. Ulcers
   b. Cysts
   c. Plaque
   d. Bruises

4. What condition appears as a white patch or area?
   a. Ulcer
   b. Candidiasis
   c. Leukoplakia
   d. Blister

5. What condition results from an infection caused by a yeast-like fungus?
   a. Plaque
   b. Ulcer
   c. Leukoplakia
   d. Candidiasis

6. What is another term for "canker sore"?
   a. Aphthous ulcer
   b. Cellulitis
   c. Leukoplakia
   d. Plaque

7. What is the condition in which inflammation causes severe pain and high fever?
   a. Glossitis
   b. Cellulitis
   c. Bruxism
   d. Candidiasis

8. What is the term for inflammation of the tongue?
   a. Aphthous ulcer
   b. Bruxism
   c. Glossitis
   d. Cellulitis

9. What is the condition in which a pattern on the tongue changes?
   a. Pseudomembranosus
   b. Candidiasis
   c. Glossitis
   d. Geographic tongue

10. What is the condition in which the body does not absorb vitamin B_{12}?
    a. Pernicious anemia
    b. Leukemia
    c. Periodontitis
    d. AIDS

11. What type of cancer affects the blood-forming organs?
    a. Carcinoma
    b. Sarcoma
    c. Leukemia
    d. Lymphoma

12. What is a common precancerous lesion among users of smokeless tobacco?
    a. Carcinoma
    b. Leukoplakia
    c. Lymphoma
    d. Leukemia

13. What is the term for a malignant lesion in the epithelial tissue of the oral cavity?
    a. Gingivitis
    b. Lymphoma
    c. Carcinoma
    d. Leukoplakia

14. What is the cause for radiation caries?
    a. Heat
    b. Harmful rays
    c. Cold
    d. Lack of saliva

15. What condition is frequently observed on the lateral border of the tongue of a patient with HIV/AIDS?
    a. Hairy leukoplakia
    b. Kaposi's sarcoma
    c. Lymphadenopathy
    d. Herpes labialis

16. What opportunistic infection is seen as bluish lesions on the skin or oral mucosa of a patient with HIV/AIDS?
    a. Leukoplakia
    b. Kaposi's sarcoma
    c. Lymphadenopathy
    d. Herpes labialis

17. What malignant condition involves the lymph nodes of patients with HIV/AIDS?
    a. Leukoplakia
    b. Kaposi's sarcoma
    c. Lymphadenopathy
    d. Herpes labialis

19. The name for bony growths in the palate is _____.
    a. Periodontitis
    b. Candidiasis
    c. Hyperplasia
    d. Torus palatinus

20. A common term for ankyloglossia is;
    a. Lisp
    b. Cleft palate
    c. Tongue-tie
    d. Warts

CASE STUDY

Tom Evans, one of your long-time patients, just noticed a large bump on his palate. He points to a torus palatinus. He is certain that it just appeared. However, you notice on Tom's chart a notation that he has a large torus palatinus. How do you respond to Tom when he asks you these questions?

1. Could it be from something I ate?

2. Could it be caused by stress?

3. Is it harmful?

4. Why did it just appear?

18 Microbiology

SHORT-ANSWER QUESTIONS

1. Explain why the study of microbiology is important for the dental assistant.

2. Give the types of bacteria according to their shape.

3. List the major groups of microorganisms.

4. Describe the differences among aerobes, anaerobes, and facultative anaerobes.

5. Identify the most resistant forms of life known, and explain how they survive.

6. Discuss specificity in relation to viruses.

7. Compare viruses to bacteria and name diseases caused by each.

8. Describe how prions differ from viruses and bacteria.

9. Name two diseases caused by prions.

10. Identify the method of transmission of Tuberculosis.

FILL-IN-THE-BLANK STATEMENTS

Select the best term from the list below and complete the following statements.

aerobes
anaerobes
Creutzfeldt–Jakob disease
facultative anaerobes
H1N1 flu virus
HAV
HBV
microbiology
MRSA

non-pathogenic
oral candidiasis
pathogenic
prions
protozoa
provirus
spore
virulent
West Nile virus

1. The study of microorganisms is _____.

2. Disease-producing microorganisms are termed _____.

3. _____ are non-disease-producing microorganisms.

4. _____ diseases are capable of causing a serious disease.

5. _____ are a variety of bacteria that require oxygen to grow.

6. Bacteria that grow in the absence of oxygen and are destroyed by oxygen are _____.

7. Organisms that can grow in the presence or the absence of oxygen are _____.

8. A(n) _____ is a single-celled microscopic animal without a rigid cell wall.

9. A(n) _____ is a hidden virus during the latency period.

10. Very tiny infectious agents that do not contain DNA or RNA are _____.

11. Some bacteria can change into a highly resistant form called _____.

12. _____ is a rare chronic brain disease with onset in middle to late life (40 to 60 years).

13. _____ is a yeast infection of the oral mucosa.

14. _____ is a virus necessary for coinfection with HDV.

15. _____ is a virus that is spread by the fecal-oral route.

16. _____ is a virus spread by mosquitoes.

17. _____ is a virus caused by A-type viruses.

18. _____ is a bacterium that is resistant to some antibiotics.

MULTIPLE-CHOICE QUESTIONS

Complete each question by circling the best answer.

1. Why is microbiology important to the dental assistant?
   a. Ability to learn to use a microscope.
   b. To gain an enhanced understanding of infection control.
   c. To better understand higher-level science concepts.
   d. To learn about the background of dental materials.

2. Who is the father of microbiology?
   a. Pierre Fauchard
   b. Joseph Lister
   c. Louis Pasteur
   d. G. V. Black

3. Who was the first to record that microorganisms are responsible for hospital-acquired infections?
   a. Pierre Fauchard
   b. Joseph Lister
   c. Louis Pasteur
   d. Lucy Hobbs

4. Who is credited for discovering the rabies vaccine?
   a. Pierre Fauchard
   b. Joseph Lister
   c. Louis Pasteur
   d. G. V. Black

5. Which is a shape of bacteria?
   a. Spherical
   b. Bacillus-like
   c. Spiral
   d. All of the above

6. The name of the staining process for separating bacteria is _____.
   a. pathology test
   b. biopsy
   c. scratch test
   d. Gram test

7. A(n)_____is an organism that is able to live in the presence of oxygen.
   a. Aerobe
   b. Anaerobe
   c. Aerated
   d. Aerial

8. The most resistant form of bacterial life is _____.
   a. Rickettsiae
   b. viruses
   c. spores
   d. fungi

9. How are prions different from other microorganisms?
   a. They contain only fat and one nucleic acid.
   b. They contain only protein and no nucleic acids.
   c. They contain no protein and only nucleic acids.
   d. They contain only carbohydrates and no phosphoric acids.

10. Which of the following oral disease is caused by bacteria?
    a. Dental caries
    b. Periodontal disease
    c. Malocclusion
    d. Both a and b

11. Which of the following forms of hepatitis is blood-borne?
    a. Hepatitis C
    b. Hepatitis D
    c. Hepatitis B
    d. All of the above

12. Pontiac fever is associated with which disease?
    a. Tuberculosis
    b. Legionnaires disease
    c. HIV
    d. Herpes simplex

13. Bacteria is the cause for which of the following diseases?
    a. Tetanus
    b. Syphilis
    c. Tuberculosis
    d. All of the above

14. The first oral indicator of syphilis is _____.
    a. a cold sore
    b. inflamed gingivae
    c. a chancre sore
    d. all of the above

15. Herpes simplex type 2 is also referred to as _____.
    a. genital herpes
    b. oral herpes
    c. chickenpox
    d. all of the above

Chapter **18 Microbiology**

Newspaper headlines and announcements at your school have released that a severe case of influenza virus is going around. Your younger sister is concerned and asks you the following questions. How do you answer her?

1. Why can't everyone just take an antibiotic and not get sick?

2. Why do we have to get a different flu vaccination every year?

3. Why can't doctors make one extra-strong vaccination?

4. How is the influenza virus spread?

19 Disease Transmission and Infection Prevention

SHORT-ANSWER QUESTIONS

1. Describe the roles of the CDC and OSHA in infection control.

2. Describe the differences between a chronic infection and an acute infection.

3. Describe the types of immunities and give examples of each.

4. Give an example of a latent infection.

5. Identify the links in the chain of infection.

6. Describe the methods of disease transmission in a dental office.

7. Discuss the infection control considerations for use of high-tech equipment.

8. List the components of an OSHA Exposure Control Plan.

9. Explain the rationale for Standard Precautions.

10. Describe the first aid necessary after an exposure incident.

11. Discuss the types of personal protective equipment (PPE) for a dental assistant.

12. Identify the various types of masks used in a dental office.

13. List the CDC recommendations regarding the use of a saliva ejector.

FILL-IN-THE-BLANK STATEMENTS

Select the best term from the list below and complete the following statements.

acquired immunity
acute infection
anaphylaxis
artificially acquired immunity
chronic infection
communicable diseases
direct contact
droplet infection
indirect contact
infection prevention

inherited immunity
latent infection
naturally acquired immunity
occupational exposure
OSHA Blood-Borne Pathogens Standard
percutaneous
permucosal
personal protective equipment
Standard Precautions

1. A(n) _____ is a persistent infection in which the symptoms come and go.

2. The symptoms of a(n) _____ are quite severe and of short duration.

3. An infection of long duration is called a(n) _____.

4. The _____ is designed to protect employees against occupational exposure to blood-borne pathogens.

5. _____ is touching or contacting a patient's blood or saliva.

6. _____ is touching or contacting a contaminated surface or instrument.

7. A(n) _____ exposure enters the mucosal surfaces of the eyes, nose, or mouth.

8. A(n) _____ exposure enters through the skin, such as through needle sticks, cuts, and human bites.

9. A(n) _____ exposure contacts mucous membranes, such as the eye or the mouth.

10. _____ is any reasonably anticipated skin, eye, or mucous membrane contact, or percutaneous injury with blood or any other potentially infectious materials, that occurs during work hours.

11. _____ is a the type of care that is designed to protect healthcare providers from pathogens that can spread by blood or any other body fluid, excretion, or secretion.

12. Items such as protective clothing, masks, gloves, and eyewear to protect employees are considered _____.

13. The most severe form of immediate allergic reaction is _____.

14. Infections that can be spread from another person or through contact with body fluids are called _____.

15. _____ is immunity that is present at birth.

16. _____ is immunity that develops during a person's lifetime.

92

17. _____ is the immunity that occurs when a person has acquired and is recovering from a disease.

18. _____ is the immunity that occurs as the result of a vaccination.

19. _____ is the ultimate goal of incorporating infection control procedures and policies.

MULTIPLE-CHOICE QUESTIONS

Complete each question by circling the best answer.

1. Which is not considered a means of direct transmission of a pathogen?
   a. Sneezing
   b. Touching a surface
   c. Spatter
   d. Infectious lesion

2. The term for acquiring an infection through a break in mucosal tissues is _____.
   a. airborne
   b. spatter
   c. droplet infection
   d. parenteral

3. What infection control measures help prevent disease transmission from the dental team to the patient?
   a. Gloves
   b. Handwashing
   c. Masks
   d. All of the above

4. The purpose of the OSHA Blood-borne Pathogens Standard is to _____.
   a. protect patients
   b. protect the community
   c. protect employees
   d. protect the Red Cross

5. How often must the practice's Exposure Control Plan be reviewed and updated?
   a. Weekly
   b. Monthly
   c. Bimonthly
   d. Annually

6. Standard Precautions are used to _____.
   a. protect healthcare providers from pathogens that can be spread by blood or any other body fluid, excretion, or secretion
   b. perform specific steps in instrument processing
   c. treat only patients without disease
   d. follow a specific routine in sterilization

7. What agency has released infection control guidelines?
   a. Centers for Disease Control and Prevention (CDC)
   b. Occupational Safety and Health Administration (OSHA)
   c. U.S. Food and Drug Administration (FDA)
   d. Environmental Protection Agency (EPA)

8. Which of the following statements about latex allergies is TRUE?
   a. The primary cause of death associated with latex allergies is anaphylaxis.
   b. There is no specific cure for latex allergies.
   c. Persons who suspect they have a latex allergy should see a physician.
   d. All of the above

9. Irritant dermatitis does not involve the immune system.
   a. True
   b. False

10. What must an employee do if he or she does not want the hepatitis B vaccine?
    a. Obtain a signature from his or her personal doctor.
    b. Sign an informed refusal form.
    c. Have a contract drawn up by his or her lawyer.
    d. All of the above

11. Long, artificial nails and rings should be avoided when working in a dental office because _____.
    a. they can stab/scratch a patient
    b. they can harbor pathogens
    c. they can contaminate items
    d. All of the above

12. An example of PPE is _____.
    a. a dental dam
    b. gloves
    c. a patient napkin
    d. a suction tip

13. What determines the type of PPE that should be worn?
    a. Risk of exposure
    b. Time of day
    c. Whether an advanced function is being performed
    d. Whether a patient has been premedicated

14. An example of protective eyewear is _____.
    a. contact lenses
    b. sunglasses
    c. glasses with side shields
    d. a magnifying glass

15. What is perhaps the most critical piece of PPE?
    a. Eyewear
    b. Mask
    c. Protective clothing
    d. Gloves

16. Sterile gloves would most commonly be worn for a(n) _____.
    a. Intra oral exam
    b. Taking radiographs
    c. Invasive surgical procedures
    d. Teeth cleaning

17. When should utility gloves be worn?
    a. When taking out the trash
    b. When disinfecting the treatment area
    c. When preparing instruments for sterilization
    d. b and c

18. What types of gloves should be worn to open drawers during a dental procedure?
    a. Sterile gloves
    b. Overgloves
    c. Powder-free latex gloves
    d. Utility gloves

LISTING EXERCISE

1. Listed are the links in the chain of infection, describe what each chain includes.
    a. Pathogenic agent
    b. Portal of entry
    c. Reservoir
    d. Portal of exit
    e. Susceptible host
    f. Mode of spread

CASE STUDY

Sheila is a dental assistant in your office and has been in the profession for 15 years. She constantly neglects to wear PPE when working in the laboratory and when breaking down and disinfecting treatment rooms. Sheila says that she never wore PPE during her first 15 years as a dental assistant and she did not get any diseases.

1. Why should Sheila start wearing PPE when she didn't wear any for 15 years?

2. Why has dentistry made such a change in its standards?

3. What type of PPE should you wear when working in the laboratory?

4. What type of PPE should you wear when breaking down and disinfecting a treatment room?

5. How should the dentist handle this situation with Sheila?

MULTIMEDIA PROCEDURES RECOMMENDED REVIEW

- Handwashing Techniques

COMPETENCY 19.1: APPLYING FIRST AID AFTER AN EXPOSURE INCIDENT

Performance Objective

By following a routine procedure that meets stated protocols, the student will role-play the proper technique for administering first aid after an exposure incident.

Evaluation and Grading Criteria

 3   Student competently met the stated criteria without assistance.

 2   Student required assistance in order to meet the stated criteria.

 1   Student showed uncertainty when performing the stated criteria.

 0   Student was not prepared and needs to repeat the step.

 N/A   No evaluation of this step.

Performance Standards

The minimum number of satisfactory performances required before final evaluation is _____.

Instructor shall identify by * those steps considered critical. If a step is missed or minimum competency is not met, the evaluated procedure fails and must be repeated.

PERFORMANCE CRITERIA	*	SELF	PEER	INSTRUCTOR	COMMENTS
1. Stopped operations immediately.					
2. Removed gloves.					
3. If the area of broken skin was bleeding, gently squeezed the site to express a small amount of visible blood.					
4. Washed hands thoroughly, using antimicrobial soap and warm water.					
5. Dried hands.					
6. Applied a small amount of antiseptic to the affected area.					
7. Applied an adhesive bandage to the area.					
8. Completed applicable postexposure follow-up steps.					
9. Notified the employer of the injury immediately after first aid was provided.					

ADDITIONAL COMMENTS

Total number of points earned _____

Grade _____ Instructor's initials _____

COMPETENCY 19.2: HANDWASHING

Performance Objective

The student will demonstrate the proper technique for handwashing before gloving.

Evaluation and Grading Criteria

3 Student competently met the stated criteria without assistance.

2 Student required assistance in order to meet the stated criteria.

1 Student showed uncertainty when performing the stated criteria.

0 Student was not prepared and needs to repeat the step.

N/A No evaluation of this step.

Performance Standards

The minimum number of satisfactory performances required before final evaluation is _____.

Instructor shall identify by * those steps considered critical. If a step is missed or minimum competency is not met, the evaluated procedure fails and must be repeated.

PERFORMANCE CRITERIA	*	SELF	PEER	INSTRUCTOR	COMMENTS
1. Removed all jewelry, including watch and rings.					
2. Used the foot or electronic control to regulate the flow of water to wet hands. (If such a control was not available, used a paper towel to grasp the faucets to turn them on and off. Discarded the towel after use.)					
3. Dispensed enough soap to cover the hand surface, using a foot-activated or electronic device.					
4. Vigorously rubbed the lathered hands together in • Circular movement • Palm on top of the other palm • In between fingers • Thumbs and nails					
5. Rinsed the hands with cool water.					
6. Used a paper towel to thoroughly dry the hands and then the forearms. (use a paper towel to turn off the facuet if foot control is not available)					
ADDITIONAL COMMENTS					

Total number of points earned _____

Grade _____ Instructor's initials _____

   Chapter **19 Disease Transmission and Infection Prevention**

COMPETENCY 19.3: APPLYING ALCOHOL-BASED HAND RUBS

Performance Objective

The student will demonstrate the proper technique for applying an alcohol-based hand rub.

Evaluation and Grading Criteria

3	Student competently met the stated criteria without assistance.
2	Student required assistance in order to meet the stated criteria.
1	Student showed uncertainty when performing the stated criteria.
0	Student was not prepared and needs to repeat the step.
N/A	No evaluation of this step.

Performance Standards

The minimum number of satisfactory performances required before final evaluation is _____.

Instructor shall identify by * those steps considered critical. If a step is missed or minimum competency is not met, the evaluated procedure fails and must be repeated.

PERFORMANCE CRITERIA	*	SELF	PEER	INSTRUCTOR	COMMENTS
1. Used enough sanitizer to cover all surfaces of hands.					
2. Rubbed the palms, in between fingers and over back of hands.					
3. Hands remained wet for minimum of 20 seconds					
ADDITIONAL COMMENTS					

Total number of points earned _____

Grade _____ Instructor's initials _____

COMPETENCY 19.4: DONNING: PUTTING ON PERSONAL PROTECTIVE EQUIPMENT (PPE)

Performance Objective

The student will demonstrate the proper technique for putting on personal protective equipment prior to providing patient care.

Evaluation and Grading Criteria

 3 Student competently met the stated criteria without assistance.

 2 Student required assistance in order to meet the stated criteria.

 1 Student showed uncertainty when performing the stated criteria.

 0 Student was not prepared and needs to repeat the step.

 N/A No evaluation of this step.

Performance Standards

The minimum number of satisfactory performances required before final evaluation is _____.

Instructor shall identify by * those steps considered critical. If a step is missed or minimum competency is not met, the evaluated procedure fails and must be repeated.

PERFORMANCE CRITERIA	*	SELF	PEER	INSTRUCTOR	COMMENTS
Gown					
1. Fully covered torso from the neck to knees, arms to end of wrists, and wrap around the back.					
2. Fasten in back of the neck and waist					
Mask					
3. Secured ties or eleastic bands at the middle of the head and neck or around the ears.					
4. Fit flexible band to nose bridge.					
5. Fit snug to the face and below the chin.					
6. Fit-check respirator.					
Goggles or Face Shield					
7. Placed over the face and eyes and adjusted to fit over the mask.					

Continued

Chapter **19 Disease Transmission and Infection Prevention**

Gloves				
8. Thoroughly washed and dried the hands. (If hands were not visibly soiled, used an alcohol-based hand rub.)				
9. Extended to cover wrist of isolation gown.				

ADDITIONAL COMMENTS

Total number of points earned _____

Grade _____ Instructor's initials _____

COMPETENCY 19.5: DOFFING: REMOVING PERSONAL PROTECTIVE EQUIPMENT (PPE)

Performance Objective

By following a routine procedure that meets stated protocols, the student will demonstrate the proper technique for removing personal protective equipment.

Evaluation and Grading Criteria

3   Student competently met the stated criteria without assistance.

2   Student required assistance in order to meet the stated criteria.

1   Student showed uncertainty when performing the stated criteria.

0   Student was not prepared and needs to repeat the step.

N/A   No evaluation of this step.

Instructor shall define grades for each point range earned on completion of each performance-evaluated task.

Performance Standards

The minimum number of satisfactory performances required before final evaluation is _____.

Instructor shall identify by * those steps considered critical. If a step is missed or minimum competency is not met, the evaluated procedure fails and must be repeated.

PERFORMANCE CRITERIA	*	SELF	PEER	INSTRUCTOR	COMMENTS
Gloves					
1. Using a gloved hand, grasped the palm area of the other gloved hand and peeled off the first glove					
2. Held the removed glove in the gloved hand, slid the fingers of the ungloved hand under the remaining glove at the wrist and peeled off the second glove over the first glove.					
3. Discarded the gloves in the appropriate waste container.					
4. Washed and thoroughly dried hands.					
Note: If no visible contamination exists and if gloves have not been torn or punctured during the procedure, an alcohol-based hand rub may be used in place of handwashing.					
Goggles Or Face Shield					
5. Removed the eyewear by touching it only on the ear rests.					
6. Placed the eyewear on a disposable towel for proper cleaning and disinfection.					

Continued

105

Gown					
7. Unfastened the gown ties, taking care that the sleeves don't contact the body when reaching for the ties					
8. Pulled the gown away from the neck and shoulders, touching inside of the gown only					
9. Turned the gown inside out					
10. Folded or rolled into a bundle and discarded in a waste container					
Mask					
11. Grasped the bottom ties or elastics of the mask/respirator, then the ones at the top, and removed without touching the front					
12. Discard in a waste container					
Wash Hands					
13. Washed hands after removing the PPE					
ADDITIONAL COMMENTS					

Total number of points earned _____

Grade _____ Instructor's initials _____

20 Principles and Techniques of Disinfection

1. List the types of surfaces in the dental office that are commonly covered with barriers.

2. Describe two methods for handling surface contamination.

3. Explain the differences between disinfection and sterilization.

4. Explain the differences between a disinfectant and an antiseptic.

5. Name the government agency that is responsible for registering a disinfectant.

6. Identify chemical products commonly used for intermediate- and low-level surface disinfection, and explain the advantages and disadvantages of each.

7. Explain the process of cleaning and disinfecting a treatment room.

8. Describe the process of precleaning contaminated dental instruments.

9. List the precautions that should be taken when using chemical sterilants or disinfectants.

10. Describe the CDC guidelines for disinfecting clinical contact surfaces.

FILL-IN-THE-BLANK STATEMENTS

Select the best term from the list below and complete the following statements.

bioburden
broad-spectrum
chlorine dioxide
disinfectant
greener infection control
glutaraldehyde
intermediate-level disinfectant
iodophor

low-level disinfectant
precleaning
residual activity
splash, spatter, and droplet surfaces
surface barrier
synthetic phenol compound
transfer surfaces
tuberculocidal

1. A(n) _____ is a fluid-impervious material that is used to cover surfaces that are likely to become contaminated.

2. _____ are surfaces that are not touched directly by the dental team, but that are often touched by contaminated instruments.

3. _____ are surfaces that do not contact the members of the dental team or the contaminated instruments or supplies.

4. _____ is the removal of bioburden before disinfection.

5. A chemical to reduce or lower the number of microorganisms is a(n) _____.

6. _____ is the action that continues long after the initial application.

7. Blood, saliva, and other body fluids are considered _____.

8. A(n) _____ agent is capable of inactivating *Mycobacterium tuberculosis*.

9. A _____ disinfectant is capable of killing a wide range of microbes.

10. A type of EPA-registered intermediate-level hospital disinfectant is _____.

11. _____ is an EPA-registered intermediate-level hospital disinfectant with a broad-spectrum disinfecting action.

12. _____ is classified as a high-level disinfectant or sterilant.

13. _____ is an effective rapid-acting environmental surface disinfectant or chemical sterilant.

14. _____ disinfectant destroys *M. tuberculosis,* viruses, fungi, and vegetative bacteria, and is used for disinfecting dental operatory surfaces.

15. A(n) _____ disinfectant destroys certain viruses and fungi, and can be used for general housecleaning purposes (e.g., walls, floors).

16. Minimizing the environmental impact of infection control products and procedures is called _____.

MULTIPLE-CHOICE QUESTIONS

Complete each question by circling the best answer.

1. Why are surfaces in dental treatment room disinfected or protected with barriers?
   a. To prevent you from injuring yourself
   b. To prevent patient-to-patient transmission of microorganisms
   c. To prevent dentist-to-patient transmission of microorganisms
   d. To prevent hygienist-to-assistant transmission of microorganisms

2. Which of the following is used to prevent surface contamination?
   a. Sterilization
   b. Disinfection
   c. Barriers
   d. b and c

3. What is the purpose of surface barriers?
   a. To prevent cross-contamination
   b. To protect surfaces from dental materials
   c. To cover the instruments
   d. To keep water from touching the unit

4. Which regulatory agency requires the use of surface disinfection?
   a. OSHA
   b. FDA
   c. ADA
   d. All of the above

5. Why is a surface precleaned?
   a. To remove the bioburden
   b. To remove the barrier
   c. To remove spilled dental materials
   d. To remove stains

6. Which item would be covered with a barrier instead of being disinfected?
   a. Operator's stool
   b. Light switch
   c. Countertop
   d. Dental assistant's stool

7. An antiseptic would be used for?
   a. Surfaces
   b. Instruments
   c. Skin
   d. Dental equipment

8. Which agency regulates disinfectants?
   a. OSHA
   b. FDA
   c. CDC
   d. EPA

9. Which of the following chemical solution(s) is recommended for items that cannot withstand heat sterilization?
   a. Glutaraldehyde
   b. Alcohol
   c. Iodophors
   d. All of the above

10. What is the name of the disinfectant that can leave a reddish or yellowish stain?
    a. Glutaraldehyde
    b. Alcohol
    c. Iodophors
    d. Sodium hypochlorite

11. What is a disadvantage of synthetic phenols?
    a. They leave a reddish stain.
    b. They can leave a residual film on surfaces.
    c. They evaporate quickly on surfaces.
    d. They are highly toxic.

12. What is a common term for sodium hypochlorite?
    a. Ammonia
    b. Vinegar
    c. Oil
    d. Bleach

13. Which product is not effective if blood or saliva is present on a surface?
    a. Alcohol
    b. Glutaraldehyde
    c. Chlorine dioxide
    d. Sodium hypochlorite

14. What is the classification of chlorine dioxide?
    a. To disinfect instruments
    b. To disinfect surfaces
    c. As a chemical sterilant
    d. b and c

15. Which is a way to practice greener infection control?
    a. Conserve water and energy.
    b. Use products with recyclable packaging.
    c. Use digital radiography.
    d. All of the above

TOPICS FOR DISCUSSION

The dentist in your office has a habit of talking alot to their patients, which always puts you behind. Today you are running 30 minutes behind and you still have not prepared the treatment room for the next patient.

1. What "corners" can you "cut" to get the room ready quickly?

2. Because this scenario happens quite frequently, would the use of disinfectants or barriers work better in this office? Why?

3. What items need to be replaced for the next patient on the dental-assisting unit?

4. What items need to be replaced for the next patient on the dental unit?

5. What personal protective equipment items need to be replaced?

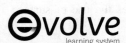

MULTIMEDIA PROCEDURES RECOMMENDED REVIEW

- Placing and Removing Surface Barriers
- Performing Treatment Room Cleaning and Disinfection

COMPETENCY 20.1: PLACING AND REMOVING SURFACE BARRIERS

Performance Objective

By following a routine procedure that meets stated protocols, the student will demonstrate the proper technique for placing and removing surface barriers.

Evaluation and Grading Criteria

<u>3</u>   Student competently met the stated criteria without assistance.

<u>2</u>   Student required assistance in order to meet the stated criteria.

<u>1</u>   Student showed uncertainty when performing the stated criteria.

<u>0</u>   Student was not prepared and needs to repeat the step.

<u>N/A</u>   No evaluation of this step.

Instructor shall define grades for each point range earned on completion of each performance-evaluated task.

Performance Standards

The minimum number of satisfactory performances required before final evaluation is _____.

Instructor shall identify by * those steps considered critical. If a step is missed or minimum competency is not met, the evaluated procedure fails and must be repeated.

PERFORMANCE CRITERIA	*	SELF	PEER	INSTRUCTOR	COMMENTS
Placement of Surface Barriers					
1. Washed and dried hands.					
2. Assembled the appropriate setup.					
3. Placed personal protective equipment according to the procedure.					
4. Selected the appropriate surface barriers.					
5. Placed each barrier over the entire surface to be protected.					
Removal of Surface Barriers					
6. Wore utility gloves to remove contaminated surface barriers.					
7. Very carefully removed each cover.					
8. Discarded the used covers into the regular waste receptacle.					
9. Washed, disinfected, and removed the utility gloves.					
10. Washed and dried hands.					
ADDITIONAL COMMENTS					

Total number of points earned _____

Grade _____ Instructor's initials _____

Performance Objective

By following the infection-control procedures, the student will demonstrate the proper technique for placing and removing surface barriers.

Evaluation and Grading Criteria

3   Student completed the listed criteria without assistance.

2   Student completed the listed criteria with some assistance.

1   Student showed uncertainty when performing the listed criteria.

0   Student was not prepared and needs to repeat the step.

N/A   The evaluation of this step is not applicable.

Instructor shall indicate, by a checkmark, whether completion of each performance criterion was achieved.

Performance Standards

The minimum number of satisfactory performances required before evaluation is ___.

Important instructions: These steps considered critical. If a step is missed or minimum competency is not met, the procedure must be repeated.

PERFORMANCE CRITERIA	SELF	PEER	INSTRUCTOR	COMMENTS
1. Placement of Surface Barriers				
Washed and dried hands.				
2. Assembled the appropriate materials.				
3. Placed required materials on the instrument tray or in the proper area.				
4. Selected the appropriate surface barriers.				
5. Placed each barrier over the entire surface to be protected.				
6. Removal of Surface Barriers				
7. Wore utility gloves, if necessary, during surface cleaning.				
8. Carefully removed each cover.				
9. Discarded used coverings in the proper waste receptacle.				
10. Washed, dried, and stored the utility gloves.				
11. Washed and dried hands.				

ADDITIONAL COMMENTS

Total number of points earned ___

Grade ___   Instructor's initials ___

COMPETENCY 20.2: PERFORMING TREATMENT ROOM CLEANING AND DISINFECTION

Performance Objective

By following a routine procedure that meets stated protocols, the student will demonstrate the proper technique for pre-cleaning and disinfecting a dental treatment room and equipment surfaces.

Evaluation and Grading Criteria

 3   Student competently met the stated criteria without assistance.

 2   Student required assistance in order to meet the stated criteria.

 1   Student showed uncertainty when performing the stated criteria.

 0   Student was not prepared and needs to repeat the step.

 N/A   No evaluation of this step.

Instructor shall define grades for each point range earned on completion of each performance-evaluated task.

Performance Standards

The minimum number of satisfactory performances required before final evaluation is _____.

Instructor shall identify by * those steps considered critical. If a step is missed or minimum competency is not met, the evaluated procedure fails and must be repeated.

PERFORMANCE CRITERIA	*	SELF	PEER	INSTRUCTOR	COMMENTS
1. Assembled the appropriate setup.					
2. Placed personal protective equipment according to the procedure.					
3. Checked to see that the precleaning and disinfecting product had been prepared correctly and was fresh. Read and followed the manufacturer's instructions.					
4. Sprayed the paper towel or gauze pad with the product and vigorously wiped the surface.					
5. Sprayed a fresh paper towel or gauze pad with the product.					
6. Allowed the surface to remain moist for the manufacturer's recommended time.					

Continued

Chapter **20** Principles and Techniques of Disinfection

7. Wiped off any excess moisture from disinfectant before seating next patient.				
8. Used water to rinse any residual disinfectant from surfaces that could come in contact with the patient's skin or mouth.				

ADDITIONAL COMMENTS

Total number of points earned _____

Grade _____ Instructor's initials _____

21 Principles and Techniques of Instrument Processing and Sterilization

SHORT-ANSWER QUESTIONS

1. List the seven steps involved in processing dental instruments.

2. Describe the necessary precautions to take when materials are packaged for sterilization.

3. List the steps required for sterilizing the high-speed dental handpiece.

4. Describe when and how biologic monitoring is done.

5. Describe the three forms of sterilization monitoring.

6. Explain how sterilization failures can occur.

7. Give the classification of instruments used to determine the type of processing that should be used.

8. List the CDC guidelines for cleaning and decontamination of instruments.

FILL-IN-THE-BLANK STATEMENTS

Select the best term from the list below and complete the following statements.

autoclave
biologic indicators
biologic monitor
chemical vapor sterilizer
clean area
contaminated area
critical instrument
dry heat sterilizer
endospore

event-related packaging
multi-parameter indicator
non-critical instruments
safety data sheet
semi-critical instruments
single-parameter indicator
ultrasonic cleaner
use-life

1. _____ means that the contents of a package will remain sterile indefinitely unless the packaging is compromised.

2. _____ is OSHA's newer term for material data sheets.

3. The _____ is a type of sterilizer that uses moist heat under pressure.

4. _____ are vials or strips, also known as *spore tests,* that contain harmless bacterial spores used to determine whether a sterilizer is operating.

5. The _____ is a type of sterilizer that uses hot formaldehyde vapors under pressure.

6. An instrument used to penetrate soft tissue or bone is classified as a(n) _____.

7. Instruments that come in contact with oral tissues, but do not penetrate soft tissue or bone, are classified as _____.

8. _____ are instruments that come into contact with intact skin only.

9. The _____ of the sterilization center stores sterilized instruments, fresh disposable supplies, and prepared trays.

10. The _____ of the sterilization center is where harmful items are brought for precleaning.

11. The _____ is a type of sterilizer that uses heated air.

12. _____ is the length of time that a germicidal solution is effective after it has been prepared for use.

13. The _____ will verify sterilization by confirming that all spore-forming microorganisms are destroyed.

14. Tapes, strips, and tabs with heat-sensitive chemicals that change color when exposed to a certain temperature are examples of a(n) _____.

15. A(n) _____ is a resistant, dormant structure that is formed inside of some bacteria and can withstand adverse conditions.

16. The _____ loosens and removes debris with the use of sound waves traveling through a liquid.

17. A(n) _____ is an indicator that reacts to time, temperature, and the presence of steam.

MULTIPLE-CHOICE QUESTIONS

Complete each question by circling the best answer.

1. The instrument classifications used to determine the method of sterilization and disinfection are _____.
   a. critical
   b. semicritical
   c. noncritical
   d. All of the above

2. Which piece of personal protective equipment is necessary when processing instruments?
   a. Goggle-type eyewear
   b. Sterile gloves
   c. Surgical scrubs
   d. Hairnet

3. The basic rule of the workflow pattern in an instrument-processing area is _____.
   a. triangular
   b. square
   c. single-loop
   d. double-loop

4. If instruments cannot be processed immediately, they should be _____.
   a. kept in the dental treatment area
   b. wrapped in aluminum foil
   c. covered with a patient napkin
   d. placed in a holding solution

5. Which is a method of precleaning instruments?
   a. Hand scrubbing
   b. Ultrasonic cleaning
   c. A thermal washer and disinfector
   d. b and c

6. Which method of precleaning instruments is not recommended?
   a. Hand scrubbing
   b. Ultrasonic cleaning
   c. Thermal washer
   d. Microwave

7. The ultrasonic cleaner works _____.
   a. by microwaves
   b. by sound waves
   c. by ultraviolet waves
   d. by light waves

8. Kitchen dishwashers cannot be used to preclean instruments because they are _____.
   a. not ADA approved
   b. not CDC approved
   c. not FDA approved
   d. not OSHA approved

9. To maintain proper opening, hinged instruments are treated with _____.
   a. disinfectant
   b. lubricant
   c. proper wrapping
   d. wax

10. Instruments should be packaged for sterilization to _____.
    a. maintain sterility
    b. identify them
    c. maintain organization
    d. make setup easier

11. Which of the following is a reason that pins, staples, and paper clips are not used on instrument packaging?
    a. The package becomes too hot to touch.
    b. You cannot record information on the package.
    c. They will damage the sterilizer.
    d. They cause holes or tears in the packaging.

12. Which is a form of sterilization monitoring?
    a. Physical
    b. Chemical
    c. Biologic
    d. All of the above

13. Where is a process indicator placed?
    a. Inside the package
    b. Outside the package
    c. Inside the sterilizer
    d. Outside the sterilizer

14. Another term for spore testing is _____.
    a. biologic monitoring
    b. single-parameter indicator
    c. multi-parameter indicator
    d. All of the above

15. Do multi-parameter indicators ensure that an item is sterile?
    a. Yes
    b. No

16. What is the best way to determine whether sterilization has occurred?
    a. Check the sterilizer.
    b. Use a process multi-parameter indicator.
    c. Use biologic monitoring.
    d. Use a single-parameter indicator.

17. What causes sterilization failures?
    a. Improper contact of the sterilizing agent
    b. Improper temperature
    c. Overloading of the sterilizer
    d. All of the above

18. Which is a method of heat sterilization used in a dental office?
    a. Steam
    b. Chemical vapor
    c. Dry heat
    d. All of the above

19. What is a primary disadvantage of "flash" sterilization?
    a. Type of sterilizer
    b. Inability to wrap items
    c. Temperature
    d. Sterilizing agent used

117

20. What is a major advantage of chemical vapor sterilization?
    a. Sterilizing time is faster.
    b. More instruments can be sterilized at one time.
    c. Instruments will not rust.
    d. The instruments do not have to be wrapped.

21. An example of dry heat sterilization is _____.
    a. static air
    b. chemical vapor
    c. autoclave
    d. microwave

22. Instruments are rinsed with _____ following a liquid chemical sterilant.
    a. hot water
    b. cold water
    c. sterile water
    d. carbonated water

23. The high-speed handpiece is prepared for sterilization by_____.
    a. placing it in a holding bath
    b. flushing water through it
    c. soaking it in soapy water
    d. taking it apart

24. What type of heat sterilizer is appropriate for high-speed handpieces?
    a. Steam
    b. Chemical vapor
    c. Liquid chemical sterilant
    d. a and b

TOPICS FOR DISCUSSION

You are the only clinical assistant in the practice and your morning has been very hectic. The contaminated instruments have not been processed for the afternoon. When you finally have a break and get back to the sterilization center, your dirty instruments are in the ultrasonic, and the trays and paper products are on the counter.

1. How could this backup have been prevented?

2. You have five trays of instruments in the ultrasonic. What can you do?

3. What could you have done immediately after performing a procedure to change this circumstance?

4. Is there anyone else in the dental office who could help keep this situation under control? If so, how could you work through this circumstance?

5. Should you discuss this experience with the dentist?

MULTIMEDIA PROCEDURES RECOMMENDED REVIEW ⊝volve
learning system

- Autoclaving Instruments
- Operating the Ultrasonic Cleaner

COMPETENCY 21.1: OPERATING THE ULTRASONIC CLEANER

Performance Objective

By following a routine procedure that meets stated protocols, when provided with the appropriate materials, the student will demonstrate the proper technique for precleaning instruments before sterilization using the ultrasonic cleaner.

Evaluation and Grading Criteria

3　　Student competently met the stated criteria without assistance.

2　　Student required assistance in order to meet the stated criteria.

1　　Student showed uncertainty when performing the stated criteria.

0　　Student was not prepared and needs to repeat the step.

N/A　　No evaluation of this step.

Instructor shall define grades for each point range earned on completion of each performance-evaluated task.

Performance Standards

The minimum number of satisfactory performances required before final evaluation is _____.

Instructor shall identify by * those steps considered critical. If a step is missed or minimum competency is not met, the evaluated procedure fails and must be repeated.

PERFORMANCE CRITERIA	*	SELF	PEER	INSTRUCTOR	COMMENTS
1. Placed personal protective equipment according to the procedure.					
2. Removed the lid from the container and checked the level of solution.					
3. Placed instruments or cassette into the basket.					
4. Replaced the lid and turned the cycle to ON.					
5. After the cleaning cycle, removed the basket and rinsed the instruments.					
6. Emptied the basket onto the towel.					
7. Replaced the lid on the ultrasonic cleaner.					

ADDITIONAL COMMENTS

Total number of points earned _____

Grade _____ Instructor's initials _____

COMPETENCY 21.2: AUTOCLAVING INSTRUMENTS

Performance Objective

By following a routine procedure that meets stated protocols, when provided with the appropriate materials, the student will demonstrate the proper technique for preparing and autoclaving instruments.

Evaluation and Grading Criteria

 3   Student competently met the stated criteria without assistance.

 2   Student required assistance in order to meet the stated criteria.

 1   Student showed uncertainty when performing the stated criteria.

 0   Student was not prepared and needs to repeat the step.

 N/A   No evaluation of this step.

Instructor shall define grades for each point range earned on completion of each performance-evaluated task.

Performance Standards

The minimum number of satisfactory performances required before final evaluation is _____.

Instructor shall identify by * those steps considered critical. If a step is missed or minimum competency is not met, the evaluated procedure fails and must be repeated.

PERFORMANCE CRITERIA	*	SELF	PEER	INSTRUCTOR	COMMENTS
1. Placed personal protective equipment according to the procedure.					
2. Properly cleaned and prepared the instruments for autoclaving.					
3. Placed the process integrator into the package.					
4. Packaged, sealed, and labeled the instruments.					
5. Placed the bagged and sealed items in the autoclave.					
6. Tilted glass or metal canisters at an angle.					
7. Placed larger packs at the bottom of the chamber.					
8. Did not overload the autoclave.					
9. Followed the manufacturer's instructions.					
10. Checked the level of water. (If necessary, added more distilled water.)					
11. Set the autoclave controls for the appropriate time, temperature, and pressure.					
12. At the end of the sterilization cycle, vented the steam into the room and allowed the contents of the autoclave to dry and cool.					

Continued

13. Checked the external process indicator for color change.					
14. Removed the instruments when they were cool and dry.					

ADDITIONAL COMMENTS

Total number of points earned _____

Grade _____ Instructor's initials _____

COMPETENCY 21.3: STERILIZING INSTRUMENTS

Performance Objective

By following a routine procedure that meets stated protocols, when provided with the appropriate materials, the student will demonstrate the proper technique for preparing and sterilizing instruments with chemical vapor.

Evaluation and Grading Criteria

 3   Student competently met the stated criteria without assistance.

 2   Student required assistance in order to meet the stated criteria.

 1   Student showed uncertainty when performing the stated criteria.

 0   Student was not prepared and needs to repeat the step.

 N/A   No evaluation of this step.

Instructor shall define grades for each point range earned on completion of each performance-evaluated task.

Performance Standards

The minimum number of satisfactory performances required before final evaluation is _____.

Instructor shall identify by * those steps considered critical. If a step is missed or minimum competency is not met, the evaluated procedure fails and must be repeated.

PERFORMANCE CRITERIA	*	SELF	PEER	INSTRUCTOR	COMMENTS
Wrapping the Instruments					
1. Placed personal protective equipment according to the procedure.					
2. Ensured that the instruments were clean and dry.					
3. Wrapped the instruments.					
4. Ensured that packages were not too large.					
Loading and Operating the Chemical Vapor Sterilizer					
5. Read and followed the manufacturer's instructions.					
6. Read the information on the MSDS for the chemical liquid.					
7. Loaded the sterilizer according to the manufacturer's instructions.					
8. Set the controls for the proper time and temperature.					
9. Followed the manufacturer's instructions for venting and cooling.					

Continued

10. Checked the external process indicator for color change.				
11. Removed the instruments when they were cool and dry.				

ADDITIONAL COMMENTS

Total number of points earned _____

Grade _____ Instructor's initials _____

COMPETENCY 21.4: STERILIZING INSTRUMENTS WITH DRY HEAT

Performance Objective

By following a routine procedure that meets stated protocols, when provided with the appropriate materials, the student will demonstrate the proper technique for preparing and sterilizing instruments with dry heat.

Evaluation and Grading Criteria

_3_   Student competently met the stated criteria without assistance.

_2_   Student required assistance in order to meet the stated criteria.

_1_   Student showed uncertainty when performing the stated criteria.

_0_   Student was not prepared and needs to repeat the step.

_N/A_   No evaluation of this step.

Instructor shall define grades for each point range earned on completion of each performance-evaluated task.

Performance Standards

The minimum number of satisfactory performances required before final evaluation is _____.

Instructor shall identify by * those steps considered critical. If a step is missed or minimum competency is not met, the evaluated procedure fails and must be repeated.

PERFORMANCE CRITERIA	*	SELF	PEER	INSTRUCTOR	COMMENTS
Wrapping the Instruments					
1. Placed personal protective equipment according to the procedure.					
2. Cleaned and dried the instruments before wrapping.					
3. Opened hinged instruments.					
4. Wrapped the instruments.					
Loading and Operating the Dry Heat Sterilizer					
5. Read and followed the manufacturer's instructions.					
6. Inserted the process integrator into the test load package.					
7. Loaded the instruments into the dry heat chamber.					
8. Set the time and temperature.					
9. Did not place additional instruments in the load once the sterilization cycle had begun.					

Continued

10. Allowed the packs to cool before handling.					
11. Checked the indicators for color change.					

ADDITIONAL COMMENTS

Total number of points earned _____

Grade _____ Instructor's initials _____

COMPETENCY 21.5: STERILIZING INSTRUMENTS WITH LIQUID CHEMICAL STERILANTS

Performance Objective

By following a routine procedure that meets stated protocols, when provided with the appropriate materials, the student will demonstrate the proper technique for preparing and sterilizing instruments with a chemical sterilant.

Evaluation and Grading Criteria

3	Student competently met the stated criteria without assistance.
2	Student required assistance in order to meet the stated criteria.
1	Student showed uncertainty when performing the stated criteria.
0	Student was not prepared and needs to repeat the step.
N/A	No evaluation of this step.

Instructor shall define grades for each point range earned on completion of each performance-evaluated task.

Performance Standards

The minimum number of satisfactory performances required before final evaluation is _____.

Instructor shall identify by * those steps considered critical. If a step is missed or minimum competency is not met, the evaluated procedure fails and must be repeated.

PERFORMANCE CRITERIA	*	SELF	PEER	INSTRUCTOR	COMMENTS
Preparing the Solution					
1. Placed personal protective equipment according to the procedure.					
2. Followed the manufacturer's instructions for preparing and activating, using, and disposing of the solution.					
3. Prepared the solution for use as a sterilant. Labeled the containers with the name of the chemical, date of preparation, and any other information relating to the hazards of the product.					
4. Covered the container and kept it closed unless putting instruments in or taking them out.					
Using the Solution					
5. Precleaned, rinsed, and dried the items to be processed.					
6. Placed the items in a perforated tray or pan. Placed the pan in the solution and covered the container—or as an alternative, used tongs.					
7. Ensured that all items were fully submerged in the solution for the entire contact time.					

Continued

127

8. Rinsed processed items thoroughly with water and dried them. Placed items in a clean package.				
Maintaining the Solution				
9. Tested the glutaraldehyde concentration of the solution with a chemical test kit (available from the manufacturer).				
10. Replaced the solution as indicated on the instructions, or when the level of the solution became low or the solution became visibly dirty.				
11. When replacing the used solution, discarded all of the used solution, cleaned the container with a detergent, rinsed it with water, dried it, and filled it with a fresh solution.				
ADDITIONAL COMMENTS				

Total number of points earned _____

Grade _____ Instructor's initials _____

COMPETENCY 21.6: FOLLOWING A STERILIZATION FAILURE

Performance Objective

By following a routine procedure that meets stated protocols, the student will demonstrate the proper technique for following up on a sterilization failure.

Evaluation and Grading Criteria

 3   Student competently met the stated criteria without assistance.

 2   Student required assistance in order to meet the stated criteria.

 1   Student showed uncertainty when performing the stated criteria.

 0   Student was not prepared and needs to repeat the step.

 N/A   No evaluation of this step.

Instructor shall define grades for each point range earned on completion of each performance-evaluated task.

Performance Standards

The minimum number of satisfactory performances required before final evaluation is _____.

Instructor shall identify by * those steps considered critical. If step is missed or minimum competency is not met, the evaluated procedure fails and must be repeated.

PERFORMANCE CRITERIA	*	SELF	PEER	INSTRUCTOR	COMMENTS
1. Take the sterilizer out of service immediately.					
2. Using the manufacturer's manual, review the proper loading and operating procedures.					
3. Determine if the times and temperatures that were used were correct.					
4. Retest and monitor the cycle. Place a chemical indicator next to the biologic indicator on the inside of a package. Check the sterilization gauges, lights, and/or the digital readouts to determine if they reach the proper sterilizing conditions.					
5. Make a decision regarding the proper operation of the sterilizer.					
ADDITIONAL COMMENTS					

Total number of points earned _____

Grade _____ Instructor's initials _____

COMPETENCY 21.7: PERFORMING BIOLOGIC MONITORING

Performance Objective

By following a routine procedure that meets stated protocols, the student will demonstrate the proper technique for performing biologic monitoring.

Evaluation and Grading Criteria

<u>3</u>   Student competently met the stated criteria without assistance.

<u>2</u>   Student required assistance in order to meet the stated criteria.

<u>1</u>   Student showed uncertainty when performing the stated criteria.

<u>0</u>   Student was not prepared and needs to repeat the step.

<u>N/A</u>   No evaluation of this step.

Instructor shall define grades for each point range earned on completion of each performance-evaluated task.

Performance Standards

The minimum number of satisfactory performances required before final evaluation is _____.

Instructor shall identify by * those steps considered critical. If a step is missed or minimum competency is not met, the evaluated procedure fails and must be repeated.

PERFORMANCE CRITERIA	*	SELF	PEER	INSTRUCTOR	COMMENTS
1. Placed personal protective equipment according to the procedure.					
2. Placed the biologic indicator (BI) strip in the bundle of instruments and sealed the package.					
3. Placed the pack with the BI strip in the center of the sterilizer load.					
4. Placed the remainder of the packaged instruments into the sterilizer and processed the load through a normal sterilization cycle.					
5. Removed the utility gloves, mask, and eyewear. Washed and dried hands.					
6. Recorded the date of the test; the type of sterilizer; the cycle, temperature, and time; and the name of the person operating the sterilizer.					

Continued

        Chapter **21 Principles and Techniques of Instrument Processing and Sterilization**

7. Removed and processed the BI strip after the load was sterilized.				
8. Mailed the processed spore test strips and the control BI strip to the monitoring service.				

ADDITIONAL COMMENTS

Total number of points earned _____

Grade _____ Instructor's initials _____

COMPETENCY 21.8: STERILIZING THE DENTAL HANDPIECE

Performance Objective

By following a routine procedure that meets stated protocols, when provided with the appropriate materials, the student will demonstrate the proper technique for preparing, cleaning, and sterilizing the dental handpiece.

Evaluation and Grading Criteria

3   Student competently met the stated criteria without assistance.

2   Student required assistance in order to meet the stated criteria.

1   Student showed uncertainty when performing the stated criteria.

0   Student was not prepared and needs to repeat the step.

N/A   No evaluation of this step.

Instructor shall define grades for each point range earned on completion of each performance-evaluated task.

Performance Standards

The minimum number of satisfactory performances required before final evaluation is _____.

Instructor shall identify by * those steps considered critical. If a step is missed or minimum competency is not met, the evaluated procedure fails and must be repeated.

PERFORMANCE CRITERIA	*	SELF	PEER	INSTRUCTOR	COMMENTS
1. Placed personal protective equipment according to the procedure.					
2. With the bur still in the chuck, wiped any visible debris from the handpiece. Operated the handpiece for approximately 10 to 20 seconds.					
3. Removed the bur from the handpiece and then removed the handpiece from the hose.					
4. Used a handpiece cleaner recommended by the manufacturer to remove internal debris and lubricated the handpiece according to the manufacturer's recommendations.					
5. Reattached the handpiece to an air hose, inserted a bur, and operated the handpiece to blow out the excess lubricant from the rotating parts.					

Continued

     Chapter **21** **Principles and Techniques of Instrument Processing and Sterilization**

6. Used a cotton-tipped applicator dampened with isopropyl alcohol to remove all excess lubricant from the fiber-optic interfaces and exposed optical surfaces.					
7. Dried the handpiece and packaged it for sterilization.					

ADDITIONAL COMMENTS

Total number of points earned _____

Grade _____ Instructor's initials _____

22 Regulatory and Advisory Agencies

SHORT-ANSWER QUESTIONS

1. Explain the differences between regulations and recommendations.

2. List four professional sources for dental information.

3. Name the leading resource for safety and infection prevention information in dentistry.

4. Describe the role of the Centers for Disease Control and Prevention.

5. Explain the primary difference between OSHA and NIOSH.

6. Describe the role of the Environmental Protection Agency in relation to dentistry.

7. Describe the role of the U.S. Food and Drug Administration in relation to dentistry.

8. Describe the role of the National Institutes of Health.

9. Describe the role of the National Institute of Dental and Craniofacial Research.

10. Describe the role of the Public Health Agency of Canada.

135

FILL-IN-THE-BLANK STATEMENTS

Select the best term from the list below and complete the following statements.

ADA   NIOSH
CDC   OSAP
EPA   OSHA
FDA   PHAC

1. The _____ is a federal regulatory agency that oversees the regulation of sterilization equipment.

2. The federal non-regulatory agency that issues recommendations on health and safety is the _____.

3. The _____ is the professional organization for dentists.

4. The federal regulatory agency that enforces regulations that pertain to employee safety is _____.

5. _____ is the global resource for safety and infection prevention information in dentistry.

6. _____ is the federal agency that is responsible for conducting research and making recommendations for the prevention of work-related disease and injury.

7. The _____ is the federal regulatory agency that deals with issues of concern to the environment or public safety.

8. The _____ is the federal agency responsible for public health in Canada.

MULTIPLE-CHOICE QUESTIONS

Complete each question by circling the best answer.

1. What is the primary role of the CDC in dentistry?
   a. Public health
   b. Research
   c. Drugs
   d. Employees

2. What is a primary role of the FDA?
   a. Fund research projects
   b. Provide public health information
   c. Regulate medical and dental devices
   d. Protect employees

3. What is the primary role of the EPA?
   a. Research
   b. Public health
   c. Employees
   d. Environment

4. What is the primary focus of OSHA in dentistry?
   a. Public health
   b. Employees
   c. Environment
   d. Research

5. What agency provides guidelines for Infection control in the Dental Health-Care Settings?
   a. Centers for Disease Control and Prevention (CDC)
   b. Occupational Safety and Health Administration (OSHA)
   c. U.S. Food and Drug Administration (FDA)
   d. Environmental Protection Agency (EPA)

6. What must an employee do if he or she does not want the hepatitis B vaccine?
   a. Obtain a signature from his or her personal doctor.
   b. Sign an informed refusal form.
   c. Have a contract drawn up by his or her lawyer.
   d. All of the above

TOPICS FOR DISCUSSION

The dentist in your office asks you to be in charge of maintaining OSHA compliance in the office and to provide training on infection prevention to the new employees. A high school student will be coming in to help with sterilization, and you must give her appropriate training. Where will you get the latest information and how will you find the newest OSHA regulations?

COMPETENCY 22.1: APPLYING FIRST AID AFTER AN EXPOSURE INCIDENT

Performance Objective

By following a routine procedure that meets stated protocols, the student will role-play the proper technique for administering first aid after an exposure incident.

Evaluation and Grading Criteria

3	Student competently met the stated criteria without assistance.
2	Student required assistance in order to meet the stated criteria.
1	Student showed uncertainty when performing the stated criteria.
0	Student was not prepared and needs to repeat the step.
N/A	No evaluation of this step.

Performance Standards

The minimum number of satisfactory performances required before final evaluation is _____.

Instructor shall identify by * those steps considered critical. If a step is missed or minimum competency is not met, the evaluated procedure fails and must be repeated.

PERFORMANCE CRITERIA	*	SELF	PEER	INSTRUCTOR	COMMENTS
1. Stopped operations immediately.					
2. Removed gloves.					
3. If the area of broken skin was bleeding, gently squeezed the site to express a small amount of visible blood.					
4. Washed hands thoroughly, using antimicrobial soap and warm water.					
5. Dried hands.					
6. Applied a small amount of antiseptic to the affected area.					
7. Applied an adhesive bandage to the area.					
8. Completed applicable postexposure follow-up steps.					
9. Notified the employer of the injury immediately after first aid was provided.					
ADDITIONAL COMMENTS					

Total number of points earned _____

Grade _____ Instructor's initials _____

23 Chemical and Waste Management

1. Describe potential short-term and long-term effects of exposure to chemicals.

2. Explain the components of the OSHA Hazard Communication Standard.

3. Describe three common methods of chemical exposure.

4. List the components of a Hazard Communication Program.

5. Explain the purpose of a safety data sheet.

6. Describe the difference between chronic and acute chemical exposure.

7. Identify four methods of personal protection against chemical exposure.

8. Describe how chemicals should generally be stored.

9. Discuss the record-keeping requirements of the Hazard Communication Standard.

10. Identify types of regulated waste generated in a dental office.

FILL-IN-THE-BLANK STATEMENTS

Select the best term from the list below and complete the following statements.

acute
chemical inventory
chronic exposure
contaminated waste
hazardous waste

infectious waste
safety data sheet (SDS)
regulated waste
toxic waste
Hazard Communication Standard

1. The _____ is a standard set in place regarding an employee's right to know about chemicals in the workplace.

2. A form that provides health and safety information regarding materials that contain chemicals is a _____.

3. _____ is repeated exposures, generally of lower levels, over a long period.

4. _____ exposure pertains to high levels of exposure over a short period.

5. Waste that has certain properties or contains chemicals that could pose a danger to human health and the environment after it is discarded is a _____.

6. A(n) _____ is a comprehensive list of every product used in the office that contains chemicals.

7. Disposable items that have had contact with blood, saliva, or other body secretions are considered _____.

8. Waste that is capable of causing an infectious disease is _____.

9. _____ is infectious waste that requires special handling, neutralization, and disposal.

10. Waste that is capable of having a poisonous effect is _____.

MULTIPLE-CHOICE QUESTIONS

Complete each question by circling the best answer.

1. In what body systems could health-related problems develop as a result of inhalation exposure to chemicals in the dental office?
   a. Neurologic
   b. Senses
   c. Respiratory
   d. Endocrine

2. What is (are) primary method(s) of chemical exposure?
   a. Inhalation
   b. Ingestion
   c. Skin contact
   d. All of the above

3. Acute chemical exposure involves _____.
   a. short-term exposure in large quantity
   b. repeated exposure in small quantity
   c. short-term exposure in small quantity
   d. long-term exposure in small quantity

4. What is a method of personal protection against chemical exposure?
   a. Ventilation
   b. Disinfected surfaces
   c. Inhalation protection
   d. Hair protection

5. What are the OSHA requirements regarding an eyewash unit?
   a. Eyewash unit in every treatment room
   b. Eyewash unit in areas where chemicals are used
   c. Eyewash unit in the building
   d. Eyewash unit on each floor

6. What could be the most likely health effect of exposure to radiographic processing solutions kept in a poorly ventilated area?
   a. Cardiac problems
   b. Reproductive problems
   c. Respiratory problems
   d. Urinary problems

7. In general, how should chemicals be stored?
   a. In a cool, dry, dark place
   b. In a locked cabinet
   c. Under water
   d. In a hot, moist place

8. Chemicals are determined to be hazardous if they are _____.
   a. ignitable
   b. corrosive
   c. reactive
   d. All of the above

9. What is another term for the Hazard Communication Standard?
   a. Employee beware law
   b. Employee right-to-know law
   c. Hazardous chemical law
   d. Chemical safety law

10. What chemicals must be included in a chemical inventory?
    a. Over-the-counter drugs
    b. Prescription drugs
    c. All chemicals
    d. Dental materials

11. What does the abbreviation SDS represent?
    a. Subscribed dental sheet
    b. Safety data sheet
    c. Materials for sterilization and dental surgery
    d. Microbiology standards and disease standards

12. What materials are exempt from labeling requirements?
    a. Food
    b. Drugs
    c. Cosmetics
    d. All of the above

13. How long must training records be kept on file?
    a. 1 year
    b. 5 years
    c. 10 years
    d. 20 years

14. An example of regulated waste is a _____.
    a. patient napkin
    b. contaminated needle
    c. dental dam
    d. 2 × 2-inch gauze

CASE STUDY

Pamela is a dental assistant who is in charge of preparing chemical labels for secondary containers in the office. While preparing a label for a new product that is highly flammable, reactive, and toxic. Pamela realizes there are missing safety data sheets for other products in the office.

1. What types of containers are considered "secondary" containers that Pamela will need to label?

2. Where can Pamela get more information about the product?

3. Where can Pamela get a safety data sheet for other products in the office?

4. What types of pictograms, or labels, will Pamela need for the new product?

COMPETENCY 23.1: CREATING AN APPROPRIATE LABEL FOR A SECONDARY CONTAINER

Performance Objective

By following a routine procedure that meets stated protocols, the student will demonstrate the proper technique for using information from a safety data sheet (SDS) to complete a chemical label for a secondary container.

Evaluation and Grading Criteria

 3   Student competently met the stated criteria without assistance.

 2   Student required assistance in order to meet the stated criteria.

 1   Student showed uncertainty when performing the stated criteria.

 0   Student was not prepared and needs to repeat the step.

 N/A   No evaluation of this step.

Instructor shall define grades for each point range earned on completion of each performance-evaluated task.

Performance Standards

The minimum number of satisfactory performances required before final evaluation is _____.

Instructor shall identify by * those steps considered critical. If a step is missed or minimum competency is not met, the evaluated procedure fails and must be repeated.

PERFORMANCE CRITERIA	*	SELF	PEER	INSTRUCTOR	COMMENTS
1. Wrote the Product Identifier on the label.					
2. Wrote the Supplier Identification.					
3. Used the appropriate Hazard Pictograms.					
4. Wrote the appropriate Precautionary Statements.					
5. Wrote the appropriate First Aid measures.					
ADDITIONAL COMMENTS					

Total number of points earned _____

Grade _____ Instructor's initials _____

24 Dental Unit Waterlines

SHORT-ANSWER QUESTIONS

1. Why would dental units have more bacteria than a faucet?

2. Explain the role of biofilm in dental unit waterline contamination.

3. Discuss why there is a concern about dental unit waterline contamination.

4. Explain the factors in bacterial contamination of dental unit water.

5. Identify the primary source of microorganisms in dental unit water.

6. Describe methods to reduce bacterial contamination in dental unit waterlines.

FILL-IN-THE-BLANK STATEMENTS

Select the best term from the list below and complete the following statements.

anti-retraction device
biofilm
colony-forming units
dental unit waterlines

Legionella
microfiltration
planktonic bacteria
self-contained water reservoir

1. _____ is a slime-producing bacterial community that can harbor fungi, algae, and protozoa.

2. The bacterium responsible for the Legionnairs' disease is _____.

3. _____ is the use of membrane filters to trap microorganisms suspended in water.

4. _____ are the minimum number of cells on the surface of a semisolid agar medium that create a visible colony.

5. _____ are plastic tubing used to deliver dental treatment water through a dental unit.

6. A(n) _____ is a container that is used to hold and supply water or other solutions to handpieces and air-water syringes attached to a dental unit.

7. _____ is a mechanism that prevents entry of fluids and microorganisms into waterlines as a result of negative water pressure, also referred to as "suck back."

8. Type of bacteria that floats in water is _____.

MULTIPLE-CHOICE QUESTIONS

Complete each question by circling the best answer.

1. Are waterborne diseases limited to dentistry?
   a. Yes
   b. No

2. When was the presence of bacteria first reported in dental unit waterlines?
   a. 5 years ago
   b. 10 years ago
   c. 20 years ago
   d. 30 years ago

3. What bacteria causes Legionnaires' pneumonia?
   a. Streptococci
   b. *Legionella* bacteria
   c. Bacilli
   d. Staphylococci

4. Where is biofilm found?
   a. Suction tips
   b. Handpiece waterlines
   c. Air-water syringe waterlines
   d. b and c

5. Should water be heated in the dental units to kill the bacteria?
   a. Yes
   b. No
   c. It doesn't matter.

6. Can biofilm in dental unit waterlines be completely eliminated?
   a. Yes
   b. No

7. If sterile water is used in a self-contained reservoir, will the water that enters the patient's mouth be sterile?
   a. Yes
   b. No

8. The recommendation for changing microfilters in waterlines is _____?
   a. Daily
   b. Weekly
   c. Bimonthly
   d. According to manufacturer's directions

9. According to CDC guidelines, who should you contact to help control biofilm in the dental unit?
   a. ADA
   b. Equipment manufacturer
   c. OSHA
   d. CDC

10. According to CDC guidelines, what type of water must be used as an irrigant for surgery involving bone?
    a. Saline water
    b. Tap water
    c. Sterile water
    d. Carbonated water

11. Will flushing dental unit waterlines remove all biofilm?
    a. Yes
    b. No

12. When should the high-volume evacuator be used to minimize aerosol?
    a. With the high-speed handpiece
    b. With the ultrasonic scaler
    c. With the air-water syringe
    d. All of the above

13. Will the use of a dental dam totally eliminate the dental assistant's exposure to microorganisms?
    a. Yes
    b. No

14. What type of personal protective equipment (PPE) is especially critical when aerosol is being generated?
    a. Eyewear
    b. Mask
    c. Gloves
    d. a and b

CASE STUDY

A patient of the practice comments on a news report she saw on television about the transmission of diseases from water in the dental office. She confides in you that she is not sure she wants to continue her treatment plan. How would you answer the following questions from your patient?

1. Is HIV transmitted from dental unit water?

2. What does the practice do to make the water safe?

3. What type of water does the practice use for surgery?

4. Is it safe to have dental treatment that requires water?

COMPETENCY 24.1: TESTING DENTAL UNIT WATERLINES

Performance Objective

By following a routine procedure that meets stated protocols, the student will demonstrate the proper technique for obtaining a water sample and preparing it for shipping.

Evaluation and Grading Criteria

3	Student competently met the stated criteria without assistance.
2	Student required assistance in order to meet the stated criteria.
1	Student showed uncertainty when performing the stated criteria.
0	Student was not prepared and needs to repeat the step.
N/A	No evaluation of this step.

Instructor shall define grades for each point range earned on completion of each performance-evaluated task.

Performance Standards

The minimum number of satisfactory performances required before final evaluation is _____.

Instructor shall identify by * those steps considered critical. If a step is missed or minimum competency is not met, the evaluated procedure fails and must be repeated.

PERFORMANCE CRITERIA	*	SELF	PEER	INSTRUCTOR	COMMENTS
1. Placed personal protective equipment according to the procedure.					
2. Placed the refrigerant pack in the Styrofoam lid and placed it in the freezer overnight.					
3. Flushed the waterlines for a minimum of 2 minutes before taking samples.					
4. Filled sterile collection vials to approximately three fourths full. *Did not touch the outlet of the waterline or the interior of the collection vial.*					
5. Used a permanent marker to label each water sample. Indicated the sample location and the type. For example, Operatory 3, air-water syringe (Op3, a-w).					
6. Filled out the sample submission form and enclosed it with the samples.					
7. Placed the refrigerant pack and water samples in a Styrofoam shipper box.					

Continued

8. Placed the Styrofoam shipper box in a mailer box.					
9. Completed U.S. Express Mail shipping label and affixed it to the box.					
ADDITIONAL COMMENTS					

Total number of points earned _____

Grade _____ Instructor's initials _____

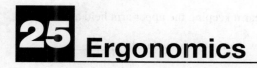

25 Ergonomics

SHORT-ANSWER QUESTIONS

1. What is the goal of ergonomics?

2. Discuss exercises that can reduce muscle fatigue and strengthen muscles.

3. Describe the neutral working position.

4. Describe exercises to reduce eyestrain.

5. Describe exercises to reduce neck strain.

6. Identify common symptoms of musculoskeletal disorders.

7. Identify three categories of risk factors that contribute to increased risk of injury.

8. List the symptoms of carpal tunnel syndrome.

FILL-IN-THE-BLANK STATEMENTS

Select the best term from the list below and complete the following statements.

carpal tunnel syndrome
cumulative trauma disorders
ergonomics
maximum horizontal reach
maximum vertical reach
musculoskeletal disorders

neutral position
normal horizontal reach
sprains
strains
thenar eminence

1. _____ is the adaptation of the work environment to the human body.

2. Pain that results from repetitive stresses to muscles, tendons, nerves, and joints are symptoms of _____.

3. _____ result from pain to the muscles and skeleton systems, such as neck and shoulder pain, back pain, and carpal tunnel syndrome.

4. _____ is the type of reach created by the sweep of the forearm keeping the upper arm held at the side.

5. The reach created by the upsweep of the forearm while keeping the elbow at mid-torso level is the _____.

6. _____ is the reach created when the upper arm is fully extended to the side.

7. Injuries caused by extreme stretching of muscles or ligaments are _____.

8. _____ are injuries caused by a sudden twisting or wrenching of a joint with stretching or tearing of ligaments.

9. _____ is the fleshy elevation of the palm side of the hand.

10. Pain associated with continued flexion and extension of the hand an arm is _____.

11. _____ is the position in which the body is properly aligned and the distribution of weight throughout the spine is equal.

MULTIPLE-CHOICE QUESTIONS

Complete each question by circling the best answer.

1. Ergonomics is the _____.
   a. prevention of air pollution
   b. adaptation of the work environment to the human body
   c. adaptation of the human body to its exercise routine
   d. foundation of team dentistry

2. The goal of ergonomics is to _____.
   a. learn proper exercises
   b. help people stay healthy
   c. perform work more effectively
   d. b and c

3. What types of disorders systematic from considered musculoskeletal disorders?
   a. Headaches
   b. Heartburn
   c. Eating
   d. Neurologic disorders

4. Which is a common risk factor that contributes to a musculoskeletal disorder?
   a. Short dental procedures
   b. Working on the maxillary arch
   c. Improper positioning
   d. Infectious patients

5. What is "neutral position"?
   a. Sitting upright
   b. Keeping weight evenly distributed
   c. Being ready for instrument transfer
   d. a and b

6. A reach that is created by the sweep of the forearm with the upper arm held at the side is _____.
   a. normal vertical reach
   b. normal horizontal reach
   c. abnormal vertical reach
   d. abnormal horizontal reach

7. What types of gloves are most likely to aggravate carpal tunnel syndrome?
   a. Sterile gloves
   b. Overgloves
   c. Ambidextrous gloves
   d. Utility gloves

8. How can eyestrain be reduced?
   a. Wear prescription glasses.
   b. Readjusting your visual distance from short to long distance.
   c. Wear side shields.
   d. Use better lighting.

9. Which exercise relieves neck strain?
   a. Sit-ups
   b. Jumping jacks
   c. Jogging
   d. Full back releases

10. What is one of the most important factor in preventing carpal tunnel syndrome?
    a. Resting the eyes
    b. Resting the back
    c. Resting the hands
    d. Resting the legs

TOPICS FOR DISCUSSION

You started working as a dental assistant in Dr. Cardono's office 2 weeks ago. Last Monday, you were the only chairside assistant, and assisted in several lengthy appointments. On Tuesday, you noticed that your neck and shoulders were stiff and sore. It hurt to turn your head, and your lower back was aching.

1. Is it likely that sleeping in an awkward position caused your stiff neck?

2. What else could have caused your pain?

3. Is there anything you can do to prevent the pain from getting worse?

4. Is there anything you can suggest to the person who schedules the patients?

5. What exercises could you do to help loosen your neck and shoulders?

MULTIMEDIA PROCEDURES RECOMMENDED REVIEW

- Body Strengthening Exercises

26 The Patient's Dental Record

SHORT-ANSWER QUESTIONS

1. Describe the rationale why each patient has his or her own patient record.

2. Name and provide a brief description of four information-gathering forms that would be completed by the patient before any clinical treatment is provided.

3. Discuss why a patient's medical and dental health history would affect the type of dental treatment they receive.

FILL-IN-THE-BLANK STATEMENTS

Select the best term from the list below and complete the following statements.

alert
assessment
chronic
chronologic

demographic
forensics
litigation
registration

1. _____ is the act of conducting legal proceedings, such as a lawsuit or trial.

2. The process of evaluating a patient's condition is known as _____.

3. An illness can be characterized as _____ if it persists over a long time and is not fatal.

4. A(n) _____ time period is one that is arranged in order of occurrence.

5. _____ information can include a person's address, phone number, and work information.

6. A(n) _____ sticker/notification is included in a patient record to bring attention to a medical condition or allergy.

7. The _____ form includes personal information, information regarding the party responsible for payment, and insurance information.

8. _____ is a scientific method used to establish the identity of an individual.

MULTIPLE-CHOICE QUESTIONS

Complete each question by circling the best answer.

1. What specific information must the dental team receive from the patient before it can provide dental treatment?
   a. Medical history, financial status, and treatment plan
   b. Patient registration, medical history, and informed consent
   c. Financial status, radiographs, and treatment plan
   d. Treatment plan, progress notes, and informed consent

2. Which term describes the collection of data to help the dentist make a correct diagnosis?
   a. Assessment
   b. Decision
   c. Recall
   d. Prescription

3. Who legally "owns" a patient's dental record?
   a. The patient
   b. The dentist
   c. A court of law
   d. The dental practice

4. Quality assurance is an important asset of a practice because _____.
   a. it describes how qualified the dental staff is
   b. it describes the financial stability of the dental practice
   c. it describes the type of care a patient is receiving
   d. it describes the location of a dental practice for a specific patient population

5. The patient should be instructed to enter his or her name on the registration form as _____.
   a. first initial and last name only
   b. first name and last initial only
   c. first initial of the first, middle, and last names
   d. first name, last name, and middle initial

6. A medical-dental history form is not complete until the _____ is entered.
   a. chart number
   b. signature and date
   c. Social Security number
   d. insurance number

7. The dental history section of a health history form provides the dental team with information concerning _____.
   a. dental procedures that are legal for the dental assistant to complete
   b. previous dental treatment and type of care received
   c. necessary dental treatment and care needed
   d. the address of the patient's previous dentist

8. Which medical condition would require an alert notification?
   a. Migraines
   b. A toothache
   c. An allergy to penicillin
   d. A broken leg

9. What dental form would a patient review and sign if referred to a dental specialist for an extensive procedure?
   a. Progress notes
   b. Treatment plan form
   c. Clinical examination form
   d. Informed consent form

CASE STUDY

Jenny Stewart is a new patient to the practice and has been asked to arrive 15 minutes before her scheduled appointment to complete new-patient forms. As you introduce yourself and call her back to the treatment area, Ms. Stewart points to a specific tooth that has been bothering her for a couple of weeks. You seat Ms. Stewart in the operatory and begin reviewing her medical-dental health history with her. You see that she has checked "yes" for having high blood pressure and is taking medication for it. She also noted that she is allergic to penicillin.

1. What dental forms does the business assistant hand to Ms. Stewart to complete?

2. Ms. Stewart indicated that she takes medication for high blood pressure. Where on the medical-dental history form would this be noted and what additional information will the dentist want to know about her high blood pressure?

3. Are there any medical alerts that should be indicated on the patient record? If so, what are they and how would they be indicated on the patient record?

4. Why would there be a question on the dental history section about who the patient's previous dentist was and how often the patient saw that dentist?

5. The dentist is ready to examine the patient clinically. What dental form is used to chart existing dental conditions?

6. Complete the progress notes for Ms. Stewart's dental visit in the following space.

7. The next time Ms. Stewart returns to the office, what dental form is used to inquire about changes in her health?

⊖volve
learning system

DENTRIX EXERCISES

Before you can begin this exercise, it will be necessary to download the Dentrix G4 Learning Edition to your computer. Please review the step-by-step installation instructions posted on the companion Evolve website (http://evolve.elsevier. com/Robinson/modern).

Practice Setup

Before you work through any Dentrix exercises, refer to the **Practice Setup** instructions posted on the Evolve website. Also refer to the Dentrix *User's Guide*, Chapter 2.

Patient Record

An important component of the practice management system is electronic storage and filing of patient records. In Dentrix, this activity is completed in the Family File. The Family File manages and stores both patient and family information, such as address, phone number, insurance coverage, and important health information. For additional information, refer to the Dentrix *User's Guide*, Chapter 3.

Exercise 1: Selecting a Patient of Record

Please refer to the information on the Evolve website on **Selecting a Patient** and **Editing a Patient's File.** Then answer the following questions for each patient listed below:

1. Sally Hayes

   a. What is her marital status?

   b. Does she have children?

   c. What is her date of birth?

   d. Does she have insurance? If so, with which provider(s)?

   e. Does she have any medical alerts? If yes, please specify.

2. Lawrence Schow

   a. What is his marital status?

   b. Does he have children?

   c. What is his date of birth?

   d. Does he have insurance? If so, with which provider(s)?

   e. Does he have any medical alerts? If yes, please specify.

3. Randall Young

   a. What is his marital status?

   b. Does he have children?

   c. What is his date of birth?

   d. Does he have insurance? If so, with which provider(s)?

   e. Does he have any medical alerts? If yes, please specify.

Exercise 2: Creating a New Patient/Family

Please refer to the information on the Evolve website on **Creating a New Family.** Then complete the following exercise:
Prepare a Family File for the Brooks family.
- Assign Gregory as the head of house.
- Add Jessica as a new family member.
- Add Christopher as a new family member.

Gregory H. Brooks

DOB	10/11/1978
Social Security #	231-47-4956
Home Address	3871 South Dockside Dr.
	Southside, NV 33333
Occupation	Sales rep for Verizon Wireless
	250 Westwood Ave.
	Southside, NV 33333
Phone	213-555-7290 (home)
	213-555-4199 (cell)
	213-972-4300 (work)
Dental Insurance	Blue Cross Blue Shield
	Group#21774
Medical Alerts	N/A
Dentist	Dennis Smith

Jessica Brooks

DOB	5/20/1984
Social Security #	342-11-7843
Home Address	3871 South Dockside Dr.
	Southside, NV 33333
Occupation	Stay-at-home mother
Phone	213-555-7290 (home)
	213-586-4198 (cell)
Dental Insurance	Blue Cross Blue Shield
	(under husband's policy) 21774
Medical Alerts	Pregnant
Dentist	Maria Cook

Christopher L. Brooks

DOB	1/22/2005
Social Security #	N/A
Home Address	3871 South Dockside Dr.
	Southside, NV 33333
Dental Insurance	Blue Cross Blue Shield
	(under father's policy) 21774
Medical Alerts	Allergic to penicillin
Dentist	Brenda Childs

COMPETENCY 26.1: REGISTERING A NEW PATIENT

Performance Objective

By following a routine procedure that meets stated protocols, the student will use the appropriate forms to gather patient registration and medical history information.

Evaluation and Grading Criteria

 3   Student competently met the stated criteria without assistance.

 2   Student required assistance in order to meet the stated criteria.

 1   Student showed uncertainty when performing the stated criteria.

 0   Student was not prepared and needs to repeat the step.

 N/A   No evaluation of this step.

Instructor shall define grades for each point range earned on completion of each performance-evaluated task.

Performance Standards

The minimum number of satisfactory performances required before final evaluation is _____.

Instructor shall identify by * those steps considered critical. If step is missed or minimum competency is not met, the evaluated procedure fails and must be repeated.

PERFORMANCE CRITERIA	*	SELF	PEER	INSTRUCTOR	COMMENTS
1. Explained each form to the patient and described the importance of providing the information.					
2. Provided the patient with a black pen and/clipboard, or iPad.					
3. Aided the patient in completing the form, if needed.					
4. Asked questions if the information on the form required clarification.					
5. Maintained an environment that was private and confidential when talking with patient and reviewing forms.					
6. Verified the patient's signature and date on the form.					
ADDITIONAL COMMENTS					

Total number of points earned _____

Grade _____ Instructor's initials _____

COMPETENCY 26.2: OBTAINING A MEDICAL-DENTAL HEALTH HISTORY

Performance Objective

By following a routine procedure that meets stated protocols, the student will obtain a completed medical and dental history.

Evaluation and Grading Criteria

<u>3</u>   Student competently met the stated criteria without assistance.

<u>2</u>   Student required assistance in order to meet the stated criteria.

<u>1</u>   Student showed uncertainty when performing the stated criteria.

<u>0</u>   Student was not prepared and needs to repeat the step.

<u>N/A</u>   No evaluation of this step.

Instructor shall define grades for each point range earned on completion of each performance-evaluated task.

Performance Standards

The minimum number of satisfactory performances required before final evaluation is _____.

Instructor shall identify by * those steps considered critical. If step is missed or minimum competency is not met, the evaluated procedure fails and must be repeated.

PERFORMANCE CRITERIA	*	SELF	PEER	INSTRUCTOR	COMMENTS
1. Explained the need for the form to be completed.					
2. Provided the patient with a pen and clipboard, or iPad.					
3. Aided the patient in completing the form, if needed.					
4. Reviewed the completed form for completeness.					
5. Asked questions about information that required clarification.					
6. Verified the patient's signature and date on the form.					
ADDITIONAL COMMENTS					

Total number of points earned _____

Grade _____ Instructor's initials _____

COMPETENCY 26.3: ENTERING TREATMENT IN A PATIENT RECORD

Performance Objective

By following a routine procedure that meets stated protocols, the student will record dental treatment and services accurately, completely, and legibly.

Evaluation and Grading Criteria

3	Student competently met the stated criteria without assistance.
2	Student required assistance in order to meet the stated criteria.
1	Student showed uncertainty when performing the stated criteria.
0	Student was not prepared and needs to repeat the step.
N/A	No evaluation of this step.

Instructor shall define grades for each point range earned on completion of each performance-evaluated task.

Performance Standards

The minimum number of satisfactory performances required before final evaluation is _____.

Instructor shall identify by * those steps considered critical. If step is missed or minimum competency is not met, the evaluated procedure fails and must be repeated.

PERFORMANCE CRITERIA	*	SELF	PEER	INSTRUCTOR	COMMENTS
1. Completed all entries in black ink.					
2. Entered date.					
3. Completed progress notes in detail: tooth number and surface, type of dental procedure, anesthetic used, and type of dental materials used.					
4. Noted how the patient tolerated the procedure.					
5. Noted what procedure is scheduled for next appointment.					
6. Signature/initials entered by dentist and dental assistant.					
ADDITIONAL COMMENTS					

Total number of points earned _____

Grade _____ Instructor's initials _____

27 Vital Signs

SHORT-ANSWER QUESTIONS

1. List the four vital signs used to detect a person's baseline health status.

2. Describe how a person's metabolism can affect vital signs.

3. Discuss three types of thermometers described in the chapter and the strengths and weaknesses of each.

4. List the common pulse sites used for taking a pulse.

5. Describe the characteristics to look for when taking a patient's pulse.

6. Give the characteristics of respiration and how they affect a patient's breathing.

7. What is the recommended way to obtain an accurate reading of a patient's respiration count?

8. Why is it important to take a patient's blood pressure in a dental office?

9. Characterize the Korotkoff sounds heard when a person's blood pressure is taken.

10. What does a pulse oximeter measure?

FILL-IN-THE-BLANK STATEMENTS

Select the best term from the list below and complete the following statements.

antecubital space	**rhythm**
arrhythmia	**sphygmomanometer**
diastolic	**stethoscope**
electrocardiogram	**temperature**
metabolism	**thermometer**
pulse	**tympanic**
radial	**volume**
respiration	

1. _____ is the term used to describe the blood pressure reading when the heart chambers are relaxed and dilated.

2. The _____ is a procedure that measures the activity of the heartbeat, and can be used in the detection and diagnosis of heart abnormalities.

3. _____ refers to the physical and chemical processes that occur within a living cell or organism that are necessary for the maintenance of life.

4. An irregularity in the force or rhythm of the heartbeat is termed _____.

5. _____ relates to the fold in the arm in front of the elbow.

6. The _____ is a rhythmic throbbing of arteries produced by regular contraction of the heart.

7. The _____ artery is located at the base of the thumb on the wrist side.

8. _____ is the act or process of inhaling and exhaling (breathing).

9. The instrument used for measuring blood pressure is the _____.

10. The instrument used for listening to sounds produced within the body is the _____.

11. _____ is the degree of hotness or coldness of a body or an environment.

12. The instrument used for measuring a person's temperature is the _____.

13. _____ is a sequence or pattern.

14. _____ relates to or resembles a drum.

15. The quantity or amount of a substance is its _____.

MULTIPLE-CHOICE QUESTIONS

Complete each question by circling the best answer.

1. The four vital signs used to detect a patient's baseline health are _____.
   a. speech, temperature, gait, and electrocardiogram
   b. height, weight, age, and race
   c. cholesterol, blood pressure, vision, and blood sugar
   d. respiration, temperature, pulse, and blood pressure

2. A thermometer is used for _____.
   a. detecting a patient's pulse
   b. taking a patient's temperature
   c. reading a patient's blood pressure
   d. counting a patient's respiration

3. Which location produces the highest temperature reading?
   a. Oral
   b. Ancillary
   c. Rectal
   d. Axillary

4. Where is the tympanic thermometer placed for a temperature reading?
   a. Orally
   b. Under the arm
   c. Rectally
   d. In the ear

5. Which artery has a pulse?
   a. Carotid
   b. Radial
   c. Brachial
   d. All of the above

6. Which artery would you normally palpate when taking a patient's pulse?
   a. Carotid
   b. Radial
   c. Brachial
   d. Any of the above

7. A normal pulse rate for an adult is _____.
   a. 25 to 65 beats per minute
   b. 40 to 80 beats per minute
   c. 60 to 100 beats per minute
   d. 75 to 115 beats per minute

8. Respiration is the process of _____.
   a. speaking
   b. breathing
   c. feeling
   d. moving

9. What breathing pattern is characteristic of a very rapid rate of breathing?
   a. Bradypnea
   b. Normal pattern
   c. Tachypnea
   d. Sighing

10. The normal respiration rate for an adult is _____.
   a. 5 to 10 breaths per minute
   b. 12 to 20 breaths per minute
   c. 18 to 30 breaths per minute
   d. 20 to 40 breaths per minute

11. What is the diastolic reading of a blood pressure?
   a. The first sound heard after pressure is released from the cuff
   b. The pulse rate taken at the brachial artery
   c. The silence between the first and last sounds after pressure is released from the cuff
   d. The last sound heard after pressure is released from the cuff

12. What instruments are used to take a patient's blood pressure?
   a. A patient record and a watch with a second hand
   b. A sphygmomanometer and a stethoscope
   c. A pen and paper to record the reading
   d. A thermometer and an electrocardiogram

13. The term for the small groove or fold on the inner arm is the _____.
   a. antecubital space
   b. brachial fold
   c. radial bend
   d. femur

14. Who discovered the series of sounds that can be heard during the taking of a blood pressure reading?
   a. G. V. Black
   b. W. B. Saunders
   c. Nicolai Korotkoff
   d. C. Edmund Kells

15. Which would be considered a normal blood pressure reading for an adult?
   a. 90/60
   b. 110/75
   c. 132/85
   d. 145/97

171

CASE STUDY

Mary Robins, a 53-year-old patient, is scheduled for a routine dental prophylaxis. You escort her back to the treatment area, review her health history update, and take her vital signs. The readings that were obtained today are temperature 99° F, pulse 75, respiration 20, and blood pressure 148/95.

1. What type of procedure is dental prophylaxis? Which dental professional would most likely be treating Mrs. Robins today?

2. As the clinical assistant in the office, what could be your role for seeing this patient today?

3. How would Mrs. Robins be positioned for taking vital signs?

4. Mrs. Robins states that she should not have her blood pressure taken on her left arm because she has had a mastectomy. She indicates that her lymph nodes were also removed on that side and the doctor told her not to have her blood pressure taken on that side. Why would a doctor say this? You may need to refer to the Internet for the reason why.

5. In addition to the rate of respiration, what characteristics of the patient's respiration should you note in her patient record?

6. Are any of the readings not within normal range? If so, which ones?

7. What is your next step when a patient's vital sign reading is abnormal?

MULTIMEDIA PROCEDURES RECOMMENDED REVIEW ⊖volve
learning system

- Taking a Patient's Blood Pressure

COMPETENCY 27.1: TAKING AN ORAL TEMPERATURE READING WITH A DIGITAL THERMOMETER

Performance Objective

By following a routine procedure that meets stated protocols, the student will obtain and record an oral temperature.

Evaluation and Grading Criteria

3   Student competently met the stated criteria without assistance.

2   Student required assistance in order to meet the stated criteria.

1   Student showed uncertainty when performing the stated criteria.

0   Student was not prepared and needs to repeat the step.

N/A   No evaluation of this step.

Instructor shall define grades for each point range earned on completion of each performance-evaluated task.

Performance Standards

The minimum number of satisfactory performances required before final evaluation is _____.

Instructor shall identify by * those steps considered critical. If a step is missed or minimum competency is not met, the evaluated procedure fails and must be repeated.

PERFORMANCE CRITERIA	*	SELF	PEER	INSTRUCTOR	COMMENTS
1. Obtained the equipment and supplies required for taking an oral temperature.					
2. Placed personal protective equipment according to the procedure.					
3. Placed a sheath over the probe of the digital thermometer.					
4. Turned the thermometer on, and, after display indicated "ready," gently placed it under the patient's tongue.					
5. Instructed the patient to close the lips over the thermometer and not to talk or move during the reading.					
6. Left the thermometer in place for the appropriate time and then removed it from the patient's mouth.					
7. Reviewed the temperature reading and recorded it in the patient record.					

Continued

8. Turned the thermometer off, removed and disposed of the sheath, and disinfected the thermometer as recommended.					
9. Documented the procedure in the patient record.					
ADDITIONAL COMMENTS					

Total number of points earned _____

Grade _____ Instructor's initials _____

COMPETENCY 27.2: TAKING A PATIENT'S PULSE

Performance Objective

By following a routine procedure that meets stated protocols, the student will take and record a patient's pulse.

Evaluation and Grading Criteria

3	Student competently met the stated criteria without assistance.
2	Student required assistance in order to meet the stated criteria.
1	Student showed uncertainty when performing the stated criteria.
0	Student was not prepared and needs to repeat the step.
N/A	No evaluation of this step.

Instructor shall define grades for each point range earned on completion of each performance-evaluated task.

Performance Standards

The minimum number of satisfactory performances required before final evaluation is _____.

Instructor shall identify by * those steps considered critical. If a step is missed or minimum competency is not met, the evaluated procedure fails and must be repeated.

PERFORMANCE CRITERIA	*	SELF	PEER	INSTRUCTOR	COMMENTS
1. Obtained the equipment and supplies required for taking a pulse.					
2. Placed personal protective equipment according to the procedure.					
3. Seated the patient in an upright position with the arm extended at the heart level.					
4. Placed the tips of index and middle fingers on the patient's radial artery.					
5. Felt for the patient's pulse before counting.					
6. Counted the pulse for 30 seconds and multiplied by 2 for a 1-minute reading.					
7. Documented the procedure in the patient record.					
ADDITIONAL COMMENTS					

Total number of points earned _____

Grade _____ Instructor's initials _____

COMPETENCY 27.3: TAKING A PATIENT'S RESPIRATION

Performance Objective

By following a routine procedure that meets stated protocols, the student will obtain and record a patient's respiration.

Evaluation and Grading Criteria

 3   Student competently met the stated criteria without assistance.

 2   Student required assistance in order to meet the stated criteria.

 1   Student showed uncertainty when performing the stated criteria.

 0   Student was not prepared and needs to repeat the step.

 N/A   No evaluation of this step.

Instructor shall define grades for each point range earned on completion of each performance-evaluated task.

Performance Standards

The minimum number of satisfactory performances required before final evaluation is _____.

Instructor shall identify by * those steps considered critical. If a step is missed or minimum competency is not met, the evaluated procedure fails and must be repeated.

PERFORMANCE CRITERIA	*	SELF	PEER	INSTRUCTOR	COMMENTS
1. Obtained the equipment and supplies required for taking a respiration.					
2. Placed personal protective equipment according to the procedure.					
3. Instructed the patient to remain seated and to maintain position while taking the pulse.					
4. Counted the rise and fall of the patient's chest for 30 seconds.					
5. Multiplied the count by 2 for a 1-minute reading.					
6. Documented the procedure in the patient record.					
ADDITIONAL COMMENTS					

Total number of points earned _____

Grade _____ Instructor's initials _____

COMPETENCY 27.4: TAKING A PATIENT'S BLOOD PRESSURE

Performance Objective

By following a routine procedure that meets stated protocols, the student will obtain and record a patient's blood pressure.

Evaluation and Grading Criteria

3	Student competently met the stated criteria without assistance.
2	Student required assistance in order to meet the stated criteria.
1	Student showed uncertainty when performing the stated criteria.
0	Student was not prepared and needs to repeat the step.
N/A	No evaluation of this step.

Instructor shall define grades for each point range earned on completion of each performance-evaluated task.

Performance Standards

The minimum number of satisfactory performances required before final evaluation is _____.

Instructor shall identify by * those steps considered critical. If a step is missed or minimum competency is not met, the evaluated procedure fails and must be repeated.

PERFORMANCE CRITERIA	*	SELF	PEER	INSTRUCTOR	COMMENTS
1. Obtained the equipment and supplies required for taking a blood pressure.					
2. Placed personal protective equipment according to the procedure.					
3. Seated the patient with the arm extended at the heart level and supported.					
4. Rolled up the patient's sleeve, if possible.					
5. Palpated the patient's brachial artery to feel for a pulse.					
6. Counted the patient's brachial pulse for 30 seconds.					
7. Multiplied the count by 2 for a 1-minute reading.					
8. Added 40 mm Hg to get inflation level.					
9. Readied the cuff by expelling any air.					
10. Placed the appropriate size cuff around the patient's arm 1 inch above antecubital space, with arrow over the brachial artery.					
11. Tightened the cuff and closed it using the Velcro tabs.					
12. Placed the earpieces of the stethoscope properly.					

Continued

13. Placed the stethoscope disc over the site of brachial artery.				
14. Grasped the rubber bulb, locked the valve, and inflated the cuff to note reading.				
15. Slowly released the valve and listened for sounds.				
16. Slowly continued to release air from the cuff until the last sound was heard.				
17. Documented the procedure in the patient record.				
18. Disinfected the diaphragm and earpieces of the stethoscope.				

ADDITIONAL COMMENTS

Total number of points earned _____

Grade _____ Instructor's initials _____

COMPETENCY 27.5: TAKING A PATIENT'S PULSE OXIMETRY (EXPANDED FUNCTION)

Performance Objective

By following a routine procedure that meets stated protocols, the student will obtain and record a patient's oximetry level.

Evaluation and Grading Criteria

_3_	Student competently met the stated criteria without assistance.
_2_	Student required assistance in order to meet the stated criteria.
_1_	Student showed uncertainty when performing the stated criteria.
_0_	Student was not prepared and needs to repeat the step.
_N/A_	No evaluation of this step.

Instructor shall define grades for each point range earned on completion of each performance-evaluated task.

Performance Standards

The minimum number of satisfactory performances required before final evaluation is _____.

Instructor shall identify by * those steps considered critical. If a step is missed or minimum competency is not met, the evaluated procedure fails and must be repeated.

PERFORMANCE CRITERIA	*	SELF	PEER	INSTRUCTOR	COMMENTS
1. Obtained the equipment and supplies required for performing oximetry.					
2. Placed personal protective equipment according to the procedure.					
3. Seated the patient with the arm extended on the chair arm.					
4. Turned the pulse oximeter on and waited for it to calibrate.					
5. Ensured that the finger was cleaned and any nail polish removed. Selected the correct size probe and positioned the probe on the finger, avoiding excess force.					
6. Allowed several seconds for the pulse oximeter to detect the pulse and calculate the oxygen saturation.					
7. Documented the procedure in the patient record.					
ADDITIONAL COMMENTS					

Total number of points earned

Grade _____ Instructor's initials _____

Chapter **27 Vital Signs**

COMPETENCY 27.6: TAKING A PATIENT'S ECG (EXPANDED FUNCTION)

Performance Objective

By following a routine procedure that meets stated protocols, the student will obtain and record a patient's electrocardiographic reading.

Evaluation and Grading Criteria

<u>3</u>   Student competently met the stated criteria without assistance.

<u>2</u>   Student required assistance in order to meet the stated criteria.

<u>1</u>   Student showed uncertainty when performing the stated criteria.

<u>0</u>   Student was not prepared and needs to repeat the step.

<u>N/A</u>   No evaluation of this step.

Instructor shall define grades for each point range earned on completion of each performance-evaluated task.

Performance Standards

The minimum number of satisfactory performances required before final evaluation is _____.

Instructor shall identify by * those steps considered critical. If a step is missed or minimum competency is not met, the evaluated procedure fails and must be repeated.

PERFORMANCE CRITERIA	*	SELF	PEER	INSTRUCTOR	COMMENTS
1. Obtained the equipment and supplies required for taking an ECG.					
2. Placed personal protective equipment according to the procedure.					
3. Explained the procedure to the patient and answered any questions.					
4. Instructed the patient to lie down on his or her back.					
5. Readied all forms and tracing paper with the patient's name, the date, the time, and any medication the patient was receiving intravenously or orally.					
6. At each location, wiped the patient's skin with an alcohol wipe and placed the electrodes at the six positions on the patient's chest.					
7. Connected the lead wires to the correct electrodes, making sure the lead wires were not crossed.					
8. At the surgeon's request, proceeded by pressing the auto button. (The machine automatically begins the tracing.)					

Continued

9. Continued the tracings until the completion of the procedure.				
10. Removed the lead wires and electrodes from the patient's chest.				
11. Turned off the electrocardiograph, properly disinfected it, and placed it in its storage area.				
12. Documented the procedure in the patient record.				

ADDITIONAL COMMENTS

Total number of points earned _____

Grade _____ Instructor's initials

28 Oral Diagnosis and Treatment Planning

SHORT-ANSWER QUESTIONS

1. List and describe the examination and diagnostic techniques used for patient assessment.

2. Discuss the role of the assistant in the clinical examination of a patient.

3. List the six Black's classification of cavities.

4. Differentiate between an anatomic diagram and a geometric diagram for charting.

5. Describe the reason for using red, blue and black for color coding when charting.

6. Define PSR and explain how the scores should be recorded.

7. Why is there a need for a soft tissue examination?

8. A treatment plan is used for what reason?

FILL-IN-THE-BLANK STATEMENTS

Select the best term from the list below and complete the following statements.

detection
extraoral
furcation
intraoral
mobility
morphology

mucogingival
palpation
probing
restoration
symmetric

1. _____ is the process of returning a tooth to being a functional permanent unit of the dentition.

2. _____ is the process of discovering decay.

3. The space or division of the roots on a tooth is termed _____.

4. _____ is a term meaning movement.

5. _____ is the branch of biology that includes the form and structure.

6. To touch or feel for abnormalities within soft tissue is _____.

7. _____ is the term that is used to mean outside the oral cavity.

8. The periodontal probe is used for _____ and for measuring the periodontal pocket.

9. _____ is the term that means within the oral cavity.

MULTIPLE-CHOICE QUESTIONS

Complete each question by circling the best answer.

1. The four reasons that a patient would seek dental care are _____.
   a. proximity to home, reasonable price, nice decor, good dentist
   b. as a new patient, for an emergency, for a consultation, as a returning patient
   c. sterile techniques, knowledgeable staff, appropriate attire, clean environment
   d. takes insurance, has flexible hours, performs specialty procedures, no waiting

2. What technique(s) could be used to diagnose decay within a tooth?
   a. Visual
   b. Instrumentation
   c. Radiographic
   d. All of the above

3. Which dental material would not be used in the restoration of a tooth?
   a. Silver
   b. Gold
   c. Brass
   d. Porcelain

4. What charting symbol would indicate that a tooth is not visible in the mouth?
   a. Circle around the tooth
   b. Outline with diagonal lines
   c. X through the tooth
   d. a and c

5. Intraoral imaging is similar to _____.
   a. use of a video camera
   b. use of a laser
   c. radiography
   d. a and c

6. Which of G. V. Black's classifications of cavities could involve the premolars and molars?
   a. Class I
   b. Class II
   c. Class III
   d. a and b

7. Which classification(s) of cavities could involve the incisors?
   a. Class I
   b. Class III
   c. Class IV
   d. All of the above

8. How would a MOD amalgam be charted for tooth number 4?
   a. The gingival one third on the facial surface would be outlined in blue/black and colored in.
   b. The mesial, occlusal, and distal surfaces would be outlined in blue/black and colored in.
   c. The occlusal surface would be outlined in blue/black, with an A placed in the center.
   d. The mesial and distal surfaces of the tooth would be outlined in red, and the occlusal portion would be colored in blue.

9. Which dental professional(s) can legally perform periodontal probing and a bleeding index for a patient?
   a. Dentist
   b. Assistant
   c. Hygienist
   d. a and c

10. Which classification of dental mobility is most severe?
    a. Class I
    b. Class II
    c. Class III
    d. Class IV

11. The cervical lymph nodes would be examined during an extraoral exam to look for _____.
    a. bruising
    b. swelling
    c. tenderness
    d. b and c

12. To avoid triggering the gag reflex during a soft tissue examination, the mouth mirror can be _____.
    a. warmed before placing it in the mouth
    b. moved from left to right in the back of the tongue
    c. placed firmly on the back of the tongue
    d. a and b

13. To examine the tongue, _____ is/are used to gently pull forward for examination.
    a. cotton pliers
    b. gauze square
    c. tongue retractor
    d. suture material

14. The abbreviation PFM stands for _____.
    a. patient fainted momentarily
    b. porcelain filling on mesial
    c. porcelain fused to metal
    d. protrusive forward movement

MULTIMEDIA PROCEDURES RECOMMENDED REVIEW ⊖volve
learning system

- Extraoral and Intraoral Photography

CHARTING EXERCISE

Chart the following findings on the diagram:

#1	impacted	#15	sealant on the occlusal surface
#2	DO amalgam	#16-17	impacted
#3	MOD amalgam	#18-21	four-unit gold bridge with #18 having a root canal
#4	porcelain crown	#24	mesial composite
#5-7	three-unit gold bridge	#25	distal composite
#8	root canal with porcelain crown	#26	fractured mesial/incisal edge
#9	root canal with porcelain crown	#27	MO composite
#10	class V facial composite	#28	missing
#11	class V facial decay	#29	MOD amalgam with recurrent decay
#12	MO decay	#30	occlusal amalgam with recurrent decay
#13	abscess	#31	impacted
#14	class I lingual pit amalgam with sealant placed on occlusal surface		

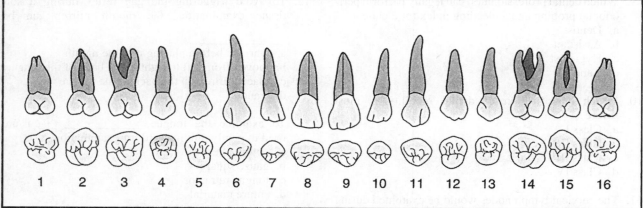

Right

Left

From your charting, answer the following questions:

1. Which teeth are missing and have been replaced by a bridge?

2. Which teeth have class II restorations?

3. Is there an area within the mouth in which drifting could take place? If so, where would it occur?

4. Why do you think the dentist chose to place composite resin material in tooth #28?

5. Which teeth would be of concern for the oral and maxillofacial surgeon?

6. What specialist would the patient be referred to for tooth #13?

DENTRIX EXERCISE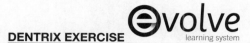

An important component of the practice management system is the Patient Chart, which makes it easy to enter electronically all existing, recommended, and completed treatments or conditions. Dentrix uses standard, easy-to-recognize textbook charting symbols. Treatment is color coded, making it easy to see at a glance whether a procedure is completed, existing, a condition, or still to be completed. Please refer to the Dentrix *User's Guide*, Chapter 4, to review how to chart within the system.

Exercise: Charting

Please refer to information on the Evolve website on **Charting.** Then chart the following conditions and completed treatment for the patient listed below:

Gregory H. Brooks

#1	Missing	#15	MO amalgam
#2	MO amalgam	#16	Missing
#3	MOD amalgam	#17	Missing
#4	PFM crown	#18	MO amalgam
#5	DO amalgam	#19	Root canal treatment with gold crown
#8	Missing	#20	MO amalgam
#11	Amalgam restoration	#30	Missing with three-unit gold bridge
#12	MOD amalgam	#32	Missing
#13	MOD amalgam		
#14	MOD amalgam		

COMPETENCY 28.1: EXTRAORAL AND INTRAORAL PHOTOGRAPHY (EXPANDED FUNCTION)

Performance Objective

By following a routine procedure that meets stated protocols, when provided with a camera, the student will demonstrate the proper technique for taking extraoral and intraoral photographs.

Evaluation and Grading Criteria

3	Student competently met the stated criteria without assistance.
2	Student required assistance in order to meet the stated criteria.
1	Student showed uncertainty when performing the stated criteria.
0	Student was not prepared and needs to repeat the step.
N/A	No evaluation of this step.

Instructor shall define grades for each point range earned on completion of each performance-evaluated task.

Performance Standards

The minimum number of satisfactory performances required before final evaluation is _____.

Instructor shall identify by * those steps considered critical. If step is missed or minimum competency is not met, the evaluated procedure fails and must be repeated.

PERFORMANCE CRITERIA	*	SELF	PEER	INSTRUCTOR	COMMENTS
1. Obtained the equipment and supplies required for the procedure.					
2. Calibrated the camera system for intraoral and extraoral photographs. For intraoral photography, set the camera to the landscape mode, and for extraoral photography, set the camera to the portrait mode.					
3. Seated the patient in the dental chair in an upright position with a neutral color background.					
4. For extraoral photographs, positioned self 5 to 6 feet from the patient.					
5. For intraoral photographs, made sure the mouth was visible and partially dried.					
6. Positioned the retractors symmetrically and then pulled them out and away from the mouth.					
7. If a mouth mirror or reflection mirror was used, it was free of fog and kept clean.					
8. Kept fingertips, mirror edges, and retractors out of the picture.					
9. Photographs of the teeth were correct and in alignment.					

Continued

10. Cleaned and disinfected all supplies and returned to case.					
11. Documented the procedure in the patient record.					

ADDITIONAL COMMENTS

Total number of points earned _____

Grade _____ Instructor's initials _____

COMPETENCY 28.2: THE SOFT TISSUE EXAMINATION (EXPANDED FUNCTION)

Performance Objective

By following a routine procedure that meets stated protocols, the student will demonstrate the proper technique for performing a soft tissue examination.

Evaluation and Grading Criteria

 3   Student competently met the stated criteria without assistance.

 2   Student required assistance in order to meet the stated criteria.

 1   Student showed uncertainty when performing the stated criteria.

 0   Student was not prepared and needs to repeat the step.

 N/A   No evaluation of this step.

Instructor shall define grades for each point range earned on completion of each performance-evaluated task.

Performance Standards

The minimum number of satisfactory performances required before final evaluation is _____.

Instructor shall identify by * those steps considered critical. If step is missed or minimum competency is not met, the evaluated procedure fails and must be repeated.

PERFORMANCE CRITERIA	*	SELF	PEER	INSTRUCTOR	COMMENTS
1. Obtained the equipment and supplies required for the procedure.					
2. Escorted the patient to the treatment area, observing patient's general appearance, speech, and behavior.					
3. Placed personal protective equipment according to the procedure.					
4. Seated the patient in the dental chair in an upright position.					
5. Explained the procedure to the patient.					
Extraoral Features					
1. Examined the patient's face, neck, and ears for asymmetry and abnormal swelling.					
2. Looked for abnormal tissue changes, skin abrasions, and discolorations.					
3. Evaluated the texture, color, and continuity of the vermilion border, commissures of the lips, philtrum, and smile line.					
4. Documented the procedure in the patient record.					

Continued

Cervical Lymph Nodes					
1. Positioned self in front and to the side of patient.					
2. Examined the right side of the neck using the fingers and thumb of the right hand to follow the chain of lymph nodes, starting in front of the ear and continuing to the collarbone.					
3. Examined the left side of the neck in the same manner.					
4. Documented the procedure in the patient record.					
Temporomandibular Joint					
1. Evaluated TMJ movement in centric, lateral, protrusive, and retrusive movements. Asked the patient to open and close the mouth normally and to move the jaw from side to side.					
2. Listened for noise in the TMJ as the patient opened and closed the mouth.					
3. Documented the procedure in the patient record.					
Indications of Oral Habits					
1. Looked for oral habits of thumb sucking, tongue-thrust swallow, mouth breathing, and tobacco use.					
2. Looked for signs of oral habits such as bruxism, grinding, and clenching.					
Interior of the Lips					
1. Examined the mucosa and the labial frenum of the patient's upper lip.					
2. Examined the mucosa and the labial frenum of the patient's lower lip.					
3. Palpated the tissues to detect lumps or abnormalities.					

Chapter **28** **Oral Diagnosis and Treatment Planning**

Oral Mucosa and Tongue					
1. Palpated the tissue of the buccal mucosa.					
2. Examined the tissue covering the hard palate.					
3. Examined the buccal mucosa and the opening of Stensen's duct.					
4. Evaluated the patient's tongue by pulling it forward and from side to side, noting color, papillae, and abnormalities.					
5. Instructed the patient to open the mouth, stick the tongue out, and say "Ahh" and examined the uvula and the base of the tongue.					
Floor of the Mouth					
1. Palpated the soft tissues of the face above and below the mandible.					
2. Palpated the interior of the floor of the mouth.					
3. Observed the quantity and consistency of the flow of the saliva.					
4. Documented the procedure in the patient record.					

ADDITIONAL COMMENTS

Total number of points earned _____

Grade _____ Instructor's initials_____

COMPETENCY 28.3: CHARTING OF TEETH

Performance Objective

By following a routine procedure that meets stated protocols, when provided with a patient chart and colored pencils, the student will demonstrate the proper technique for recording the dentist's findings as dictated during an examination.

Evaluation and Grading Criteria

 3   Student competently met the stated criteria without assistance.

 2   Student required assistance in order to meet the stated criteria.

 1   Student showed uncertainty when performing the stated criteria.

 0   Student was not prepared and needs to repeat the step.

 N/A   No evaluation of this step.

Instructor shall define grades for each point range earned on completion of each performance-evaluated task.

Performance Standards

The minimum number of satisfactory performances required before final evaluation is _____.

Instructor shall identify by * those steps considered critical. If step is missed or minimum competency is not met, the evaluated procedure fails and must be repeated.

PERFORMANCE CRITERIA	*	SELF	PEER	INSTRUCTOR	COMMENTS
1. Obtained the equipment and supplies required for the procedure.					
2. Placed personal protective equipment according to the procedure.					
3. Seated the patient in the dental chair in a supine position and draped him/her with a patient napkin.					
4. If using paper chart, had red/black pen and clinical examination form readily available.					
5. Recorded specific notations the operator called out for each tooth.					
6. Throughout the procedure, used the air syringe to dry the mouth mirror.					
7. Adjusted the operating light as necessary.					
8. Documented the procedure in the patient record.					
9. Accurately read back the operator's findings.					
ADDITIONAL COMMENTS					

Total number of points earned _____

Grade _____ Instructor's initials _____

Chapter **28 Oral Diagnosis and Treatment Planning**

COMPETENCY 28.4: PERIODONTAL SCREENING: EXAMINATION OF THE GINGIVAL TISSUES

Performance Objective

By following a routine procedure that meets stated protocols, the student will assist the dentist or the dental hygienist in the examination and charting of gingival tissues.

Evaluation and Grading Criteria

 3   Student competently met the stated criteria without assistance.

 2   Student required assistance in order to meet the stated criteria.

 1   Student showed uncertainty when performing the stated criteria.

 0   Student was not prepared and needs to repeat the step.

 N/A   No evaluation of this step.

Instructor shall define grades for each point range earned on completion of each performance-evaluated task.

Performance Standards

The minimum number of satisfactory performances required before final evaluation is _____.

Instructor shall identify by * those steps considered critical. If step is missed or minimum competency is not met, the evaluated procedure fails and must be repeated.

PERFORMANCE CRITERIA	*	SELF	PEER	INSTRUCTOR	COMMENTS
1. Obtained the equipment and supplies required for the procedure.					
2. Placed personal protective equipment according to the procedure.					
3. Seated the patient in the dental chair in a supine position and draped him/her with a patient napkin.					
4. Provided air from the air-water syringe on the mirror during the examination.					
5. Transferred the instruments as needed.					
6. Recorded probing depths correctly on the examination form.					
7. Charted bleeding.					
8. Noted sensitivity, calculus, mobility, saliva changes, and furcation involvement.					

Continued

9. Documented the procedure in the patient record.					
10. Accurately read back the operator's findings.					

ADDITIONAL COMMENTS

Total number of points earned _____

Grade _____ Instructor's initials _____

29 The Special Needs and Medically Compromised Patient

SHORT-ANSWER QUESTIONS

1. Give three categories in which older adults can be defined throughout their aging process. Explain how they differ with regard to their dental care.

2. List the five most common oral health conditions that affect the older patient.

3. What is important to obtain from a medically compromised patient in addition to the medical-dental history?

4. You are scheduling a patient with early onset Alzheimer's. What clinical considerations should be taken into consideration for this patient?

5. You will be transferring a patient from a wheelchair to the patient chair. What will you need to have on hand to help in the moving process?

FILL-IN-THE-BLANK STATEMENTS

Select the best term from the list below and complete the following statements.

aging
Alzheimer's
anemia
angina
arthritis
asthma
atrophy
bacteremia
bronchitis
diabetes

epilepsy
hemophilia
hyperthyroidism
hypothyroidism
leukemia
myocardial infarction
seizure
stroke
xerostomia

1. A person with a deficiency in the oxygen-carrying component of blood is said to have _____.

2. A term for wasting away or deterioration is _____.

3. A(n) _____ is a sudden episode, spasm, or convulsion that occurs in specific disorders.

4. The presence of bacteria in the blood is termed _____.

5. _____ is a term for the loss of saliva production that causes a dry mouth.

201

6. _____ is severe pain in the chest that results from an insufficient supply of blood to the heart.

7. _____ is a neurological disorder that includes sudden recurring seizures of motor, sensory, or psychological function.

8. _____ refers to the changes that occur with becoming mature or older.

9. _____ is a disorder in which progressive mental deterioration occurs in middle to old age.

10. A blood coagulation disorder in which the blood fails to clot normally is _____.

11. _____ is a chronic disorder in which the inflammation of the mucous membrane of the bronchial tubes occurs.

12. A condition that results from excessive activity of the thyroid gland is _____.

13. A disease of the bone marrow in which an abnormal development of white blood cells occurs is _____.

14. _____ is also known as a heart attack.

15. Inflammation, pain, and swelling of the joints are symptoms of _____.

16. _____ is a chronic respiratory disease that is often associated with allergies and is characterized by sudden recurring attacks of labored breathing, chest constriction, and coughing.

17. _____ is a condition that results from severe thyroid insufficiency.

18. A sudden loss of brain function caused by a blockage or rupture of a blood vessel to the brain is a _____.

19. _____ is a metabolic disorder that is characterized by having high blood glucose and insufficient insulin.

MULTIPLE-CHOICE QUESTIONS

Complete each question by circling the best answer.

1. The fastest-growing segment of the population is _____.
   a. infants
   b. young adults
   c. middle-aged adults
   d. older adults

2. What characteristic below might fit a frail older adult?
   a. Better educated
   b. Beginning to have multiple health problems
   c. Having fewer natural teeth
   d. a and c

3. Xerostomia is a condition of _____.
   a. excessive saliva
   b. eye infection
   c. loss of hearing
   d. dry mouth

4. What oral health condition(s) affect(s) the aging population?
   a. Periodontal disease
   b. Root caries
   c. Bone resorption
   d. All of the above

5. Dementia is a condition of _____.
   a. bone loss
   b. deterioration of mental capacity
   c. aging
   d. body senses

6. What common oral adverse effect results from taking Dilantin?
   a. Xerostomia
   b. Allergies
   c. Endocarditis
   d. Anxiety

7. A medical disorder used to describe a cerebrovascular accident is _____.
   a. angina
   b. stroke
   c. seizure
   d. Alzheimer's

8. An example of a neurologic disorder is _____.
   a. emphysema
   b. multiple sclerosis
   c. Parkinson's disease
   d. b and c

9. The leading cause of death in the United States is _____.
   a. emphysema
   b. Alzheimer's disease
   c. heart disease
   d. drug abuse

10. Hypertension is also known as _____.
    a. high blood pressure
    b. seizure
    c. depression
    d. anemia

11. What organ in the body is affected by pulmonary disorders?
    a. Heart
    b. Brain
    c. Lungs
    d. Kidneys

12. The abbreviation COPD stands for _____.
    a. common older population disorders
    b. category of pulmonary diseases
    c. cardiovascular patients in dentistry
    d. chronic obstructive pulmonary disease

13. What body system would be affected if a patient has an overactive thyroid gland?
    a. Digestive
    b. Endocrine
    c. Pulmonary
    d. Neurologic

14. A patient with type I diabetes is classified as _____.
    a. diet dependent
    b. exercise dependent
    c. insulin dependent
    d. non-insulin dependent

15. What is the psychological disorder in which a patient experiences alternating, prolonged episodes of extreme elation followed by depression?
    a. Bulimia
    b. Angina
    c. Bipolar disorder
    d. Schizophrenia

16. Which developmental disorder causes difficulties with social interaction, communication, and repetitive behaviors?
    a. Autism
    b. Epilepsy
    c. Arthritis
    d. Angina

17. Which category best describes a modification of care made by the dental team for a patient requiring scheduling changes or shorter appointments?
    a. Category I
    b. Category II
    c. Category III
    d. Category IV

Josh Allen is a 37-year-old patient of the practice who has been diagnosed with multiple sclerosis. His condition has deteriorated so that he now uses a wheelchair. He has called the office to schedule an appointment to have two teeth restored.

1. How would you categorize this patient with regard to how treatment is to proceed?

2. Do you think a certain time of day would be better for the dental team to see Josh? If so, what would be the best time for his appointment?

3. As you are reviewing the health history update, Josh indicates that he has recently been diagnosed with trigeminal neuralgia. What is this disorder and how will it affect his dental care?

4. Are there any specific drugs that Josh may be taking that should be noted before the time of treatment? If so, what would they be?

5. Your dental treatment area is not designed to treat a patient in a wheelchair. Where should Josh be seen by the dentist?

6. Describe specific techniques that help when moving a patient from a wheelchair to the dental chair.

7. Describe specific ergonomic techniques that will keep you from injuring yourself while moving a patient from a wheelchair to the dental chair.

8. Based on his disease, should Josh be put in an upright or supine position?

COMPETENCY 29.1: TRANSFERRING A PATIENT FROM A WHEELCHAIR

Performance Objective

By following a routine procedure that meets stated protocols, the student will demonstrate the proper technique for transferring a patient from a wheelchair.

Evaluation and Grading Criteria

<u>3</u>   Student competently met the stated criteria without assistance.

<u>2</u>   Student required assistance in order to meet the stated criteria.

<u>1</u>   Student showed uncertainty when performing the stated criteria.

<u>0</u>   Student was not prepared and needs to repeat the step.

<u>N/A</u>   No evaluation of this step.

Instructor shall define grades for each point range earned on completion of each performance-evaluated task.

Performance Standards

The minimum number of satisfactory performances required before final evaluation is _____.

Instructor shall identify by * those steps considered critical. If a step is missed or minimum competency is not met, the evaluated procedure fails and must be repeated.

PERFORMANCE CRITERIA	*	SELF	PEER	INSTRUCTOR	COMMENTS
1. Cleared all items from the pathway of the wheelchair.					
2. Determined whether it was best for the wheelchair to enter the treatment room forward or backward.					
3. Moved the wheelchair as close to the dental chair as possible.					
4. Locked the wheelchair.					
5. Brought the patient to the edge of the wheelchair.					
6. Positioned the gait belt around the waist, with the clip in front.					
7. Placed the fingers between the gait belt and the patient, using an underhand motion to grasp the gait belt.					
8. Assisted the patient to stand slowly.					
9. Pivoted the patient so that the back side was closest to the dental chair.					

Continued

Chapter **29** **The Special Needs and Medically Compromised Patient**

10. Lowered the patient into the dental chair.					
11. Swung the patient's legs over and onto the dental chair.					
ADDITIONAL COMMENTS					

Total number of points earned _____

Grade _____ Instructor's initials _____

30 Principles of Pharmacology

SHORT-ANSWER QUESTIONS

1. Differentiate between a drug's chemical, generic, and trade names.

2. Describe the stages a drug goes through once it enters the body.

3. Identify each section of a prescription.

4. Describe the various methods of administering a medication.

5. Define the DEA and explain why drugs are categorized in the five schedules of the Controlled Substance Act.

6. Describe the negative effects of drug use.

7. Describe why drug reference materials would be located in a dental office.

8. Describe the classification of prescription drugs and their effects.

9. Explain why a drug would be prescribed for a patient in the dental office.

FILL-IN-THE-BLANK STATEMENTS

Select the best term from the list below and complete the following statements.

absorption	**inscription**
antibiotic prophylaxis	**patent**
distribution	**pharmacology**
dosage	**prescription**
dose	**signature**
drug	**superscription**
excretion	**systemic**
generic	

1. _____ is the action by which a drug leaves the body.

2. The action by which the body takes in or receives a drug is _____.

3. The _____ includes the drugs's name, strength, dose and number of tablets to dispense.

4. The term _____ relates to a drug that affects a specific system of the body.

5. A specified quantity or volume of a drug or medicine is termed a(n) _____.

6. A substance that is used in the diagnosis, treatment, or prevention of a disease is a(n) _____.

7. _____ is the process or action of a drug when it is released throughout the body.

8. The _____ refers to specific instructions on a prescription about how to take a prescribed medicine.

9. _____ is the amount of drug to be administered according to time and specific body weight.

10. A drug that can be obtained without a prescription is referred to as a(n) _____ drug.

11. _____ is the science of drugs.

12. A(n) _____ is a written order to the pharmacist for a specific drug.

13. A patient may be prescribed a(n) _____ for the prevention of infective endocarditis.

14. The _____ are the patients name, address date and Rx symbol.

15. A(n) _____ name of a drug does not have a brand name or a trademark.

MULTIPLE-CHOICE QUESTIONS

Complete each question by circling the best answer.

1. Where do drugs come from?
   a. Plants
   b. Animals
   c. Laboratories
   d. All of the above

2. What type of drug name is *Advil*?
   a. Generic name
   b. Brand name
   c. Chemical name
   d. Company name

3. The slowest route of absorption for a drug is

   _____.
   a. intramuscular
   b. rectal
   c. oral
   d. intravenous

4. Who is responsible for regulating the sale of medicines?
   a. Pharmaceutical companies
   b. U.S. Department of Public Health
   c. Centers for Disease Control and Prevention
   d. U.S. Food and Drug Administration

5. Within the dental profession, who can prescribe drugs to a patient?
   a. Oral surgeon
   b. General dentist
   c. Dental hygienist
   d. a and b

6. What part of the prescription includes the name and the quantity of the drug?
   a. Subscription
   b. Inscription
   c. Superscription
   d. Description

7. If a medication were placed sublingually, where would it be placed?
   a. Into a vein
   b. Rectally
   c. Under the tongue
   d. On the surface of the skin

8. By which route is a subcutaneous injection given?
   a. Muscular
   b. Intravenous
   c. Nerve
   d. Under the skin

9. What schedule of drug is Tylenol with codeine?
   a. I
   b. II
   c. III
   d. IV

10. Which of the following is the term used to describe the body's negative reaction to a drug?
   a. Adverse effect
   b. Response
   c. Symptom
   d. Sign

11. An analgesic could be prescribed for _____.
   a. treatment of seizure
   b. treatment of a fungus
   c. pain relief
   d. b and c

12. Which of the following is an example of an antibiotic?
   a. Aspirin
   b. Codeine
   c. Erythromycin
   d. Meperidine

13. A drug that is prescribed to slow the clotting of blood is _____.
   a. epinephrine
   b. Valium
   c. Coumadin
   d. Monistat

14. _____ could be prescribed to a patient with a cold.
   a. Dilantin
   b. Prozac
   c. Sudafed
   d. Ventolin

15. The main reason that Ritalin is considered a Schedule II drug is its _____.
   a. hallucinogenic effects
   b. high potential for abuse
   c. depressant effects
   d. high cost

ACTIVITY

Listed below are different types of prescription drugs. Give the body system it affects.

DRUG	BODY SYSTEM AFFECTED (CARDIOVASCULAR, RESPIRATORY, GASTROINTESTINAL, NEUROLOGIC, PSYCHOACTIVE, ENDOCRINE)
1. Prozac	
2. Zocor	
3. Tagamet	
4. Dilantin	
5. Bronchodilator	
6. Metformin	
7. Valium	
8. Nitroglycerin	
9. Albuterol	
10. HCTZ	

ABBREVIATION IDENTIFICATION

List the meaning of each abbreviation.

ABBREVIATION	MEANING
a.a.	
a.c.	
a.m.	
b.i.d.	
disp.	
H	
h.s.	
NPO	
p.c.	
prn	
q.	
q.d.	
q.i.d.	
SL	
t, tsp	
T, tbs	
t.i.d.	

CASE STUDY

John Miller is scheduled for a gingivectomy on the lower right quadrant. In setting up the treatment area, you upload the patient's radiographic images and health history on the screen for the dentist to review. While assembling the documents, you notice an alert notification indicating that Mr. Miller has a history of congenital heart disease and is allergic to penicillin.

1. What is an alert notification in an electronic record?

2. Where would you find the alert notification?

3. Is there any significance to Mr. Miller's heart disease in terms of today's procedure? If so, what is it?

4. What type of procedure is Mr. Miller having today?

5. Is this procedure considered high risk? If so, what does that mean?

6. Why is it important to know that Mr. Miller is allergic to penicillin?

7. What classification of antibiotic could be chosen when penicillin is contraindicated?

8. According to the American Heart Association, should a prophylactic antibiotic be prescribed for Mr. Miller before the time of his appointment?

9. Following the procedure, Mr. Miller will receive postoperative instructions, and a prescription for Tylenol with codeine. Why would this drug be prescribed for Mr. Miller?

31 Assisting in a Medical Emergency

SHORT-ANSWER QUESTIONS

1. Define *medical emergency*.

2. Give the specific role each staff member should be responsible for during a medical emergency.

3. List the basic items to be included in an emergency kit.

4. Explain how the use of an AED can benefit the person in an emergency.

5. What are common physical changes often seen in a patient during a medical emergency?

6. What are the most common causes of hypoglycemia in a patient?

FILL-IN-THE-BLANK STATEMENTS

Select the best term from the list below and complete the following statements.

acute
allergen
allergy
anaphylaxis
antibodies
antigen
aspiration
asthma
cardiopulmonary resuscitation

convulsion
erythema
gait
hyperglycemia
hyperventilating
hypoglycemia
hypotension
myocardial infarction
syncope

1. A(n) _____ is a sudden, irregular, uncontrollable movement of a limb or body.

2. _____ is a redness that is most likely caused by inflammation or infection.

3. _____ is an emergency procedure used to restore a heartbeat and life.

4. Rapid onset of a symptom can be termed _____.

213

5. A person who is highly sensitive to a certain substance has a(n) _____ to that substance.

6. A(n) _____ can trigger an allergic state.

7. _____ is the loss of consciousness caused by lack of blood going to the brain.

8. A person's _____ is his or her way or manner of moving by foot.

9. _____ is a chronic respiratory disease.

10. _____ is a life-threatening hypersensitivity to a substance.

11. _____ are the immunoglobulins produced by lymphoid tissue in response to a foreign substance.

12. A substance that is introduced into the body to stimulate the production of an antibody is an _____.

13. _____ is the action of inhaling something by mouth.

14. An abnormally low level of glucose in the blood is the condition of _____.

15. _____ is a condition that is diagnosed in a patient with an abnormally low blood pressure.

16. A(n) _____ can occur when an area of heart tissue undergoes necrosis as a result of obstruction of blood supply.

17. An abnormally high presence of glucose in the blood is the condition diagnosed as _____.

18. When a patient is breathing abnormally fast or deeply, they are said to be _____.

MULTIPLE-CHOICE QUESTIONS

Complete each question by circling the best answer.

1. The best way to prevent an emergency is to _____.
   a. have the drug kit placed by the dental chair and ready for all procedures
   b. know your patient
   c. call the patient's physician before the appointment
   d. take vital signs before seating the patient in the dental treatment area

2. Most medical emergencies occur because a person is _____.
   a. overweight
   b. not taking his or her medication
   c. stressed
   d. not active

3. What member of the dental team is ultimately responsible for a patient's safety in the dental office?
   a. Dental assistant
   b. Dental hygienist
   c. Business assistant
   d. Dentist

4. Which member of the dental team would most likely oversee calling the emergency medical services?
   a. Dentist
   b. Business assistant
   c. Dental laboratory technician
   d. Another patient

5. Emergency phone numbers should be kept _____.
   a. next to each phone
   b. in each treatment area
   c. in the business area
   d. all of the above

6. What minimum credentials must a dental assistant have to meet emergency care standards?
   a. RN license
   b. CPR, Heimlich, and AED certification
   c. EMT certification
   d. DDS

7. In emergency care, the acronym *CAB* signifies _____.
   a. certified assisted breathing
   b. continue airway breathing
   c. chest compressions, airway, breathing
   d. call ambulance before

8. What is the ratio of breaths to compressions when CPR is performed on an adult?
   a. 5 compressions/1 breath
   b. 7 compressions/2 breaths
   c. 15 compressions/1 breath
   d. 30 compressions/2 breaths

9. The most commonly used drug for a medical emergency is _____.
   a. an ammonia capsule
   b. nitroglycerin
   c. epinephrine
   d. oxygen

10. In emergency care, the acronym *AED* represents _____.
    a. automated external defibrillator
    b. auxiliary examination device
    c. acute emergency drill
    d. airway that is externally directed

11. What does the AED provide to the heart?
    a. Oxygen
    b. Jolt of an electrical current
    c. Blood
    d. Heat

12. If a patient tells you how he or she is feeling, the patient is referring to a(n) _____.
    a. diagnosis
    b. sign
    c. explanation
    d. symptom

13. When a patient is not responsive to sensory stimulation, he or she is said to be _____.
    a. agitated
    b. unconscious
    c. comatose
    d. paralyzed

14. The medical term for fainting is _____.
    a. stroke
    b. seizure
    c. syncope
    d. senile

15. _____ is the medical term for chest pain.
    a. angioplasty
    b. angina
    c. angiogram
    d. anemia

16. A stroke is also a _____.
    a. cerebrovascular accident
    b. cardiovascular accident
    c. cardiopulmonary obstruction
    d. obstructed airway

17. The medication that an asthmatic patient would most commonly carry with them is _____.
    a. nitroglycerin
    b. insulin
    c. a bronchodilator
    d. an analgesic

18. What type of allergic response is considered life-threatening?
    a. Grand mal seizure
    b. Anaphylaxis
    c. Myocardial infarction
    d. Airway obstruction

19. An abnormal increase of glucose in the blood can cause _____.
    a. angina
    b. hypoglycemia
    c. seizure
    d. hyperglycemia

20. The universal sign that someone is choking is _____.
    a. wheezing
    b. placement of the hands to the throat
    c. turning blue
    d. screaming

Renee Miller is a 26-year-old woman in her third trimester of pregnancy. Renee is scheduled to have a root canal on tooth #12. Her health history and treatment record show no indication of adverse reactions to prior treatment. Renee is seated in the dental chair and pretreatment instructions have been provided. The procedure goes well and you are repositioning the chair in an upright position while the dentist is discussing posttreatment steps. Renee comments that she feels faint.

1. How was the dental chair positioned for Renee during the procedure?

2. Should Renee have dental care while she is pregnant? If so, what is your reasoning?

3. What might be the cause for Renee's feeling faint?

4. What type of medical emergency may Renee be experiencing?

5. How do you respond to this medical emergency?

6. What drug should be retrieved from the emergency medical kit?

7. Could anything else have been done to prevent Renee from feeling this way?

COMPETENCY 31. 1: ADMINISTERING OXYGEN DURING AN EMERGENCY

Performance Objective

By following a routine procedure that meets stated protocols, the student will demonstrate the proper technique for preparing an oxygen system for use in an emergency.

Evaluation and Grading Criteria

3	Student competently met the stated criteria without assistance.
2	Student required assistance in order to meet the stated criteria.
1	Student showed uncertainty when performing the stated criteria.
0	Student was not prepared and needs to repeat the step.
N/A	No evaluation of this step.

Instructor shall define grades for each point range earned on completion of each performance-evaluated task.

Performance Standards

The minimum number of satisfactory performances required before final evaluation is _____.

Instructor shall identify by * those steps considered critical. If a step is missed or minimum competency is not met, the evaluated procedure fails and must be repeated.

PERFORMANCE CRITERIA	*	SELF	PEER	INSTRUCTOR	COMMENTS
1. Obtained the equipment and supplies required for the procedure.					
2. Confirmed that the oxygen cylinder had an adequate level of oxygen.					
3. Turned the unit on and adjusted the flow according to the oxygen use.					
4. Veryified the oxygen flow by listening and feeling through the delivery device.					
5. Positioned the device comfortably.					
6. Monitored the patient.					
7. Documented the procedure in the patient record.					
ADDITIONAL COMMENTS					

Total number of points earned _____

Grade _____ Instructor's initials _____

COMPETENCY 31.2: RESPONDING TO THE UNCONSCIOUS PATIENT

Performance Objective

By following a routine procedure that meets stated protocols, the student will physically and verbally respond to loss of consciousness in a patient.

Evaluation and Grading Criteria

3   Student competently met the stated criteria without assistance.

2   Student required assistance in order to meet the stated criteria.

1   Student showed uncertainty when performing the stated criteria.

0   Student was not prepared and needs to repeat the step.

N/A   No evaluation of this step.

Instructor shall define grades for each point range earned on completion of each performance-evaluated task.

Performance Standards

The minimum number of satisfactory performances required before final evaluation is _____.

Instructor shall identify by * those steps considered critical. If a step is missed or minimum competency is not met, the evaluated procedure fails and must be repeated.

PERFORMANCE CRITERIA	*	SELF	PEER	INSTRUCTOR	COMMENTS
1. Placed the patient in a supine / subsupine position,					
2. Completed a head tilt/jaw thrust to open air way.					
3. Loosened any binding clothing.					
4. Evaluated the oxygen level and had an ammonia inhalant ready to administer under the patient's nose.					
5. Had oxygen ready for use.					
6. Monitored and recorded the vital signs.					
7. Documented the procedure in the patient record.					
ADDITIONAL COMMENTS					

Total number of points earned _____

Grade _____ Instructor's initials _____

COMPETENCY 31.3: RESPONDING TO THE PATIENT WITH CHEST PAIN

Performance Objective

By following a routine procedure that meets stated protocols, the student will physically and verbally respond to a patient with chest pain.

Evaluation and Grading Criteria

3   Student competently met the stated criteria without assistance.

2   Student required assistance in order to meet the stated criteria.

1   Student showed uncertainty when performing the stated criteria.

0   Student was not prepared and needs to repeat the step.

N/A   No evaluation of this step.

Instructor shall define grades for each point range earned on completion of each performance-evaluated task.

Performance Standards

The minimum number of satisfactory performances required before final evaluation is _____.

Instructor shall identify by * those steps considered critical. If a step is missed or minimum competency is not met, the evaluated procedure fails and must be repeated.

PERFORMANCE CRITERIA	*	SELF	PEER	INSTRUCTOR	COMMENTS
1. Called for medical assistance.					
2. Placed the patient in an semi up-right position.					
3. Obtained nitroglycerin from the patient or emergency kit.					
4. Administered oxygen as directed by the dentist.					
5. Monitored and recorded the vital signs.					
6. Documented the procedure in the patient record.					
ADDITIONAL COMMENTS					

Total number of points earned _____

Grade _____ Instructor's initials _____

COMPETENCY 31.4: RESPONDING TO THE PATIENT WHO IS EXPERIENCING A CEREBROVASCULAR ACCIDENT (STROKE)

Performance Objective

By following a routine procedure that meets stated protocols, the student will physically and verbally respond to a patient who is experiencing a stroke (CVA).

Evaluation and Grading Criteria

3	Student competently met the stated criteria without assistance.
2	Student required assistance in order to meet the stated criteria.
1	Student showed uncertainty when performing the stated criteria.
0	Student was not prepared and needs to repeat the step.
N/A	No evaluation of this step.

Instructor shall define grades for each point range earned on completion of each performance-evaluated task.

Performance Standards

The minimum number of satisfactory performances required before final evaluation is _____.

Instructor shall identify by * those steps considered critical. If a step is missed or minimum competency is not met, the evaluated procedure fails and must be repeated.

PERFORMANCE CRITERIA	*	SELF	PEER	INSTRUCTOR	COMMENTS
1. Called for medical assistance.					
2. Positoned the patient in a semi-sitting position with the head elevated.					
3. Monitored and recorded the vital signs.					
4. Initiated CPR if the patient became unconscious.					
5. Documented the procedure in the patient record.					
ADDITIONAL COMMENTS					

Total number of points earned _____

Grade _____ Instructor's initials _____

COMPETENCY 31.5: RESPONDING TO THE PATIENT WITH BREATHING DIFFICULTY

Performance Objective

By following a routine procedure that meets stated protocols, the student will physically and verbally respond to a patient with a breathing problem.

Evaluation and Grading Criteria

 3   Student competently met the stated criteria without assistance.

 2   Student required assistance in order to meet the stated criteria.

 1   Student showed uncertainty when performing the stated criteria.

 0   Student was not prepared and needs to repeat the step.

 N/A   No evaluation of this step.

Instructor shall define grades for each point range earned on completion of each performance-evaluated task.

Performance Standards

The minimum number of satisfactory performances required before final evaluation is _____.

Instructor shall identify by * those steps considered critical. If a step is missed or minimum competency is not met, the evaluated procedure fails and must be repeated.

PERFORMANCE CRITERIA	*	SELF	PEER	INSTRUCTOR	COMMENTS
1. Postion the patient in a comfortable upright position.					
2. Used a quiet voice to calm and reassure the patient.					
3. If the breathing problem was associated with asthma, had the patient self-medicate with an inhaler.					
4. If the patient was hyperventilating, instructed the patient to cup the hands and breathe into them.					
5. Monitored and recorded the vital signs.					
6. Documented the procedure in the patient record.					

ADDITIONAL COMMENTS

Total number of points earned _____

Grade _____ Instructor's initials _____

COMPETENCY 31.6: RESPONDING TO THE PATIENT WHO IS EXPERIENCING AN ALLERGIC REACTION

Performance Objective

By following a routine procedure that meets stated protocols, the student will physically and verbally respond to a patient who is experiencing an allergic reaction.

Evaluation and Grading Criteria

3	Student competently met the stated criteria without assistance.
2	Student required assistance in order to meet the stated criteria.
1	Student showed uncertainty when performing the stated criteria.
0	Student was not prepared and needs to repeat the step.
N/A	No evaluation of this step.

Instructor shall define grades for each point range earned on completion of each performance-evaluated task.

Performance Standards

The minimum number of satisfactory performances required before final evaluation is _____.

Instructor shall identify by * those steps considered critical. If a step is missed or minimum competency is not met, the evaluated procedure fails and must be repeated.

PERFORMANCE CRITERIA	*	SELF	PEER	INSTRUCTOR	COMMENTS
Localized Rash					
1. Identified the area of rash.					
2. Monitored and recorded the vital signs.					
3. Readied an antihistamine or epinephrine autoinjector (EpiPen) for administration if needed.					
4. Initiated basic life support if needed.					
5. Referred the patient for medical consultation.					
6. Documented the procedure in the patient record.					
Anaphylaxis					
1. Called for emergency assistance.					
2. Placed the patient in a supine position.					
3. If the patient became unconscious, started basic life support (CPR).					
4. Prepared epinephrine autoinjector (EpiPen) for administration.					
5. Administered oxygen.					

Continued

6. Monitored and recorded the vital signs.				
7. Documented the procedure in the patient record.				

ADDITIONAL COMMENTS

Total number of points earned _____

Grade _____ Instructor's initials _____

COMPETENCY 31.7: RESPONDING TO THE PATIENT WHO IS EXPERIENCING A CONVULSIVE SEIZURE

Performance Objective

By following a routine procedure that meets stated protocols, the student will physically and verbally respond to a patient who is experiencing a convulsive seizure.

Evaluation and Grading Criteria

 3   Student competently met the stated criteria without assistance.

 2   Student required assistance in order to meet the stated criteria.

 1   Student showed uncertainty when performing the stated criteria.

 0   Student was not prepared and needs to repeat the step.

 N/A   No evaluation of this step.

Instructor shall define grades for each point range earned on completion of each performance-evaluated task.

Performance Standards

The minimum number of satisfactory performances required before final evaluation is _____.

Instructor shall identify by * those steps considered critical. If a step is missed or minimum competency is not met, the evaluated procedure fails and must be repeated.

PERFORMANCE CRITERIA	*	SELF	PEER	INSTRUCTOR	COMMENTS
Grand Mal Seizure (General Seizure)					
1. Called for medical assistance.					
2. If the patient was in the dental chair, quickly removed all materials from the mouth and placed the patient in a supine position.					
3. Protected the patient from self-injury during the seizure.					
4. Readied the anticonvulsant from the drug kit if needed.					
5. Initiated basic life support if needed.					
6. Monitored and recorded the vital signs.					
7. Documented the procedure in the patient record.					
Focal Seizure (Partial Seizure)					
1. Position in comfortable position.					
2. Monitored and recorded the vital signs.					

Continued

3. Referred the patient for medical consultation.				
4. Documented the procedure in the patient record.				

ADDITIONAL COMMENTS

Total number of points earned _____

Grade _____ Instructor's initials _____

COMPETENCY 31.8: RESPONDING TO THE PATIENT WHO IS EXPERIENCING A DIABETIC EMERGENCY

Performance Objective

By following a routine procedure that meets stated protocols, the student will physically and verbally respond to a patient who is experiencing a diabetic emergency.

Evaluation and Grading Criteria

3   Student competently met the stated criteria without assistance.

2   Student required assistance in order to meet the stated criteria.

1   Student showed uncertainty when performing the stated criteria.

0   Student was not prepared and needs to repeat the step.

N/A   No evaluation of this step.

Instructor shall define grades for each point range earned on completion of each performance-evaluated task.

Performance Standards

The minimum number of satisfactory performances required before final evaluation is _____.

Instructor shall identify by * those steps considered critical. If a step is missed or minimum competency is not met, the evaluated procedure fails and must be repeated.

PERFORMANCE CRITERIA	*	SELF	PEER	INSTRUCTOR	COMMENTS
1. Called for medical assistance if necessary.					
2. If patient was conscious, inquired about when the patient last ate or took insulin.					
3. Retrieved the patient's insulin if the patient was hyperglycemic, or provided concentrated carbohydrate if the patient was hypoglycemic.					
4. If the patient was unconscious, provided basic life support.					
5. Monitored and recorded the vital signs.					
6. Documented the procedure in the patient record.					
ADDITIONAL COMMENTS					

Total number of points earned _____

Grade _____ Instructor's initials _____

32 The Dental Office

SHORT-ANSWER QUESTIONS

1. Describe how the dental office environment should be maintained in a professional style.

2. What are the important features of a reception area?

3. Describe the goals to be met when designing the dental operatory.

4. List the main clinical equipment required for the dental operatory.

5. Discuss the basic function of the dental unit.

FILL-IN-THE-BLANK STATEMENTS

Select the best term from the list below and complete the following statements.

air/water syringe
amalgamator
compressor
condensation
consultation
curing light
dental operatory
dental unit

high-volume evacuator
rheostat
saliva ejector
subsupine
supine
triturate
upright

1. Of the two types of suction systems, the _____ is the least powerful.

2. In the _____ position, commonly used in emergency situations, the patient's head is below the heart.

3. To mechanically mix something is to _____.

4. The _____ provides the necessary electrical power, water, and air to the high-speed handpiece.

5. The _____ provides compacted air to the dental unit.

233

6. The _____ is a means of delivering air and water to the oral cavity.

7. A(n) _____ is a type of meeting held to discuss a diagnosis or treatment.

8. A _____ is a wand-like attachment used to harden dental materials.

9. When the physical state of matter changes from water vapor to liquid, this is called _____.

10. A patient is sitting in the _____ position when their head and chest are vertical to the floor.

11. The _____ is used to remove fluid and debris from the oral cavity during a dental procedure.

12. A room designed for the treatment of dentistry is referred to as the _____.

13. A foot-controlled device used to operate the dental handpiece is a _____.

14. A _____ is an electrical machine used to mechanically mix encapsulated dental materials.

15. When a patient is in the _____ position, the head, chest, and knees are at the same level.

MULTIPLE-CHOICE QUESTIONS

Complete each question by circling the best answer.

1. The ideal temperature for the reception area of a dental practice is _____.
   a. 68° F
   b. 72° F
   c. 75° F
   d. 78° F

2. What type of flooring would not be suitable for the clinical areas?
   a. Carpet
   b. Wood
   c. Laminate
   d. Tile

3. What items are important to have in the reception area?
   a. Seating
   b. Lighting
   c. Reading material
   d. All the above

4. Where would money transactions take place in the dental office?
   a. The operatory
   b. The dental laboratory
   c. The administrative area
   d. The dentist's private office

5. Another term for operatory is _____.
   a. rheostat
   b. treatment area
   c. radiography
   d. laboratory

6. The dental chair is positioned in the _____ position for most dental procedures.
   a. upright
   b. subsupine
   c. supine
   d. flat

7. Which two items would be found on the dental assistant's stool that are not found on the operator's stool?
   a. Light switch and up-and-down button
   b. Back cushion and wheeled coasters
   c. Headrest and armrests
   d. Footrest and abdominal bar

8. What foot-controlled device is used to operate the dental handpiece?
   a. Dental unit
   b. Amalgamator
   c. Rheostat
   d. Central air compressor

9. The acronym HVE stands for _____?
   a. High-volume evacuator
   b. Hose vacuum evacuator
   c. Hinged-velocity evacuator
   d. Handle volume evacuator

10. Where are dental materials placed to be triturated?
   a. In the dental unit
   b. In the amalgamator
   c. In the rheostat
   d. In the central air compressor

CASE STUDY

You are responsible for showing the new staff member around the office. Nancy has been in dentistry for 14 years and is familiar with her role as a professional clinical dental assistant. She has conveyed to you that she really likes the design and setup of the dental office, and is excited about adding her personal touches with the goal of making the office more functional.

1. Why would you need to show Nancy the office, since she has been dental assistant for so long?

2. Your office has four dental operatory's with three full-time dental assistants and one dental hygienist. Describe how each member can incorporate a personal touch and still maintain a professional setting.

3. What types of items can be placed in the dental office to show a team-type atmosphere?

4. How would you feel about a new employee wanting to make changes so quickly?

5. Nancy has requested that the temperature be turned up in the clinical area because she is "cold natured" and does not want to have to wear multiple layers of clothing to stay warm. How should the office manager handle this concern? Why is the temperature set differently throughout the office?

COMPETENCY 32.1: PERFORMING THE MORNING ROUTINE (OPENING THE OFFICE)

Performance Objective

By following a routine procedure that meets stated protocols, the student will open and prepare the dental office for patients.

Evaluation and Grading Criteria

 3 Student competently met the stated criteria without assistance.

 2 Student required assistance in order to meet the stated criteria.

 1 Student showed uncertainty when performing the stated criteria.

 0 Student was not prepared and needs to repeat the step.

 N/A No evaluation of this step.

Instructor shall define grades for each point range earned on completion of each performance-evaluated task.

Performance Standards

The minimum number of satisfactory performances required before final evaluation is _____.

Instructor shall identify by * those steps considered critical. If a step is missed or minimum competency is not met, the evaluated procedure fails and must be repeated.

PERFORMANCE CRITERIA	*	SELF	PEER	INSTRUCTOR	COMMENT
1. Conveyed that staff arrive 30 minutes before the first scheduled patient.					
2. Turned on the master switches for the central air compressor and vacuum units.					
3. Turned on the master switches for the dental and radiographic units.					
4. Confirmed that the dental treatment area is ready for patient care.					
5. Checked the appointment schedule.					
6. Laid out the setup in the treatment room for the first patient.					
ADDITIONAL COMMENTS					

Total number of points earned _____

Grade _____ Instructor's initials _____

COMPETENCY 32.2: PERFORMING THE EVENING ROUTINE (CLOSING THE OFFICE)

Performance Objective

By following a routine procedure that meets stated protocols, the student will close the dental office at the end of the day.

Evaluation and Grading Criteria

3   Student competently met the stated criteria without assistance.

2   Student required assistance in order to meet the stated criteria.

1   Student showed uncertainty when performing the stated criteria.

0   Student was not prepared and needs to repeat the step.

N/A   No evaluation of this step.

Instructor shall define grades for each point range earned on completion of each performance-evaluated task.

Performance Standards

The minimum number of satisfactory performances required before final evaluation is _____.

Instructor shall identify by * those steps considered critical. If a step is missed or minimum competency is not met, the evaluated procedure fails and must be repeated.

PERFORMANCE CRITERIA	*	SELF	PEER	INSTRUCTOR	COMMENT
1. Completed the treatment room exposure control cleanup and preparation protocols.					
2. Turned off all equipment.					
3. Restocked the treatment rooms.					
4. Posted appointment schedules for the next day.					
5. Checked the appointment schedules to ensure that instruments, patient records, and laboratory work were ready for the next day.					
6. Ensured that all contaminated instruments had been processed and sterilized.					
7. Ensured that the treatment rooms were ready for use.					
8. Placed any soiled PPE in the appropriate container.					
ADDITIONAL COMMENTS					

Total number of points earned _____

Grade _____ Instructor's initials _____

33 Delivering Dental Care

SHORT-ANSWER QUESTIONS

1. Describe how a dental operatory is prepared prior to seating a patient.

2. What specific items are set out for patient treatment?

3. Describe how the operator is positioned for treatment.

4. Describe how the assistant is positioned for treatment.

5. Explain the single-handed instrument transfer technique.

6. Describe the three grasps used by the operator or assistant when carrying out an expanded function.

7. Identify five areas in which the dental assistant must become proficient when performing an expanded function.

FILL-IN-THE-BLANK STATEMENTS

Select the best term from the list below and complete the following statements.

classification of motions	**fulcrum**
delegate	**grasp**
direct supervision	**indirect supervision**
expanded function	**indirect vision**
four-handed dentistry	**operating zones**

1. The dentist is said to provide _____ when he or she is physically in the same treatment area overseeing an expanded-function procedure.

2. By following the clock concept, the dental team is using the four _____ of positioning when implementing four-handed dentistry.

3. _____ is the method of viewing a tooth using a mirror.

4. The _____ involves the five categories that describe the range of movement by the clinical assistant when he or she is assisting.

5. A(n) _____ is a procedure that is delegated to the dental assistant by the dentist that requires advanced knowledge, skill, and credentials.

6. A(n) _____ is a finger rest used to stabilize a dental instrument or handpiece.

7. The process by which a skilled dental assistant and dentist work together as a team to perform clinical tasks is termed _____.

8. A(n) _____ is the way a specific instrument or handpiece is held.

9. The dentist provides _____ when he or she is present in the immediate area to oversee the dental assistant's expanded function.

10. To _____ is when the dentist assigns or entrusts a specific procedure to the dental assistant.

MULTIPLE-CHOICE QUESTIONS

Complete each question by circling the best answer.

1. What can increase productivity in a dental office?
   a. Patient comfort
   b. Minimization of stress and fatigue
   c. Delegation of expanded functions
   d. All of the above

2. When using the clock concept for a right-handed operator, where is the static zone located?
   a. Twelve o'clock to two o'clock
   b. Two o'clock to four o'clock
   c. Four o'clock to seven o'clock
   d. Seven o'clock to twelve o'clock

3. According to the clock concept, instruments are to be exchanged during a procedure in the _____.
   a. static zone
   b. assistant's zone
   c. transfer zone
   d. operator's zone

4. Besides the assistant, what could be in the assistant's zone?
   a. Mobile dental unit
   b. Patient light
   c. Assistant's stool
   d. a and c

5. In relation to the seated operator, how is the assistant positioned?
   a. At the same height
   b. 4 to 6 inches higher than the operator
   c. Level with the patient's head
   d. 4 to 6 inches lower than the operator

6. How should the operator maintain his or her posture while performing intraoral functions?
   a. Upright
   b. Elbows at the side
   c. Feet flat on the ground
   d. All of the above

7. The chairside assistant should use _____ hand(s) in the transfer of an explorer.
   a. both
   b. one
   c. varying
   d. a or c

8. What hand does the assistant use primarily to transfer instruments to a right-handed dentist?
   a. Left
   b. Right
   c. Either

9. Depending on the operator's position, indirect vision could be used for which of the following tooth surface(s)?
   a. Lingual area of tooth #7
   b. Facial area of tooth #25
   c. Occlusal area of tooth #3
   d. All of the above

10. Another term for finger rest is _____.
   a. rheostat
   b. intraoral
   c. fulcrum
   d. tactile

11. When recreiving scissors from the operator, the assistant should grasp _____ _____.
    a. the beaks of the scissors
    b. the henge of the scissors
    c. finger slots
    d. a and c

12. During instrument transfer, the working end of an instrument is positioned _____ for tooth #13.
    a. Downward toward the mandibular
    b. Upward toward the maxillary
    c. It does not matter; the dentist will position the instrument
    d. Facing to the right

13. The exchange of surgical instruments is best executed with the use of a _____ transfer.
    a. single-handed
    b. two-handed
    c. pen-grasp
    d. reverse palm-thumb

14. During instrument transfer, the handles of the instruments are held parallel to avoid _____.
    a. injuring the patient
    b. injuring the dental team
    c. tangling
    d. All of the above

15. During a procedure, the assistant transfers instruments using their left hand and holds the _____ in their right hand.
    a. next instrument to transfer
    b. air-water syringe
    c. HVE
    d. anesthetic syringe

TOPIC FOR DISCUSSION

Dr. Williams is a general dentist who has been practicing dentistry for 35 years. She identifies her clinical team as an important part of the practice and recognizes everyone as a contributor to patient care. Dr. Williams advocates advanced functions and believes that dental assistants should be allowed to practice procedures that they are legally permitted to perform.

1. How can you find out what procedures are legal for you to practice in your state and of territory?

2. As you begin your clinical training, describe specific skills that you should review and practice to help you become more proficient in expanded functions.

3. What preparation could you use to maintain a high level of competency when performing advanced functions?

4. If a new clinical procedure became an advanced function in your state, how would you acquire the knowledge and skill to practice the procedure?

5. Are there any procedures that you believe dental assistants could perform but are not legal to perform in your state?

LABELING EXERCISE

Label the operating zones for a right-handed operator.

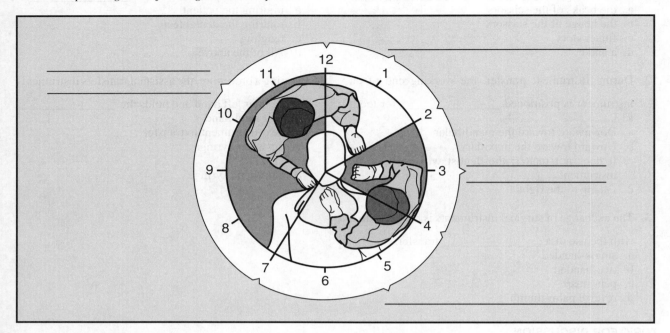

MULTIMEDIA PROCEDURES RECOMMENDED REVIEW

⊖volve learning system

■ Transferring Instruments (Single-Handed)

COMPETENCY 33.1: ADMITTING AND SEATING OF THE PATIENT

Performance Objective

By following a routine procedure that meets stated protocols, the student will admit, seat, and prepare the patient for treatment.

Evaluation and Grading Criteria

_3_	Student competently met the stated criteria without assistance.
_2_	Student required assistance in order to meet the stated criteria.
_1_	Student showed uncertainty when performing the stated criteria.
_0_	Student was not prepared and needs to repeat the step.
_N/A_	No evaluation of this step.

Instructor shall define grades for each point range earned on completion of each performance-evaluated task.

Performance Standards

The minimum number of satisfactory performances required before final evaluation is _____.

Instructor shall identify by * those steps considered critical. If a step is missed or minimum competency is not met, the evaluated procedure fails and must be repeated.

PERFORMANCE CRITERIA	*	SELF	PEER	INSTRUCTOR	COMMENT
1. Ensured that the treatment room was properly cleaned and prepared, with the chair properly positioned and the patient's path clear.					
2. Performed instrument setup and placed materials.					
3. Identified and greeted the patient appropriately.					
4. Escorted the patient to the treatment area.					
5. Placed the patient's personal items in a safe place within the treatment room.					
6. Properly seated the patient.					
7. Placed the napkin around the patient's neck.					
8. Properly positioned the dental chair for the procedure.					
9. Adjusted the operating light to focus on the patient's chest and then turned it on.					

Continued

10. Initiated conversation with the patient. Asked whether the patient had any questions about the procedure.				
11. Maintained patient comfort throughout these preparations.				
ADDITIONAL COMMENTS				

Total number of points earned _____

Grade _____ Instructor's initials _____

COMPETENCIES 33.2 AND 33.3: TRANSFERRING INSTRUMENTS WITH SINGLE-HANDED AND TWO-HANDED TECHNIQUES

Performance Objective

By following a routine procedure that meets stated protocols, the student will perform single-handed and specialized instrument transfer in a safe and efficient manner.

Evaluation and Grading Criteria

 3   Student competently met the stated criteria without assistance.

 2   Student required assistance in order to meet the stated criteria.

 1   Student showed uncertainty when performing the stated criteria.

 0   Student was not prepared and needs to repeat the step.

 N/A   No evaluation of this step.

Instructor shall define grades for each point range earned on completion of each performance-evaluated task.

Performance Standards

The minimum number of satisfactory performances required before final evaluation is _____.

Instructor shall identify by * those steps considered critical. If a step is missed or minimum competency is not met, the evaluated procedure fails and must be repeated.

PERFORMANCE CRITERIA	*	SELF	PEER	INSTRUCTOR	COMMENT
Single-Handed Transfer and Exchange					
1. Placed personal protective equipment according to the procedure.					
2. Retrieved the instrument from the instrument tray using the left hand, grasping the instrument with the thumb and index and middle fingers, opposite the working end.					
3. Held the instrument in the transfer zone, in a ready position 8 to 10 inches away from the dentist.					
4. Anticipated the dentist's transfer signal and positioned the new instrument parallel to the instrument in the dentist's hand.					
5. Retrieved the used instrument using the last two fingers, tucking it into the palm.					
6. Delivered the new instrument to the dentist.					
7. Maintained safety throughout the transfer.					

Continued

Non-locking Cotton Pliers Transfer				
1. Placed personal protective equipment according to the procedure.				
2. Retrieved the cotton pliers, grasping a cotton pellet securely by pinching the beaks together.				
3. Delivered the instrument to the transfer zone and positioned the pliers for transfer.				
4. Delivered the pliers so the dentist could grasp it correctly and hold the beaks together.				
5. Retrieved the pliers without dropping the cotton pellet.				
Forceps Transfer				
1. Placed personal protective equipment according to the procedure.				
2. Used the right hand to retrieve the forceps from the tray. Carried the forceps to the transfer zone in the position of use.				
3. Used the left hand to retrieve the used instrument from the dentist.				
4. Delivered the new instrument to the dentist in a palm grasp in the appropriate position of use.				
5. Returned the used instrument to its proper position on the tray.				
Handpiece Exchange				
1. Placed personal protective equipment according to the procedure.				
2. Used the left hand to retrieve the handpiece, holding it for delivery in the position of use in the transfer zone.				
3. Used the right hand to take the used instrument from the dentist.				
4. Delivered the handpiece to the dentist in the appropriate position.				
5. When exchanging two handpieces, did not tangle the cords.				

Air-Water Syringe Transfer					
1. Placed personal protective equipment according to the procedure.					
2. Held the nozzle of the air-water syringe in the delivery position, holding the tip in between the fingers.					
3. Retrieved the instrument the dentist was using, and then delivered the syringe.					
Scissors Transfer					
1. Placed personal protective equipment according to the procedure.					
2. Retrieved the scissors from the tray, holding them near the working end with the beaks slightly open.					
3. Positioned the handle of the scissors over the dentist's fingers.					
4. Retrieved the used instrument with the right hand.					
ADDITIONAL COMMENTS					

Total number of points earned _____

Grade _____ Instructor's initials _____

COMPETENCY 33.4: USING THE DENTAL MIRROR INTRAORALLY

Performance Objective

By following a routine procedure that meets stated protocols, the student will demonstrate the proper technique for using the dental mirror intraorally.

Evaluation and Grading Criteria

 3 Student competently met the stated criteria without assistance.

 2 Student required assistance in order to meet the stated criteria.

 1 Student showed uncertainty when performing the stated criteria.

 0 Student was not prepared and needs to repeat the step.

 N/A No evaluation of this step.

Instructor shall define grades for each point range earned on completion of each performance-evaluated task.

Performance Standards

The minimum number of satisfactory performances required before final evaluation is _____.

Instructor shall identify by * those steps considered critical. If a step is missed or minimum competency is not met, the evaluated procedure fails and must be repeated.

PERFORMANCE CRITERIA	*	SELF	PEER	INSTRUCTOR	COMMENT
1. Placed personal protective equipment according to the procedure.					
2. Placed the patient in a supine position.					
3. Positioned self as the operator.					
4. Used patient light and illuminated the oral cavity.					
5. Asked the patient to position the head with mandibular incisors vertical to the floor.					
6. Grasped the dental mirror in the left hand using a pen grasp.					
7. Positioned the dental mirror for indirect vision of the lingual surfaces of the maxillary anterior.					
8. Positioned the dental mirror for light illumination on the lingual aspects of the mandibular anterior.					

Continued

9. Positioned the dental mirror for retraction.					
10. Maintained patient comfort throughout these steps.					

ADDITIONAL COMMENTS

Total number of points earned _____

Grade _____ Instructor's initials _____

COMPETENCY 33.5: USING AN INSTRUMENT INTRAORALLY (EXPANDED FUNCTION)

Performance Objective

By following a routine procedure that meets stated protocols, the student will demonstrate the proper technique for using an instrument intraorally.

Evaluation and Grading Criteria

_3_   Student competently met the stated criteria without assistance.

_2_   Student required assistance in order to meet the stated criteria.

_1_   Student showed uncertainty when performing the stated criteria.

_0_   Student was not prepared and needs to repeat the step.

_N/A_   No evaluation of this step.

Instructor shall define grades for each point range earned on completion of each performance-evaluated task.

Performance Standards

The minimum number of satisfactory performances required before final evaluation is _____.

Instructor shall identify by * those steps considered critical. If a step is missed or minimum competency is not met, the evaluated procedure fails and must be repeated.

PERFORMANCE CRITERIA	*	SELF	PEER	INSTRUCTOR	COMMENT
1. Placed personal protective equipment according to the procedure.					
2. Seated the patient and placed the patient in the supine position.					
3. Positioned self as the operator.					
4. Instructed the patient to open the mouth.					
5. Adjusted the dental light to illuminate the oral cavity.					
6. Retrieved the dental mirror in the left hand and the explorer in the right hand, using a pen grasp for both instruments.					
7. With the tip of the instrument, followed around each tooth beginning with #1 and continuing through #32.					
8. With the mirror and explorer, examined all surfaces using visualization and touch.					
9. Using a fulcrum and indirect vision, adapted the instruments to all areas of the mouth.					

Continued

10. Identified specific dental landmarks through the dentition.					
11. Maintained patient comfort throughout these steps.					

ADDITIONAL COMMENTS

Total number of points earned _____

Grade _____ Instructor's initials _____

34 Dental Hand Instruments

SHORT-ANSWER QUESTIONS

1. Give the three parts of a dental hand instrument.

2. Provide the rationale of the instrument formula designed by G. V. Black.

3. List the examination instruments and their use.

4. List the types of hand cutting instruments set out for a restorative procedure.

5. List the types of restorative instruments and their uses.

6. Describe additional accessory instruments used in restorative dentistry.

7. List the reasons for using preset trays and tubs in dentistry.

8. Discuss the theory of placing instruments in a specific sequence.

FILL-IN-THE-BLANK STATEMENTS

Select the best term from the list below and complete the following statements.

beveled	point
blade	serrated
handle	shank
nib	tactile
plane	working end

1. _____ means to have a sense of touch or feeling.

2. The _____ is the portion of a dental instrument that is used directly on the tooth surface or for mixing dental materials.

3. The portion of a dental instrument that the operator grasps is the _____.

4. An angled or slanted working end of an instrument is referred to as being _____.

5. A flat edge of the working end of an instrument that is sharp enough to cut is a _____.

6. The working end of an explorer has a _____.

7. A _____ instrument has a notch like projection that extends from a flat surface.

8. A flat or level surface is a _____.

9. The _____ is the portion of a dental instrument that attaches the handle to the working end.

10. A _____ is a blunt point or tip on the working end.

MULTIPLE-CHOICE QUESTIONS

Complete each question by circling the best answer.

1. Which dental instruments are commonly referred to by a number than by their name?
   a. Mirrors
   b. Restorative instruments
   c. Pliers
   d. Excavators

2. What part of the instrument is located between the handle and the working end?
   a. Nib
   b. Shank
   c. Blade
   d. Plane

3. What classification of instruments are used to manually remove decay from a prepared tooth structure?
   a. Examination
   b. Hand cutting
   c. Restorative
   d. Accessory

4. Besides indirect vision, the mouth mirror is used for _____.
   a. moisture control
   b. anesthesia
   c. retraction
   d. placement of restorations

5. The main characteristic of the working end of an explorer is that it is _____.
   a. dull
   b. flat
   c. serrated
   d. pointed

6. Which instrument is part of the basic setup?
   a. Spoon excavator
   b. Cotton pliers
   c. Condenser
   d. Carver

7. Which instrument is used to measure the sulcus of a tooth?
   a. Spoon excavator
   b. Cotton pliers
   c. Explorer
   d. Periodontal probe

8. Which instrument is similar to the spoon excavator in appearance and use?
   a. Explorer
   b. Black spoon
   c. Discoid-cleoid
   d. Gingival margin trimmer

9. Which instrument is used to carve the interproximal portion of the restoration?
   a. Black spoon
   b. Discoid-cleoid
   c. Explorer
   d. Hollenback

10. Which instrument is used to pack a restorative material into the tooth preparation?
    a. Cotton pliers
    b. Amalgam knife
    c. Condenser
    d. Burnisher

11. What kind of instrument is a discoid-cleoid?
    a. Carver
    b. Examination
    c. Hand cutting
    d. Packing

12. What type of scissors would commonly be seen on a restorative tray setup?
    a. Tissue
    b. Suture
    c. Crown and bridge
    d. Surgical

13. Howe pliers are also referred to as _____.
    a. cotton pliers
    b. 110 pliers
    c. articulating pliers
    d. chisel pliers

14. Newly triturated amalgam is placed in the _____ before it is packed in the amalgam carrier.
    a. syringe
    b. cotton pliers
    c. spoon excavator
    d. amalgam well

15. On which tooth surface(s) would the Hollenback carver be used to carve a restorative material?
    a. Occlusal
    b. Facial
    c. Distal
    d. Lingual

ACTIVITY

You are assisting with a class II amalgam procedure on tooth #29. In order of use, list the instruments you would place in the setup, beginning from the left and working toward the right of the tray. Next to the name of each instrument, describe its use for the procedure.

COMPETENCIES 34.1 THROUGH 34.4: IDENTIFYING DENTAL INSTRUMENTS FOR A RESTORATIVE PROCEDURE

Performance Objective

By following a routine procedure that meets stated protocols, the student will retrieve and organize the appropriate examination, hand cutting, restorative, and accessory instruments and supplies for a specified restorative procedure.

Evaluation and Grading Criteria

3	Student competently met the stated criteria without assistance.
2	Student required assistance in order to meet the stated criteria.
1	Student showed uncertainty when performing the stated criteria.
0	Student was not prepared and needs to repeat the step.
N/A	No evaluation of this step.

Instructor shall define grades for each point range earned on completion of each performance-evaluated task.

Performance Standards

The minimum number of satisfactory performances required before final evaluation is _____.

Instructor shall identify by * those steps considered critical. If a step is missed or minimum competency is not met, the evaluated procedure fails and must be repeated.

PERFORMANCE CRITERIA	*	SELF	PEER	INSTRUCTOR	COMMENTS
1. Reviewed the patient record and determined the type of procedure and setup.					
2. Selected correct instruments for the procedure.					
3. Placed the instruments in the appropriate order of use on the tray.					
4. Stated verbally or recorded the use for each instrument and item placed on the tray setup.					
ADDITIONAL COMMENTS					

Total number of points earned _____

Grade _____ Instructor's initials _____

35 Dental Handpieces and Accessories

SHORT-ANSWER QUESTIONS

1. Give the use of the low-speed handpiece in dentistry.

2. List the three attachments used on the low-speed motor.

3. Give the use of the high-speed handpiece in dentistry.

4. Provide a brief description of other types of handpieces used in dentistry.

5. Describe rotary instruments and explain their use.

6. List the parts of a bur.

7. Give the composition, shape, and uses of carbide and diamond burs.

FILL-IN-THE-BLANK STATEMENTS

Select the best term from the list below and complete the following statements.

fiber optic	**rotary**
flutes	**shank**
friction grip	**torque**
laser	**tungsten carbide**
latch-type	**ultrasonic**
mandrel	

1. A(n) _____ bur has no retention grooves in the shank end to lock it into the handpiece.

2. The _____ handpiece uses a beam of light to vaporize hard and soft tissue.

3. A(n) _____ is defined as a part or device that rotates around an axis.

4. The _____ or grooves in the cutting portion of a bur resemble pleats.

5. A(n) _____ bur is rigid and stronger than a steel bur and remains sharper for longer periods.

6. The narrow portion of the bur that fits into the handpiece is called a(n) _____.

7. The _____ bur has a shank with a small groove at the end that mechanically locks into a contra-angle attachment.

8. The high-speed handpiece has a(n) _____ lighting system to direct light on the tooth during use.

9. A(n) _____ handpiece provides mechanical energy that creates water and sound vibrations.

10. The twisting or turning of the internal components of a handpiece is referred to as _____.

11. Sandpaper discs are mounted onto a _____ for use.

MULTIPLE-CHOICE QUESTIONS

Complete each question by circling the best answer.

1. How did the first dental handpiece operate?
   a. Operated with a hand pedal
   b. Operated with electricity
   c. Driven by a belt
   d. Powered by water

2. Which dental handpiece is the most versatile?
   a. Low-speed
   b. High-speed
   c. Laboratory
   d. Air abrasion

3. How fast will the low-speed handpiece rotate?
   a. 30,000 rpm
   b. 60,000 rpm
   c. 300,000 rpm
   d. 450,000 rpm

4. What attachment on the low-speed handpiece motor is used to hold a latch-type bur?
   a. Prophy angle
   b. Contra-angle
   c. Straight
   d. Mandrel

5. How fast does the high-speed handpiece rotate?
   a. 250,000 rpm
   b. 400,000 rpm
   c. 650,000 rpm
   d. 950,000 rpm

6. During cavity preparation, how does the high-speed handpiece keep the tooth at a proper temperature and free of debris?
   a. Air
   b. Suction system
   c. Water coolant
   d. Application of a dental material

7. A bur is held in place in the high-speed handpiece using a _____.
   a. friction grip
   b. locking key
   c. latch-type lock
   d. twist and lock

8. On the high-speed handpiece, the _____ helps illuminate the working field.
   a. water
   b. air
   c. fiber-optic light
   d. suction

9. What type of handpiece resembles a sandblaster?
   a. Laser
   b. Low-speed
   c. Air abrasion
   d. High-speed

10. A _____ shank bur fits into the lab handpiece.
   a. friction grip
   b. mandrel
   c. latch-type
   d. long

11. Restorative burs are commonly manufactured from what material?
   a. Stainless steel
   b. Tungsten carbide
   c. Gold
   d. Nickel

12. What design of bur is a 33½?
   a. Round
   b. Tapered
   c. Inverted cone
   d. Pear

13. _____ is an advantage of a diamond bur.
   a. Cutting ability
   b. Fineness
   c. Polishing ability
   d. Non-abrasive ability

14. A finishing bur is commonly used for what type of restorative material?
   a. Amalgam
   b. Intermediate restorative material
   c. Gold
   d. Composite resin/esthetic materials

15. The low-speed handpiece would be equipped with a _____ to hold a sandpaper disc.
   a. Contra-angle attachment
   b. Bur
   c. Mandrel
   d. Prophy angle

CASE STUDY

You are setting up the treatment area for a patient who will be receiving a class II composite resin on tooth #5. Your tray setup includes a high-speed handpiece, low-speed motor, contra-angle attachment, #169 friction grip bur, #4 round latch-type bur, mandrel, sandpaper discs, and rubber points.

1. Which hose will the highspeed handpiece be attached to on the dental unit?

2. Which handpiece will you attach to the contra-angle attachment?

3. In which handpiece will you insert the #169 bur?

4. In which handpiece will you insert the #4 round bur?

5. At what step in the procedure would the operator use the #4 bur?

6. At what step in the procedure would the operator use the #169 bur?

7. What handpiece would the mandrel be attached to?

263

8. When would the discs and points be used during the procedure?

9. At the completion of the procedure, how are the dental handpieces and rotary instruments removed from the dental unit and prepared for the next procedure?

MULTIMEDIA PROCEDURES RECOMMENDED REVIEW Θvolve
learning system
_____

■ Identifying and Attaching Handpieces

COMPETENCIES 35.1 AND 35.2: IDENTIFYING AND ATTACHING HANDPIECES AND ROTARY INSTRUMENTS

Performance Objective

By following a routine procedure that meets stated protocols, given instructions for which size or type to select, the student will place and remove burs in high-speed and low-speed handpieces.

Evaluation and Grading Criteria

 3   Student competently met the stated criteria without assistance.

 2   Student required assistance in order to meet the stated criteria.

 1   Student showed uncertainty when performing the stated criteria.

 0   Student was not prepared and needs to repeat the step.

 N/A   No evaluation of this step.

Note: The student is provided with an appropriate assortment of burs and handpieces with which to work.

Instructor shall define grades for each point range earned on completion of each performance-evaluated task.

Performance Standards

The minimum number of satisfactory performances required before final evaluation is _____.

Instructor shall identify by * those steps considered critical. If a step is missed or minimum competency is not met, the evaluated procedure fails and must be repeated.

PERFORMANCE CRITERIA	*	SELF	PEER	INSTRUCTOR	COMMENT
1. Attached the high-speed handpiece to the correct receptor on the dental unit.					
2. Attached the low-speed handpiece to the correct receptor on the dental unit.					
3. Attached the straight attachment, contra-angle attachment, and prophylaxis angle to the low-speed handpiece.					
4. Identified varying shapes of burs for the low-speed and high-speed handpieces.					
5. Selected the specified size and type of bur for the high-speed handpiece.					
6. Placed burs in the handpiece in accordance with the manufacturer's instructions.					
7. Removed burs from the handpiece in accordance with the manufacturer's instructions.					
8. Selected the specified size and type of bur for the low-speed handpiece.					

Continued

9. Placed the bur in the handpiece in accordance with the manufacturer's instructions.				
10. Removed the bur from the handpiece in accordance with the manufacturer's instructions.				
ADDITIONAL COMMENTS				

Total number of points earned _____

Grade _____ Instructor's initials _____

36 Moisture Control

SHORT-ANSWER QUESTIONS

1. List three isolation techniques used to decrease moisture during a dental procedure.

2. Define the two types of oral evacuation systems used in dentistry.

3. Describe the grasp and positioning of the high-volume oral evacuator (HVE) tip.

4. Define the use of the air-water syringe.

5. Explain how the dental dam works and its role in moisture control.

6. List the set-up for the dental dam application.

7. Give a unique situation where the preparation and placement of the dental dam would change.

FILL-IN-THE-BLANK STATEMENTS

Select the best term from the list below and complete the following statements.

aspirate	jaw
beveled	malaligned
bow	septum
exposed	stylus
inverted	universal

1. The _____ is the curved part of the dental dam clamp visible in the mouth once the dam material has been placed.

2. The end of the HVE tip is _____ so that it can be positioned parallel to the site for better suction.

3. The dental dam is _____ around each tooth to create a seal to prevent the leakage of saliva.

4. The _____ is the part of the dental dam clamp that is stabilized around the anchor tooth.

5. The dam punch has a _____, which is a sharp pointed tool used for cutting.

6. An instrument is said to be _____ when it can be adapted or adjusted to multiple areas of the dentition.

7. When tooth #4 is overlapping tooth #5, it is considered to be _____.

8. A(n) _____ is the piece of the dental dam placed between each pair of punched holes.

9. When a tooth is visible in the dental dam, it becomes _____.

10. _____ means to inhale an object or material.

MULTIPLE-CHOICE QUESTIONS

Complete each question by circling the best answer.

1. The two types of evacuation systems used in dental procedures are
   a. Cotton rolls and saliva ejector
   b. High-volume suction and saliva ejector
   c. Dental dam and high-volume suction
   d. Air-water syringe and saliva ejector

2. The main function of the saliva ejector is to _____.
   a. remove dental materials
   b. remove blood
   c. remove saliva and water
   d. remove tooth fragments

3. HVE suction tips are made from _____.
   a. surgical steel
   b. stainless steel
   c. plastic
   d. b and c

4. The type of rinsing technique used throughout a dental procedure is the _____.
   a. Limited
   b. Full
   c. Breath freshener
   d. Spray

5. What method of isolation could be used for sealant placement?
   a. Dry angles
   b. Cotton roll
   c. Cheek retractors
   d. a and b

6. Which technique provides a moisture-free isolation for the restoration of a class IV composite resin?
   a. Dental dam
   b. Cotton roll
   c. Gauze squares
   d. Saliva ejector

7. Why is it important to moisten a cotton roll before removing it from the mouth?
   a. The cotton roll may interfere with the setting of the dental materials.
   b. The cotton roll may stick to the teeth.
   c. The cotton roll may irritate the lining mucosa.
   d. The cotton roll may be sucked up in the suction tip.

8. Teeth that become visible after the dam material is placed are referred to as being _____.
   a. open
   b. exposed
   c. revealed
   d. inverted

9. What piece of equipment stabilizes and stretches the dam away from the face?
   a. Dental dam frame
   b. Dental dam clamp
   c. Ligature tie
   d. Dental dam forceps

10. If you are unable to slide the dam material interproximal, what can be used on the underside of the dam to help in the application?
    a. Water
    b. Petroleum jelly
    c. Water-soluble lubricant
    d. Powder

11. What hole size is punched in the dental dam for the anchor tooth?
    a. 2
    b. 3
    c. 4
    d. 5

12. Which cavity classification would indicate the use of an anterior dental dam clamp?
    a. class I on tooth #4
    b. class II on tooth #18
    c. class V on tooth #7
    d. class VI on tooth #28

13. The assistant uses the _____ grasp when holding the HVE.
    a. pen
    b. thumb-to-nose
    c. reverse-palm
    d. a or b

14. The right-handed dentist is preparing a class V restoration on the buccal surface of tooth #5; the HVE tip would be positioned on the _____.
    a. mesial lingual surface of the tooth
    b. mesial facial surface of the tooth
    c. distal lingual surface of the tooth
    d. distal facial surface of the tooth

15. The rationale for inverting the dental dam is to _____.
    a. prevent saliva leakage
    b. remove excess material
    c. stabilize the restoration
    d. all of the above

16. The working end of the HVE tip should be positioned _____ for the preparation of the occlusal surface of tooth # 20.
    a. mesially
    b. distally
    c. gingivally
    d. directly on

17. The _____ is used to create holes in the dental dam to expose the teeth for isolation.
    a. dental dam clamp
    b. dental dam punch
    c. dental dam frame
    d. dental dam forceps

18. What is secured on the dental dam clamp before positioning on the patient's tooth?
    a. Dental dam material
    b. Cotton roll
    c. Compound wax
    d. Dental floss

19. The equipment used to perform a limited rinse includes _____.
    a. Dry-angle
    b. Air-water syringe
    c. HVE
    d. b and c

20. The operator has positioned the high-speed handpiece on the occlusal surface of tooth #4. Where should the HVE be positioned?
    a. Lingual surface of tooth #3
    b. Occlusal surface of tooth #5
    c. Buccal surface of tooth #15
    d. Lower right buccal vestibule

CASE STUDY

Candy Allen is scheduled to have a class III composite resin placed on the mesial surface of tooth #8. Candy has had several restorations and is comfortable with the dental treatment she will be receiving today. Throughout the procedure, it will be your responsibility to maintain moisture control.

1. After administration of anesthesia, what type of moisture control would be used to rinse her mouth?

2. The dentist has indicated that you should place the dental dam. At what point in the procedure will you do so?

3. Which teeth are to be isolated? What size hole will be punched for each tooth?

4. When placing the dam, you find that the contacts are very tight, which is making it difficult to slide the dam interproximally. What surfaces of the teeth are involved in the contact area? How can you adapt the dam to fit interproximally?

5. How is the dental dam held away from the working area?

6. At what stage of the procedure will you remove the dental dam?

7. When the dam is removed, you see that a piece of the dam has been torn away and is missing. How do you retrieve this missing piece?

ACTIVITY

Tooth #29 will be receiving a class II amalgam restoration today. The dentist would like the dam to be prepared for one tooth distal of tooth #29 to the opposite canine.

Give the tooth numbers of each tooth exposed, and beside the tooth number, give the size of the hole to be punched.

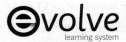

MULTIMEDIA PROCEDURES RECOMMENDED REVIEW

- Positioning the High-Volume Evacuator During a Procedure
- Preparing, Placing, and Removing the Dental Dam

COMPETENCY 36.1: POSITIONING THE HIGH-VOLUME EVACUATOR DURING A PROCEDURE

Performance Objective

By following a routine procedure that meets stated protocols, the student will maintain moisture control, access, and visibility during patient care by appropriately positioning the high-volume oral evacuator (HVE).

Evaluation and Grading Criteria

 3   Student competently met the stated criteria without assistance.

 2   Student required assistance to meet the stated criteria.

 1   Student showed uncertainty when performing the stated criteria.

 0   Student was not prepared and needs to repeat the step.

 N/A   No evaluation of this step.

Instructor shall define grades for each point range earned on completion of each performance-evaluated task.

Performance Standards

The minimum number of satisfactory performances required before final evaluation is _____.

Instructor shall identify by * those steps considered critical. If a step is missed or minimum competency is not met, the evaluated procedure fails and must be repeated.

PERFORMANCE CRITERIA	*	SELF	PEER	INSTRUCTOR	COMMENTS
1. Placed personal protective equipment according to the procedure.					
2. Attached the HVE tip and air-water syringe tip on the correct receptacle and readied them for the procedure.					
3. Assumed the correct seated position to accommodate a left-handed or a right-handed dentist.					
4. Used the proper grasp when holding the HVE.					
5. Grasped the air-water syringe in the left hand during HVE placement.					
6. Positioned the HVE correctly for the maxillary left posterior treatment.					
7. Positioned the HVE correctly for the maxillary right posterior treatment.					
8. Positioned the HVE correctly for the mandibular left posterior treatment.					
9. Positioned the HVE correctly for the mandibular right posterior treatment.					

Continued

10. Positioned the HVE correctly for the anterior treatment with lingual access.				
11. Positioned the HVE correctly for the anterior treatment with facial access.				
12. Maintained patient comfort and followed appropriate infection control measures throughout the procedure.				

ADDITIONAL COMMENTS

Total number of points earned _____

Grade _____ Instructor's initials _____

COMPETENCY 36.2: PERFORMING A MOUTH RINSE

Performance Objective

By following a routine procedure that meets stated protocols, the student will perform a limited-area rinse and a complete mouth rinse using the high-volume oral evacuator (HVE) and air-water syringe.

Evaluation and Grading Criteria

 3   Student competently met the stated criteria without assistance.

 2   Student required assistance to meet the stated criteria.

 1   Student showed uncertainty when performing the stated criteria.

 0   Student was not prepared and needs to repeat the step.

 N/A   No evaluation of this step.

Instructor shall define grades for each point range earned on completion of each performance-evaluated task.

Performance Standards

The minimum number of satisfactory performances required before final evaluation is _____.

Instructor shall identify by * those steps considered critical. If a step is missed or minimum competency is not met, the evaluated procedure fails and must be repeated.

PERFORMANCE CRITERIA	*	SELF	PEER	INSTRUCTOR	COMMENTS
Limited-Area Rinse					
1. Placed personal protective equipment according to the procedure.					
2. Grasped the air-water syringe with the left hand.					
3. Grasped the HVE in the right hand using the pen or thumb-to-nose grasp.					
4. Correctly positioned the HVE on the tooth/teeth being worked on, and maintained a clean and visible environment for the dentist.					
5. Maintained patient comfort and followed appropriate infection control measures throughout the procedure.					
Complete Mouth Rinse					
1. Held the air-water syringe in the left hand.					
2. Held the HVE in the right hand using a proper grasp.					
3. Instructed the patient to turn toward assistant.					

Continued

4. Positioned the HVE in the vestibule of the mouth and, starting at one area, rinsed the mouth thoroughly, suctioning the accumulated water and debris.				
5. Maintained patient comfort and followed appropriate infection control measures throughout the procedure.				

ADDITIONAL COMMENTS

Total number of points earned _____

Grade _____ Instructor's initials _____

COMPETENCY 36.3: PLACING AND REMOVING COTTON ROLLS

Performance Objective

By following a routine procedure that meets stated protocols, the student will place and properly remove cotton roll isolation for each area of the mouth.

Evaluation and Grading Criteria

 3 Student competently met the stated criteria without assistance.

 2 Student required assistance to meet the stated criteria.

 1 Student showed uncertainty when performing the stated criteria.

 0 Student was not prepared and needs to repeat the step.

 N/A No evaluation of this step.

Instructor shall define grades for each point range earned on completion of each performance-evaluated task.

Performance Standards

The minimum number of satisfactory performances required before final evaluation is _____.

Instructor shall identify by * those steps considered critical. If a step is missed or minimum competency is not met, the evaluated procedure fails and must be repeated.

PERFORMANCE CRITERIA	*	SELF	PEER	INSTRUCTOR	COMMENTS
Maxillary Placement					
1. Placed personal protective equipment according to the procedure.					
2. Positioned the patient with the head turned toward the assistant and the chin raised.					
3. Used cotton pliers to transfer cotton rolls to the mouth.					
4. Positioned the cotton rolls securely in the mucobuccal fold.					
5. Positioned the cotton rolls close to the working field.					
Mandibular Placement					
1. Positioned the patient with the head turned toward the assistant and the chin lowered.					
2. Used cotton pliers to transfer cotton rolls to the mouth.					
3. Positioned one cotton roll securely in the mucobuccal fold.					
4. Positioned the second cotton roll in the floor of the mouth between the working field and the tongue.					
5. Positioned the cotton rolls close to the working field.					

Continued

Cotton Roll Removal					
1. If cotton rolls were dry, moistened them with water from the air-water syringe.					
2. Removed cotton rolls with cotton pliers.					
3. Performed a limited rinse.					
4. Maintained patient comfort and followed appropriate infection control measures throughout the procedure.					
ADDITIONAL COMMENTS					

Total number of points earned _____

Grade _____ Instructor's initials _____

COMPETENCY 36.4: PREPARING, PLACING, AND REMOVING THE DENTAL DAM (EXPANDED FUNCTION)

Performance Objective

By following a routine procedure that meets stated protocols, the student will prepare, place, stabilize, and remove the dental dam.

Evaluation and Grading Criteria

 3   Student competently met the stated criteria without assistance.

 2   Student required assistance to meet the stated criteria.

 1   Student showed uncertainty when performing the stated criteria.

 0   Student was not prepared and needs to repeat the step.

 N/A   No evaluation of this step.

Instructor shall define grades for each point range earned on completion of each performance-evaluated task.

Performance Standards

The minimum number of satisfactory performances required before final evaluation is _____.

Instructor shall identify by * those steps considered critical. If a step is missed or minimum competency is not met, the evaluated procedure fails and must be repeated.

PERFORMANCE CRITERIA	*	SELF	PEER	INSTRUCTOR	COMMENTS
1. Placed personal protective equipment according to the procedure.					
2. Selected instrument setup for the procedure.					
3. Used a mouth mirror and explorer to examine the site to be isolated.					
4. Flossed all contacts involved in the placement of dental dam.					
5. Correctly punched the dam for the teeth to be isolated.					
6. Selected the correct size of clamp and tied a ligature to it.					
7. Placed the prepared clamp in the dental dam forceps in the position of use.					
8. Prepared the dental dam material and clamp for placement.					
9. Seated the clamp so that it was secure around the anchor tooth.					
10. Slid the dam over the clamp, making sure to pull the ligature through the keyhole of the dam.					
11. Positioned the dental dam frame correctly, making sure to fasten all notches to the dam.					

Continued

277

12. Slid the dam through all contacts, using floss to push the dam interproximally.				
13. Inverted the dental dam using floss, air, or a blunted instrument.				
14. Ensured that the dam was ligated and stabilized for the procedure.				
15. When removing the dental dam, removed the stabilization ligature.				
16. Cut the dental dam septum with scissors.				
17. Removed the dental dam clamp, dental dam frame, and dental dam.				
18. Examined the dental dam for tears or missing pieces.				
19. Used the air-water syringe and HVE tip to rinse the patient's mouth.				
20. Gently wiped debris from the area around the patient's mouth.				
21. Maintained patient comfort and followed appropriate infection control measures throughout the procedure.				

ADDITIONAL COMMENTS

Total number of points earned _____

Grep Grade _____ Instructor's initials _____

37 Anesthesia and Pain Control

SHORT-ANSWER QUESTIONS

1. Discuss the importance of pain control in dentistry.

2. Give the chemical makeup and application of topical anesthetic agents.

3. Give the chemical makeup and application of local anesthetic agents.

4. Describe the use of nitrous oxide/oxygen (N_2O/O_2) sedation and explain its use in dentistry.

5. Discuss the importance of reducing the dental team's exposure to N_2O/O_2.

6. Discuss intravenous sedation and its use in dentistry.

7. Discuss general anesthesia and its use in dentistry.

FILL-IN-THE-BLANK STATEMENTS

Select the best term from the list below and complete the following statements.

analgesia	lumen
anesthesia	oximetry
anesthetic	permeate
duration	porous
gauge	tidal volume
induction	titration
innervation	vasoconstrictor

1. A type of drug used in dentistry that produces a temporary loss of feeling or sensation is a(n) _____.

2. _____ is a method to determine the measurement of the oxygen concentration in the blood.

3. The time from induction of an anesthetic to its complete reversal is its _____

4. The _____ is the standard dimension or measurement of the thickness of an injection needle.

5. The _____ is a measurement of the amount of air inhaled and exhaled with each breath during N_2O/O_2 sedation.

6. _____ is a temporary loss of feeling or sensation.

7. A(n) _____ is a type of drug to prolong anesthetic action and constrict blood vessels.

8. To spread or flow throughout is to _____.

9. _____ is determining the exact amount of drug to use to achieve a desired level of sedation.

10. Something that is _____ will have openings to allow gas or fluid to pass through.

11. _____ is the supply or distribution of nerves to the jaw or a specific body part.

12. The _____ is the hollow center of the injection needle.

13. The time from injection to the point at which anesthesia takes effect is the _____.

14. _____ is the absence of feeling pain without being unconscious.

MULTIPLE-CHOICE QUESTIONS

Complete each question by circling the best answer.

1. Topical anesthetics are used in dentistry for _____.
   a. sedating the patient
   b. numbing localized nerves
   c. numbing surface tissue
   d. inhalation sedation

2. The most frequently selected form of pain control used in dentistry is _____.
   a. prescribed drugs
   b. local anesthesia
   c. N_2O/O_2 sedation
   d. intravenous sedation

3. Local anesthetics are injected near _____ to create a numbing effect.
   a. an artery
   b. a vein
   c. a nerve
   d. the pulp

4. What is added to a local anesthetic solution to prolong its physiologic effect?
   a. Alcohol
   b. Ammonia
   c. Nitrous oxide
   d. Epinephrine

5. What type of injection technique would the dentist most frequently use for a small area of maxillary teeth?
   a. Nerve block
   b. Infiltration
   c. Intraosseous
   d. Intravenous

6. What needle sizes are most commonly used in dentistry?
   a. $\frac{1}{2}$-inch and $\frac{3}{4}$-inch needles
   b. 1-inch and 2-inch needles
   c. $1\frac{1}{2}$-inch and $1\frac{5}{8}$-inch needles
   d. 1-inch and $1\frac{5}{8}$-inch needles

7. Is it common for a patient with an acute infection to not feel the numbing sensation of local anesthesia?
   a. No
   b. Only when the anesthesia has a vasoconstrictor
   c. Yes
   d. Only with a block injection

8. What type of condition is paresthesia?
   a. A localized toxic reaction
   b. An injection into a blood vessel
   c. Numbness that lasts longer than normal
   d. An infected area

9. The first dentist to offer N_2O/O_2 to his patients was

_____.

    a. G. V. Black
    b. Horace Wells
    c. C. Edmund Kells
    d. Pierre Fauchard

10. The dental team can be at risk for exposure to N_2O/O_2 in a dental office because of;
    a. Leaking or escaping of gases from the nasal mask
    b. Patients' exhalation of gases
    c. Leaking of gases from the hoses
    d. All of the above

11. A patient would receive _____ at the beginning and end of an N_2O/O_2 sedation procedure.
    a. Local anesthesia
    b. Oxygen
    c. Gauze to bite down on
    d. A drink of water

12. At what level or stage of anesthesia would a patient reach if he or she is relaxed and fully conscious?
    a. Analgesia
    b. Excitement
    c. General anesthesia
    d. Respiratory failure

13. What stage of consciousness should a patient reach during general anesthesia?
    a. stage I
    b. stage II
    c. stage III
    d. stage IV

14. General anesthesia is best provided in what type of environment to be most safely administered?
    a. Dental office
    b. Health department
    c. Hospital or surgical center
    d. a and b

15. The tank or cylinder of _____ is always color coded green.
    a. topical anesthetic
    b. vasoconstrictor
    c. nitrous oxide
    d. oxygen

16. Anesthetic cartridges should be _____.
    a. refrigerated before use
    b. enclosed in their packaging before use
    c. heated before use
    d. soaked in disinfectant before use

17. _____ anesthesia is achieved by injecting the anesthetic into the posterior superior alveolar nerve.
    a. IV sedation
    b. General
    c. Block
    d. Infiltration

18. A _____ size needle is used for infiltration injections.
    a. 1-inch
    b. $^5/_8$-inch
    c. 2-inch
    d. $2^5/_8$-inch

19. The recommended form of topical anesthetic for controlling a gag reflex is _____.
    a. ointment
    b. liquid
    c. spray
    d. a patch

20. A used or contaminated needle is to be discarded in the _____.
    a. medical waste
    b. sharps container
    c. sterilization center
    d. general garbage

CASE STUDY

Meredith Smith is scheduled to begin treatment for a fixed bridge on teeth #3, #4, and #5. She is apprehensive about the procedure. Ms. Smith has discussed the option of receiving N_2O/O_2. analgesia during the procedure and seems reassured that this will help alleviate her anxiety.

1. What methods or types of anesthesia will most likely be given to Ms. Smith throughout the procedure today?

2. Could any contraindications prevent Ms. Smith from receiving any of the anesthesia methods you have mentioned? If so, give examples.

3. Where would you find these contraindications?

4. In what order would Ms. Smith receive the methods of anesthesia?

5. What specific supplies and equipment would be placed out for the pain control procedures?

6. At the completion of the procedure, what postoperative instructions will you give Meredith regarding the type of anesthesia received?

7. How would you write up the anesthetics used today in the patient's chart?

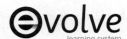

MULTIMEDIA PROCEDURES RECOMMENDED REVIEW

- Applying a Topical Anesthetic
- Assembling the Local Anesthetic Syringe

COMPETENCY 37.1: APPLYING A TOPICAL ANESTHETIC

Performance Objective

By following a routine procedure that meets stated protocols, the student will select the necessary setup, identify the injection site, and apply topical anesthetic.

Evaluation and Grading Criteria

 3   Student competently met the stated criteria without assistance.

 2   Student required assistance in order to meet the stated criteria.

 1   Student showed uncertainty when performing the stated criteria.

 0   Student was not prepared and needs to repeat the step.

 N/A   No evaluation of this step.

Instructor shall define grades for each point range earned on completion of each performance-evaluated task.

Performance Standards

The minimum number of satisfactory performances required before final evaluation is _____.

Instructor shall identify by * those steps considered critical. If a step is missed or minimum competency is not met, the evaluated procedure fails and must be repeated.

PERFORMANCE CRITERIA	*	SELF	PEER	INSTRUCTOR	COMMENT
1. Placed personal protective equipment according to the procedure.					
2. Gathered the appropriate setup.					
3. Used a sterile cotton-tipped applicator to remove a small amount of topical anesthetic ointment from the container; replaced the cover immediately.					
4. Explained the procedure to the patient.					
5. Determined the injection site.					
6. Wiped the injection site dry using a sterile 2 × 2-inch gauze pad.					
7. Applied topical anesthetic ointment to the injection site only.					
8. Left the topical anesthetic ointment in contact with the oral tissues for 2 to 5 minutes.					
9. Removed the cotton-tipped applicator just before the injection was made by the dentist.					

Continued

10. Maintained patient comfort and followed appropriate infection control measures throughout the procedure.				
11. Documented the procedure in the patient record.				

ADDITIONAL COMMENTS

Total number of points earned _____

Grade _____ Instructor's initials _____

COMPETENCIES 37.2 AND 37.3: ASSISTING IN THE ASSEMBLY AND ADMINISTRATION OF LOCAL ANESTHETIC INJECTION

Performance Objective

By following a routine procedure that meets stated protocols, the student will select the necessary setup, prepare an aspirating-type syringe for local anesthetic injection, and assist in its administration.

Evaluation and Grading Criteria

<u>3</u>   Student competently met the stated criteria without assistance.

<u>2</u>   Student required assistance in order to meet the stated criteria.

<u>1</u>   Student showed uncertainty when performing the stated criteria.

<u>0</u>   Student was not prepared and needs to repeat the step.

<u>N/A</u>   No evaluation of this step.

Instructor shall define grades for each point range earned on completion of each performance-evaluated task.

Performance Standards

The minimum number of satisfactory performances required before final evaluation is _____.

Instructor shall identify by * those steps considered critical. If a step is missed or minimum competency is not met, the evaluated procedure fails and must be repeated.

PERFORMANCE CRITERIA	*	SELF	PEER	INSTRUCTOR	COMMENT
1. Placed personal protective equipment according to the procedure.					
2. Gathered the necessary instruments and supplies.					
3. Inspected the syringe, needle, and anesthetic cartridge, and prepared the syringe out of the patient's sight.					
4. Double-checked the anesthetic cartridge to confirm that the anesthetic was the type the dentist had indicated.					
5. Retracted the piston using the thumb ring, and inserted the anesthetic cartridge with the rubber stopper end first.					
6. Released the piston and gently engaged the harpoon.					
7. Gently pulled back on the thumb ring to confirm the harpoon was securely in place.					
8. Removed the plastic cap from the syringe end of the needle, and screwed the needle onto the syringe.					

Continued

9. Loosened the colored plastic cap from the injection end of the needle.				
10. Transferred the syringe below the patient's chin or behind the patient's head as instructed.				
11. Took appropriate safety precaution measures while transferring the syringe.				
12. When disassembling the syringe, retracted the piston of the syringe by pulling back on the thumb ring.				
13. While still retracting the piston, removed the anesthetic cartridge from the syringe.				
14. Unscrewed and removed the needle from the syringe.				
15. Disposed of the needle in an appropriate sharps container.				
16. Disposed of the used cartridge in the appropriate waste container.				
17. Followed appropriate infection control measures throughout the procedure.				
18. Documented the procedure in the patient record.				

ADDITIONAL COMMENTS

Total number of points earned _____

Grade _____ Instructor's initials _____

COMPETENCY 37.4: ASSISTING IN THE ADMINISTRATION AND MONITORING OF NITROUS OXIDE/OXYGEN SEDATION (EXPANDED FUNCTION)

Performance Objective

By following a routine procedure that meets stated protocols, the student will assist with the administration of nitrous oxide analgesia by monitoring the patient's reactions and recording appropriate information in the patient's record.

Evaluation and Grading Criteria

 3   Student competently met the stated criteria without assistance.

 2   Student required assistance in order to meet the stated criteria.

 1   Student showed uncertainty when performing the stated criteria.

 0   Student was not prepared and needs to repeat the step.

 N/A   No evaluation of this step.

Instructor shall define grades for each point range earned on completion of each performance-evaluated task.

Performance Standards

The minimum number of satisfactory performances required before final evaluation is _____.

Instructor shall identify by * those steps considered critical. If a step is missed or minimum competency is not met, the evaluated procedure fails and must be repeated.

PERFORMANCE CRITERIA	*	SELF	PEER	INSTRUCTOR	COMMENT
1. Placed personal protective equipment according to the procedure.					
2. Checked the nitrous oxide and oxygen tanks for adequate supply.					
3. Gathered appropriate supplies and placed a sterile mask of the appropriate size on the tubing.					
4. Updated the patient's health history, and then took and recorded the patient's vital signs.					
5. Instructed the patient on the procedure of nitrous oxide analgesia and what to expect.					
6. Placed the patient in a supine position.					
7. Assisted the patient with placement of the mask.					
8. Made necessary adjustments to the mask and tubing to ensure proper fit.					
9. At the dentist's direction, adjusted the flow of oxygen to the established tidal volume.					
10. At the dentist's direction, adjusted the flow of nitrous oxide and oxygen.					

Continued

11. Noted on the patient's chart the times and volumes of gas needed to achieve baseline.					
12. Monitored the patient's status throughout the procedure.					
13. At the dentist's direction, turned off the flow of nitrous oxide and increased the flow of oxygen.					
14. After oxygenation was complete, removed the nosepiece and then slowly returned the patient to the upright position.					
15. Recorded in the patient record the concentrations of gases administered and any patient reaction to the analgesia.					
16. Maintained patient comfort and followed appropriate infection control measures throughout the procedure.					

ADDITIONAL COMMENTS

Total number of points earned _____

Grade _____ Instructor's initials _____

Foundations of Radiography, Radiographic Equipment, and Radiologic Safety

38

SHORT-ANSWER QUESTIONS

1. How is dental imaging applied in the dental setting?

2. Describe the discovery of x-radiation.

3. List the properties of x-radiation.

4. Describe the effect of kilovoltage on the quality of the x-ray beam.

5. What are the types of effects of radiation exposure on the human body?

6. What are the risks versus benefits of dental images?

7. What critical organs are sensitive to radiation?

8. What is the ALARA concept?

9. What methods are used to protect the patient from excess radiation?

10. What methods are used to protect the operator from excess radiation?

Select the best term from the list below and complete the following statements.

ALARA	**kilovoltage peak**
anode	**latent period**
cathode	**matter**
contrast	**milliampere**
density	**penumbra**
dental radiography	**photon**
digital imaging	**primary beam**
dose	**radiation**
electrons	**radiograph**
energy	**radiology**
genetic effects	**somatic effects**
image	**tungsten target**
image receptor	**x-radiation**
ion	**x-ray**
ionizing radiation	

1. _____ is the emission of energy in the form of waves through space or a material.

2. _____ is a high-energy ionizing electromagnetic radiation.

3. A form of ionizing radiation is the _____.

4. _____ is the science or study of radiation used in medicine.

5. A(n) _____ is an image produced on a photosensitive film by exposing the film to x-rays and then processing it.

6. The exposing of images of teeth and adjacent structures through exposure to x-rays is _____.

7. _____ is radiation that produces ionization.

8. The positive electrode in the x-ray tube is the _____.

9. The negative electrode in the x-ray tube is the _____.

10. The _____ is the most penetrating beam produced at the target of the anode.

11. An electrically charged particle is a(n) _____.

12. The _____ is the x-ray tube peak voltage used during an x-ray exposure.

13. A(n) _____ is 1/1000 of an ampere, a unit of measurement used to describe the intensity of an electric current.

14. Tiny negatively charged particles found in the atom are _____.

15. The _____ is a focal spot in the anode.

16. _____ is the difference in degrees of blackness on a radiograph.

17. _____ is the overall darkness or blackness of a radiograph.

18. The amount of energy absorbed by tissues is its _____.

19. _____ are effects of radiation that are passed on to future generations through genetic cells.

20. Effects of radiation that cause illness that is responsible for poor health are _____.

21. The time between exposure to ionizing radiation and the appearance of symptoms is the _____.

22. _____ is a concept of radiation protection holding that all exposures should be kept "as low as reasonably achievable."

23. A(n) _____ is a minute bundle of pure energy that has no weight or mass.

24. Anything that occupies space and has form or shape is _____.

25. _____ is a filmless method of capturing an image and displaying it by using an image sensor, an electronic signal, and a computer to process and store the image.

26. The blurred or indistinct area that surrounds an image is _____.

27. A film-based or digitally produced recording of an anatomic structure is a(n) _____.

28. A(n) _____ is a recording medium for images such as a film or sensor.

29. The ability to do work takes _____.

LABELING EXERCISE

1. Label the components of the dental x-ray tubehead.

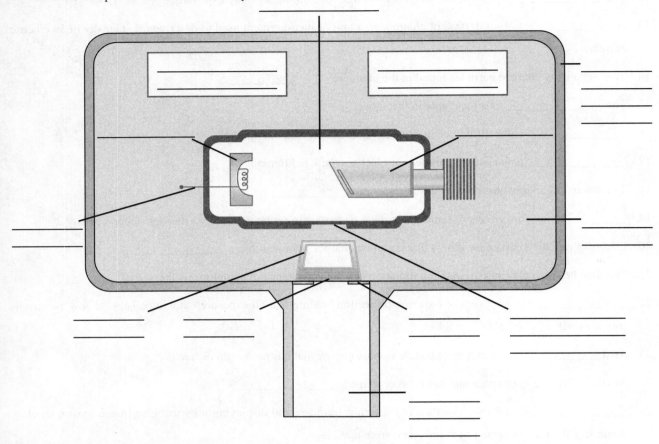

(From Iannucci J, Jansen Howerton L: Dental radiography: principles and techniques, ed 4, St Louis, 2012, Saunders.)

a. X-ray tube
b. Metal housing of x-ray tubehead
c. Insulating oil
d. Unleaded glass window of x-ray tube
e. Lead collimator
f. Position-indicating device
g. Aluminum discs

h. Tubehead seal
i. Filament circuit
j. Cathode (−)
k. Anode (+)
l. Step-up transformer
m. Step-down transformer

MULTIPLE-CHOICE QUESTIONS

Complete each question by circling the best answer.

1. Who discovered x-rays?
   a. G. V. Black
   b. W. C. Roentgen
   c. Pierre Fauchard
   d. Horace Wells

2. Who was the first person to expose a dental radiograph?
   a. C. Edmund Kells
   b. G. V. Black
   c. Otto Walkhoff
   d. Horace Wells

3. _____ is the process by which electrons are removed from electrically stable atoms.
   a. Physics
   b. Radiation
   c. Ionization
   d. Roentgen

4. The primary components of a dental x-ray machine are the _____.
   a. tubehead
   b. PID
   c. extension arm
   d. all of the above

5. The name of the negative electrode inside the x-ray tube is the _____.
   a. cathode
   b. nucleus
   c. anode
   d. photon

6. The name of the positive electrode inside the x-ray tube is the _____.
   a. cathode
   b. nucleus
   c. anode
   d. neutron

7. What is located on the x-ray machine control panel?
   a. Filter
   b. Collimator
   c. Milliamperage (mA) selector
   d. Tubehead

8. During the production of x-rays, how much energy is lost as heat?
   a. 5%
   b. 25%
   c. 50%
   d. 99%

9. What are the types of radiation?
   a. Primary
   b. Secondary
   c. Scatter
   d. All of the above
   e. a and b

10. A structure that appears dark on a processed radiograph is termed _____.
    a. radiopaque
    b. radiolucent
    c. contrast
    d. density

11. A structure that appears light on a processed radiograph is termed _____.
    a. radiopaque
    b. density
    c. contrast
    d. radiolucent

12. What exposure factor controls contrast?
    a. mA
    b. kVp
    c. Time
    d. Distance

13. Density is the _____.
    a. overall lightness of a processed radiograph
    b. structure that appears light on a processed radiograph
    c. overall darkness of a processed radiograph
    d. structure that appears dark on a processed radiograph

14. The name of the process for the harmful effects of x-rays is _____.
    a. radiation
    b. ionization
    c. ultraviolet rays
    d. infrared rays

15. The time between x-ray exposure and the appearance of symptoms is the _____.
    a. exposure time
    b. primary radiation
    c. development
    d. latent period

16. Radiation that is passed on to future generations is the _____.
    a. cumulative effect
    b. somatic effect
    c. genetic effect
    d. exposure effect

17. _____ is a system that is used to measure radiation.
    a. The traditional or standard system
    b. The metric system
    c. Système Internationale
    d. a and c

18. The maximum permissible dose of radiation for occupationally exposed persons is _____.
    a. 5.0 rems/year
    b. 15 rems/year
    c. 50 rems/year
    d. 0.05 rems/year

Chapter **38** Foundations of Radiography, Radiographic Equipment, and Radiologic Safety

19. The purpose of the collimator is to _____.
   a. filter the primary beam
   b. reduce the exposure of the primary beam
   c. restrict the size of the primary beam
   d. both b and c

20. The purpose of the aluminum filter is to _____.
   a. reduce the exposure of the primary beam
   b. remove the low-energy, long-wavelength rays
   c. restrict the size of the primary beam
   d. remove the high-energy, short-wavelength rays

21. Which patient should wear a lead apron and thyroid collar?
   a. Patients with a pacemaker
   b. Patients with lung cancer
   c. Children
   d. All patients

22. What is the purpose of personnel monitoring?
   a. To record the amount of radiation a patient receives
   b. To record the amount of radiation the operator receives
   c. To record the amount of radiation that is produced
   d. To check for radiation leakage

23. What is the purpose of equipment monitoring?
   a. To record the amount of radiation a patient receives
   b. To determine the amount of radiation produced during exposure of a radiograph
   c. To record the amount of radiation that reaches a body
   d. To check for radiation leakage

24. Which rule states that "all exposure to radiation should be kept to a minimum" or "as low as reasonably achievable"?
   a. Right to Know Law
   b. ALARA concept
   c. Patient's Bill of Rights
   d. Dental Assistant Creed

25. What is the purpose of using a position indicator device (PID)?
   a. To increase the contrast on the radiograph
   b. To direct the x-ray beam
   c. To increase the density on the radiograph
   d. All of the above

26. What is the primary type of radiation produced in the dental x-ray tubehead?
   a. Roentgen radiation
   b. Bavarian radiation
   c. Tungsten radiation
   d. Bremsstrahlung radiation

TOPICS FOR DISCUSSION

Your next patient is a 37-year-old woman who is new to the practice. She is scheduled today for a series of radiographs, but she appears apprehensive, asking a lot of questions and making nervous statements. How would you respond to her questions and statements?

1. "I don't know why the dentist wants x-rays; my teeth look fine."

2. "Why are you putting that heavy thing on my lap?"

3. "Why do you leave the room?"

4. "How do you know how many pictures you are going to take?"

5. "Are dental x-rays really safe?"

INTERACTIVE DENTAL OFFICE PATIENT CASE EXERCISE

Access the *Interactive Dental Office* on the Evolve website and click on the patient case file for Margaret Brown.

- Review Margaret's record.
- Answer the following question.

1. Would it be better if the dental assistant held the film in the proper position for the child? It would be for only one film.

39 Digital Imaging, Dental Film, and Processing Radiographs

SHORT-ANSWER QUESTIONS

1. List the types of dental image receptor holding devices.

2. Describe the composition of a dental x-ray film.

3. What film-processing problems result from time and temperature errors?

4. What film-processing problems result from chemical contamination errors?

5. What film-processing problems result from film-handling errors?

6. What film-processing problems result from lighting errors?

7. List the three types of dental images and the indications for their use.

8. Give the five basic sizes of intraoral dental x-ray film.

9. Describe the differences between direct and indirect digital imaging.

10. Describe the advantages and disadvantages of digital radiography.

297

Select the best term from the list below and complete the following statements.

beam alignment devices	**film speed**
bitewing radiograph	**intraoral film**
charge-coupled device (CCD)	**label side**
digital image	**manual processing**
duplicating film	**occlusal radiograph**
emulsion	**periapical radiograph**
extraoral film	**processing errors**
film cassette	**tube side**
film-holding devices	

1. A(n) _____ is an electronic signal captured by sensors and displayed on computer monitors.

2. A coating on the x-ray film that contains energy-sensitive crystals is the _____.

3. The _____ is the solid white side of the film that should face the x-ray tube.

4. The _____ is the colored side of the film that should face away from the x-ray tube.

5. _____ is a method of film processing that uses film racks and processing tanks.

6. _____ are used to stabilize the film in position in the patient's mouth.

7. _____ are used to indicate the location of the position indicator device (PID) in relation to the tooth and film.

8. _____ is a type of film that is placed within the mouth.

9. Film designed for use in cassettes is _____.

10. Film designed for use in film-duplicating machines is _____.

11. A radiograph that shows the crown, root tip, and surrounding structures is a(n) _____.

12. A(n) _____ shows the crowns of both arches on one film.

13. A radiograph that shows the anterior area of the maxilla or mandible is the _____.

14. The _____ is used to encase extraoral films during exposure.

15. The _____ is determined by the sensitivity of the emulsion on the film to radiation.

16. _____ is a solid-state image sensor used in intraoral digital imaging.

17. _____ are mistakes that occur on the radiograph during processing.

MULTIPLE-CHOICE QUESTIONS

Complete each question by circling the best answer.

1. How does positioning instruments protect the patient from unnecessary radiation?
   a. It filters the scatter radiation.
   b. It keeps the patient's hands and fingers from being exposed to x-radiation.
   c. It speeds up the process.
   d. It shows the correct teeth.

2. Describe a basic style of film holder.
   a. Hemostat device
   b. Clothespin device that holds the film
   c. Square pad with adhesive on the back
   d. Bite-block with a backing plate and a slot for the film

3. Which is a component of an intraoral film?
   a. Film emulsion
   b. Aluminum foil
   c. Plastic
   d. Alginate

4. The image on a film before it is processed is the

   _____.
   a. density
   b. latent image
   c. contrast
   d. mirror image

5. Which side of the film faces toward the tube?
   a. Envelope-looking side
   b. Silver side
   c. White side

6. What size film is used for posterior periapical radiographs on an adult patient?
   a. 0
   b. 1
   c. 2
   d. 3

7. What size film is used for occlusal radiographs?
   a. 2
   b. 3
   c. 4
   d. 5

8. Name the types of extraoral film cassettes.
   a. Flexible
   b. Rigid
   c. Expandable
   d. a and b

9. What converts x-ray energy into visible light?
   a. Aluminum foil
   b. Cardboard
   c. Intensifying screen
   d. Collimator

10. Why would you duplicate a radiograph?
    a. To get a second opinion
    b. To send to an insurance company
    c. To refer a patient to a specialist
    d. b and c

11. How should x-ray film be stored?
    a. Away from light
    b. In heat
    c. In a moist environment
    d. Submersed in chemicals

12. Where is the expiration date on a package of x-ray film?
    a. On the film
    b. Outside the box
    c. On the package insert
    d. On the bar code

13. What is the second step in the manual processing of dental radiographs?
    a. Developing
    b. Fixing
    c. Rinsing
    d. Washing

14. Indirect digital imaging involves the use of a(n)

    _____.
    a. digital sensor
    b. phosphor storage plate (PSP)
    c. intraoral film
    d. extraoral film

15. How often should processing solution be replenished?
    a. Daily
    b. Weekly
    c. Bimonthly
    d. Monthly

16. What low-intensity light is composed of long wavelengths in the red-orange spectrum?
    a. X-rays
    b. Safelight
    c. Intensifying screen
    d. Filter

17. The minimum distance between a safelight and the working area is _____.
    a. 1 foot
    b. 2 feet
    c. 3 feet
    d. 4 feet

18. What is the optimum temperature for the water in the manual processing tanks?
    a. 65° F
    b. 68° F
    c. 72° F
    d. 75° F

19. The major advantage of automatic film processing is _____.
    a. The quality of the radiograph is better.
    b. It saves time.
    c. It uses fewer chemicals.
    d. It is safer.

20. Are manual processing solutions and automatic processing solutions interchangeable?
    a. Yes
    b. No

ACTIVITY

You are scheduled to expose radiographs of the following patients. Listed are the areas of the mouth of which you will be taking films. For each area, give the size of the film that you will need to set up for the procedure.

Patient One: 28 Years Old

Maxillary right molar: _____

Maxillary left molar: _____

Maxillary central: _____

Mandibular right molar: _____

Mandibular left molar: _____

Mandibular central: _____

Right bitewing: _____

Left bitewing: _____

Patient Two: 8 years old

Maxillary right molar: _____

Maxillary left molar: _____

Maxillary central: _____

Mandibular right molar: _____

Mandibular left molar: _____

Mandibular central: _____

Right bitewing: _____

Left bitewing: _____

Patient Three: 4 years old

Maxillary occlusal: _____

Mandibular occlusal: _____

MULTIMEDIA PROCEDURES RECOMMENDED REVIEW

Θvolve
learning system

- Automatic Processing of Dental Radiographs
- Duplicating Radiographs
- Manual Processing of Radiographs
- Digital Imaging (4 videos)

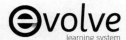

Access the *Interactive Dental Office* on the *Evolve* website and click on the patient case file for Miguel Ricardo.
- Review Mr. Ricardo's record.
- Mount his radiographs.
- Answer the following questions.

1. Is the dark area below the roots of the mandibular molars a processing error?

2. What size film was used for the bitewings?

Access the *Interactive Dental Office* on the Evolve website and click on the patient case file for Mrs. Harriet Ross.
- Review Mrs. Ross's record.
- Mount her radiographs.
- Answer the following questions.

3. Why were only 13 films taken?

4. Are there any processing errors on her FMX?

Access the *Interactive Dental Office* on the Evolve website and click on the patient case file for Lee Wong.
- Review Mr. Wong's record.
- Mount his radiographs.
- Answer the following questions.

5. Is the dark area around the roots caused by a processing error?

6. Did a processing error cause the round circle at the bottom on the right side of the film?

COMPETENCY 39.1: ASSEMBLING THE EXTENSION-CONE PARALLELING (XCP) INSTRUMENTS

Performance Objective

By following a routine procedure that meets stated protocols, the student will demonstrate the proper technique for assembling a localizer ring film- or sensor-holding instrument.

Evaluation and Grading Criteria

3   Student competently met the stated criteria without assistance.

2   Student required assistance in order to meet the stated criteria.

1   Student showed uncertainty when performing the stated criteria.

0   Student was not prepared and needs to repeat the step.

N/A   No evaluation of this step.

Instructor shall define grades for each point range earned on completion of each performance-evaluated task.

Performance Standards

The minimum number of satisfactory performances required before final evaluation is _____.

Instructor shall identify by * those steps considered critical. If a step is missed or minimum competency is not met, the evaluated procedure fails and must be repeated.

PERFORMANCE CRITERIA	*	SELF	PEER	INSTRUCTOR	COMMENT
1. Placed personal protective equipment according to the procedure.					
2. Assembled the instruments for the area to be radiographed.					
3. Placed the film or sensor into the backing plate.					
4. Used the entire horizontal length of the bite-block.					
5. Placed the anterior edge of the bite-block on the incisal or occlusal surfaces of the teeth being radiographed.					
6. Instructed the patient to close the mouth slowly but firmly.					
7. Placed a cotton roll between the bite-block and the teeth of the opposite arch.					

Continued

303

8. Moved the localizer ring down the indicator rod into position.				
9. Aligned the position indicator device.				
10. Exposed the image and then removed the film- or sensor-holding device from the patient's mouth.				

ADDITIONAL COMMENTS

Total number of points earned _____

Grade _____ Instructor's initials _____

COMPETENCY 39.2: DUPLICATING DENTAL RADIOGRAPHS

Performance Objective

By following a routine procedure that meets stated protocols, the student will demonstrate the proper technique for duplicating dental radiographs.

Evaluation and Grading Criteria

 3   Student competently met the stated criteria without assistance.

 2   Student required assistance in order to meet the stated criteria.

 1   Student showed uncertainty when performing the stated criteria.

 0   Student was not prepared and needs to repeat the step.

 N/A   No evaluation of this step.

Instructor shall define grades for each point range earned on completion of each performance-evaluated task.

Performance Standards

The minimum number of satisfactory performances required before final evaluation is _____.

Instructor shall identify by * those steps considered critical. If a step is missed or minimum competency is not met, the evaluated procedure fails and must be repeated.

PERFORMANCE CRITERIA	*	SELF	PEER	INSTRUCTOR	COMMENT
1. Turned on the safelight and turned off the white light.					
2. Placed the radiographs on the duplicator machine glass.					
3. Placed the duplicating film on top of the radiographs with the emulsion side against the radiograph.					
4. Turned on the light in the duplicating machine for the manufacturer's recommended time.					
5. Removed the duplicating film from the machine and processed it normally, using manual or automatic techniques.					
6. Accurately documented the procedure in the patient record.					

ADDITIONAL COMMENTS

Total number of points earned _____

Grade _____ Instructor's initials _____

COMPETENCY 39.3: PROCESSING DENTAL FILMS MANUALLY

Performance Objective

By following a routine procedure that meets stated protocols, the student will demonstrate the proper technique for processing films manually.

Evaluation and Grading Criteria

 3   Student competently met the stated criteria without assistance.

 2   Student required assistance in order to meet the stated criteria.

 1   Student showed uncertainty when performing the stated criteria.

 0   Student was not prepared and needs to repeat the step.

 N/A   No evaluation of this step.

Instructor shall define grades for each point range earned on completion of each performance-evaluated task.

Performance Standards

The minimum number of satisfactory performances required before final evaluation is _____.

Instructor shall identify by * those steps considered critical. If a step is missed or minimum competency is not met, the evaluated procedure fails and must be repeated.

PERFORMANCE CRITERIA	*	SELF	PEER	INSTRUCTOR	COMMENT
1. Followed all infection control steps.					
2. Stirred the solutions and checked the solution levels and temperature. The temperature was 65° F to 70° F.					
3. Labeled the film rack with the patient's name and the date of exposure.					
4. Turned on the safelight and then turned off the white light.					
5. Washed and dried hands and put on gloves.					
6. Opened the film packets and allowed the films to drop onto a clean paper towel. Used care not to touch the films.					
7. Removed the contaminated gloves and washed and dried the hands.					
8. Attached each film to the film rack so that films were parallel and not touching.					
9. Agitated the rack slightly while inserting it into the solution.					
10. Started the timer after setting it according to the manufacturer's instructions based on the temperature of the solutions.					

Continued

11. Removed the rack of films after the timer went off and rinsed it in running water in the center tank for 20 to 30 seconds.				
12. Determined the fixation time and set the timer. Immersed the rack of films in the fixer tank.				
13. Returned the rack of films to the center tank with circulating water for a minimum of 20 minutes.				
14. Removed the rack of films from the water and allowed it to dry.				
15. When the rack of films was completely dry, removed the films from the rack and mounted them in an appropriately labeled mount.				

ADDITIONAL COMMENTS

Total number of points earned _____

Grade _____ Instructor's initials _____

COMPETENCY 39.4: PROCESSING DENTAL FILMS IN AN AUTOMATIC FILM PROCESSOR

Performance Objective

By following a routine procedure that meets stated protocols, the student will demonstrate the proper technique for processing dental radiographs in an automatic film processor.

Evaluation and Grading Criteria

3	Student competently met the stated criteria without assistance.
2	Student required assistance in order to meet the stated criteria.
1	Student showed uncertainty when performing the stated criteria.
0	Student was not prepared and needs to repeat the step.
N/A	No evaluation of this step.

Instructor shall define grades for each point range earned on completion of each performance-evaluated task.

Performance Standards

The minimum number of satisfactory performances required before final evaluation is _____.

Instructor shall identify by * those steps considered critical. If a step is missed or minimum competency is not met, the evaluated procedure fails and must be repeated.

PERFORMANCE CRITERIA	*	SELF	PEER	INSTRUCTOR	COMMENT
1. Before the machine was operational, turned it on and allowed the chemicals to warm up (according to manufacturer's recommendations for proper temperature).					
2. Followed infection control steps.					
3. Opened the lid on the daylight loader, placed a paper towel over the bottom, and then placed two disposable cups on the paper towel.					
4. Put on gloves and slid the gloved hands through the sleeves of the daylight loader.					
5. Opened the film packet and removed the black paper and lead foil. Placed the films in the processor.					
6. Fed the films slowly into the machine and kept them straight. Allowed at least 10 seconds between film insertions. Alternated the slots within the processor when possible.					

Continued

7. After the last film was inserted into the machine, removed the gloves and dropped them into the center of the paper towel. Wrapped the paper towel over the contaminated film packets and gloves, touching only the corners and underside of the paper towel. Placed the paper towel into the second cup.				
8. Removed the cup containing the lead foil and took it to the recycling container.				
9. Removed the processed radiographs from the film recovery slot on the outside of the automatic processor and allowed 4 to 6 minutes for the automated process to be completed.				

ADDITIONAL COMMENTS

Total number of points earned _____

Grade _____ Instructor's initials _____

40 Compliance Control in Dental Radiology

1. Describe what is included on an informed consent form regarding dental imaging.

2. What laws affect the practice of dental radiography?

3. Describe what is included in the Consumer-Patient Radiation Health and Safety Act.

4. Who "owns" the patient's dental images?

5. What is the purpose of a quality assurance program?

6. Give the components of a quality assurance program.

7. Explain the use of a stepwedge.

8. Describe infection control protocol when preparing an x-ray operatory.

9. Describe the infection control protocol for exposures using digital sensors.

10. Describe the infection control protocol for exposures using conventional dental x-ray film.

FILL-IN-THE-BLANK STATEMENTS

Select the best term from the list below and complete the following statements.

stepwedge
disclosure
quality control tests

liable
informed consent
quality assurance

1. _____ is the process of informing the patient about dental imaging procedures.

2. _____ is permission granted by a patient after he or she has been informed about the particulars of the procedure.

3. _____ means that a person is accountable, or legally responsible.

4. _____ ensures that high-quality diagnostic radiographs are produced.

5. Specific criteria used to ensure quality in dental x-ray equipment, supplies, and film processing are _____.

6. A(n) _____ is used to demonstrate film densities and contrasts.

MULTIPLE-CHOICE QUESTIONS

Complete each question by circling the best answer.

1. What federal act requires persons who expose radiographs to be trained and certified?
   a. Hazard Communication Standard
   b. Blood-Borne Pathogen Standard
   c. Consumer-Patient Radiation Health and Safety Act
   d. Bill of Rights Act

2. What type of agreement is obtained before exposing radiographs on a patient?
   a. Liability agreement
   b. Dentist's signature
   c. Informed consent
   d. Medical approval

3. Under state laws, who would prescribe dental images in a general practice?
   a. Radiologist
   b. Specialist
   c. Physician
   d. Dentist

4. Who legally owns a patient's dental images?
   a. The patient
   b. The radiologist
   c. The dentist
   d. The physician

5. A way to ensure that high-quality diagnostic radiographs are produced is by the addition of _____.
   a. the best type of film
   b. quality assurance
   c. certified dental assistants
   d. Kodak approval

6. Quality control tests are _____.
   a. specific tests that are used to monitor dental x-ray equipment, supplies, and film processing
   b. specific tests that dental personnel must take and pass
   c. national board examinations for dentists
   d. radiology certification

7. When should you check a box of film for freshness?
   a. Daily
   b. Monthly
   c. Every Monday morning
   d. Each time you open a new box

8. Will a scratched film cassette affect the image?
   a. Yes
   b. No

9. Which of the following is a critical area in a quality control testing?
   a. Patient consent
   b. Film mounting
   c. Film processing
   d. Use of PPE

10. What is the purpose of the coin test?
   a. To check the x-ray machine
   b. To check the safelight
   c. To check the processor
   d. To check the technique

11. How often should processing solutions be replenished?
   a. Daily
   b. Weekly
   c. Monthly
   d. Twice a year

12. Why would a reference radiograph and a stepwedge be used?
   a. To check the absorbed dose
   b. To check the processing technique
   c. To check the densities and contrast
   d. To check the radiolucency and radiopacity

13. How can you tell when the fixer is losing its strength?
   a. Films take longer to clear.
   b. Films appear dark.
   c. Films are black.
   d. Films appear light.

14. The purpose of quality administration procedures is to deal with _____.
   a. Credentialing
   b. Management
   c. Who takes the x-rays in the office
   d. Being compensated for exposing the x-rays

15. Which member of the dental team is responsible for the quality administration program?
   a. Office manager
   b. Dental assistant
   c. Dental hygienist
   d. Dentist

16. What surfaces involved in radiographic exposure are covered with a barrier?
   a. All surfaces
   b. Surfaces that cannot be easily cleaned and disinfected
   c. No surfaces should be covered with a barrier
   d. Surfaces the patient will touch

17. What precautions should NOT be taken when handling contaminated phosphor storage plates (PSPs)?
   a. Wearing overgloves
   b. Placing the films in a paper cup
   c. Soaking the plates in a liquid sterilant
   d. Wiping saliva off the film as soon as the film is removed from the mouth

18. What is the minimum personal protective equipment the operator should wear while exposing radiographs?
   a. Mask
   b. Eyewear
   c. Gloves
   d. Hair cover

19. How should sensors be sterilized?
   a. Heat
   b. Moisture
   c. Vapor
   d. You cannot sterilize sensors.

MULTIMEDIA PROCEDURES RECOMMENDED REVIEW

Evolve
learning system

■ Preparing Operatory/Equipment to Take Radiographs

TOPICS FOR DISCUSSION

A series of films has just been processed in the automatic processor and something has happened to them. You take them to the view box and all the films are dark. Dark films can be the result of a variety of processing errors. Explain how the following factors can affect the processing of a film:

Time:

Solution strength:

Temperature:

Light leaks:

Improper fixation:

Paper left on the film:

COMPETENCY 40.1: PRACTICING INFECTION CONTROL DURING FILM EXPOSURE

Performance Objective

By following a routine procedure that meets stated protocols, the student will demonstrate the proper technique for implementing appropriate infection control procedures during film exposure.

Evaluation and Grading Criteria

 3   Student competently met the stated criteria without assistance.

 2   Student required assistance in order to meet the stated criteria.

 1   Student showed uncertainty when performing the stated criteria.

 0   Student was not prepared and needs to repeat the step.

 N/A   No evaluation of this step.

Instructor shall define grades for each point range earned on completion of each performance-evaluated task.

Performance Standards

The minimum number of satisfactory performances required before final evaluation is _____.

Instructor shall identify by * those steps considered critical. If a step is missed or minimum competency is not met, the evaluated procedure fails and must be repeated.

PERFORMANCE CRITERIA	*	SELF	PEER	INSTRUCTOR	COMMENT
1. Washed and dried hands and placed barriers.					
2. Set out the packaged positioning device, film, labeled container for exposed film, paper towel, and other miscellaneous items needed.					
3. Seated the patient and positioned the lead apron.					
4. Washed and dried hands and put on gloves.					
5. Placed each exposed film into the container, being careful not to touch the external surface.					
6. Wiped the exposed packet on the paper towel.					
7. After exposures were complete, removed the lead apron and dismissed the patient.					
8. When finished exposing films and while still gloved, discarded the barriers and paper towel.					

Continued

9. Removed gloves and washed the hands before leaving the treatment room.				
10. Carried the cup or bag of exposed films to the processing area.				

ADDITIONAL COMMENTS

Total number of points earned _____

Grade _____ Instructor's initials _____

COMPETENCY 40.2: PRACTICING INFECTION CONTROL IN THE DARKROOM

Performance Objective

By following a routine procedure that meets stated protocols, the student will demonstrate the proper technique for implementing proper infection control in the darkroom.

Evaluation and Grading Criteria

  3   Student competently met the stated criteria without assistance.

  2   Student required assistance in order to meet the stated criteria.

  1   Student showed uncertainty when performing the stated criteria.

  0   Student was not prepared and needs to repeat the step.

 N/A   No evaluation of this step.

Instructor shall define grades for each point range earned on completion of each performance-evaluated task.

Performance Standards

The minimum number of satisfactory performances required before final evaluation is _____.

Instructor shall identify by * those steps considered critical. If a step is missed or minimum competency is not met, the evaluated procedure fails and must be repeated.

PERFORMANCE CRITERIA	*	SELF	PEER	INSTRUCTOR	COMMENT
1. Placed a paper towel and a clean cup on the counter near the processor.					
2. Washed hands and put on a new pair of gloves.					
3. Opened the film packets and allowed each exposed film to drop onto the paper towel. Ensured that unwrapped films did not come into contact with gloves.					
4. Removed the lead foil from the packet and placed it into the foil container.					
5. Placed the empty film packets into the clean cup.					
6. Discarded the cup and removed the gloves with the insides turned out and discarded them.					
7. Placed the films into the processor.					
ADDITIONAL COMMENTS					

Total number of points earned _____

Grade _____ Instructor's initials _____

COMPETENCY 40.3: PRACTICING INFECTION CONTROL WITH USE OF DAYLIGHT LOADER

Performance Objective

By following a routine procedure that meets stated protocols, the student will demonstrate proper infection control techniques while using the daylight loader.

Evaluation and Grading Criteria

 3   Student competently met the stated criteria without assistance.

 2   Student required assistance in order to meet the stated criteria.

 1   Student showed uncertainty when performing the stated criteria.

 0   Student was not prepared and needs to repeat the step.

 N/A   No evaluation of this step.

Instructor shall define grades for each point range earned on completion of each performance-evaluated task.

Performance Standards

The minimum number of satisfactory performances required before final evaluation is _____.

Instructor shall identify by * those steps considered critical. If a step is missed or minimum competency is not met, the evaluated procedure fails and must be repeated.

PERFORMANCE CRITERIA	*	SELF	PEER	INSTRUCTOR	COMMENT
1. Washed and dried hands and placed a paper towel or piece of plastic as a barrier inside the bottom of the daylight loader.					
2. Placed the cup with the contaminated film, a clean pair of gloves, and a second paper cup on the barrier and closed the top.					
3. Put the clean hands through the sleeves and put on the gloves.					
4. Opened the packets and allowed the films to drop onto the clean barrier. Placed the contaminated packets into the second cup and the lead foil into the foil container.					
5. After opening the last packet, removed the gloves with the insides turned out and inserted the films into the developing slots.					
6. After inserting the last film, pulled the ungloved hands through sleeves.					
7. Opened the top of the loader and carefully pulled the ends of the barrier over the paper cup that contains the used gloves and empty film packets, and then discarded the cup. Used care not to touch the contaminated parts of the barrier with bare hands.					

Continued

Chapter **40 Compliance Control in Dental Radiology**

8. Washed and dried the hands.					
9. Labeled a film mount, paper cup, or envelope with the patient's name and used it to collect the processed films.					

ADDITIONAL COMMENTS

Total number of points earned _____

Grade _____ Instructor's initials _____

COMPETENCY 40.4: PRACTICING INFECTION CONTROL WITH DIGITAL SENSORS

Performance Objective

By following a routine procedure that meets stated protocols, the student will demonstrate all infection control practices using digital sensors.

Evaluation and Grading Criteria

3	Student competently met the stated criteria without assistance.
2	Student required assistance in order to meet the stated criteria.
1	Student showed uncertainty when performing the stated criteria.
0	Student was not prepared and needs to repeat the step.
N/A	No evaluation of this step.

Instructor shall define grades for each point range earned on completion of each performance-evaluated task.

Performance Standards

The minimum number of satisfactory performances required before final evaluation is _____.

Instructor shall identify by * those steps considered critical. If a step is missed or minimum competency is not met, the evaluated procedure fails and must be repeated.

PERFORMANCE CRITERIA	*	SELF	PEER	INSTRUCTOR	COMMENT
1. Washed and dried hands and then placed surface barriers on equipment, computer keyboard and mouse, and work area.					
2. Set out the packaged positioning device, barriers for the sensor and cable, and a paper towel or gauze squares.					
3. Secured the barrier around the digital sensor.					
4. Seated the patient and positioned the lead apron.					
5. Washed and dried the hands and donned gloves.					
6. After all exposures were complete, removed the lead apron using appropriate aseptic techniques and dismissed the patient.					
7. Put on utility gloves and removed barriers from the x-ray equipment, keyboard, and mouse, taking care not to touch the surfaces underneath.					
8. Disposed the barriers and paper towels.					
9. Placed the positioning device on a tray to be returned to the instrument processing area.					

Continued

10. Disinfected the lead apron and any surfaces that may have become contaminated during the removal of surface barriers.				
11. Washed and dried the hands.				

ADDITIONAL COMMENTS

Total number of points earned _____

Grade _____ Instructor's initials _____

COMPETENCY 40.5: PRACTICING INFECTION CONTROL WITH PHOSPHOR STORAGE PLATES (PSPS)

Performance Objective

By following a routine procedure that meets stated protocols, the student will demonstrate all infection control practices when using phosphor storage plates.

Evaluation and Grading Criteria

 3   Student competently met the stated criteria without assistance.

 2   Student required assistance in order to meet the stated criteria.

 1   Student showed uncertainty when performing the stated criteria.

 0   Student was not prepared and needs to repeat the step.

 N/A   No evaluation of this step.

Instructor shall define grades for each point range earned on completion of each performance-evaluated task.

Performance Standards

The minimum number of satisfactory performances required before final evaluation is _____.

Instructor shall identify by * those steps considered critical. If a step is missed or minimum competency is not met, the evaluated procedure fails and must be repeated.

PERFORMANCE CRITERIA	*	SELF	PEER	INSTRUCTOR	COMMENT
Preparation for Exposure					
1. Turned on the computer and logged on to link the patient's images to his or her chart. Chose the image layout.					
2. Washed and dried hands.					
3. Placed surface barriers on the equipment and work area.					
4. Slid the phosphor plates into barrier envelopes.					
5. Sealed each barrier envelope by removing the protective strip and gently pressed to seal the edge.					
6. Set out the packaged positioning device, transfer box, paper towel, and any other miscellaneous items necessary.					
Exposures					
7. Seated the patient and positioned the lead apron.					
8. Washed and dried the hands and donned gloves.					
9. Placed a PSP into the film holder for each exposure.					
10. After each exposure, wiped the excess saliva from the PSP using a paper towel or gauze.					

Continued

11. Placed each exposed PSP into a paper cup that had been labeled with the patient's name.				
12. After exposures were complete, removed the lead apron and dismissed the patient.				
13. Removed the barriers, taking care not to touch the surfaces underneath.				
14. Disposed of barriers and placed the positioning devices on the tray to be returned to the instrument processing area.				
Preparation for Scanning				
15. While gloved, removed PSPs from the paper cup.				
16. Carefully opened the sealed envelope and allowed each PSP to drop into the black transfer box.				
17. Disposed of the contaminated envelopes.				
18. Removed the gloves and washed the hands.				
Scanning				
19. Followed the manufacturer's directions for insertion of PSPs into the scanner.				
20. When imaging was complete, logged off the system.				
21. Accurately documented the procedure in the patient record.				

ADDITIONAL COMMENTS

Total number of points earned _____

Grade _____ Instructor's initials _____

41 Intraoral Imaging

SHORT-ANSWER QUESTIONS

1. Name the two primary types of projections used in an intraoral radiograph.

2. What are the advantages and disadvantages of the paralleling and bisection of the angle technique?

3. Why is a film or sensor holder necessary with the paralleling technique?

4. What are the five basic rules of the paralleling technique?

5. What is the recommended vertical angulation for all bitewing exposures?

6. State the basic principle for the bitewing technique.

7. Give the main concept of the bisecting technique.

8. Describe correct vertical angulation.

9. Describe incorrect vertical angulation.

10. What type of methods can be used for managing a patient with a hypersensitive gag reflex?

FILL-IN-THE-BLANK STATEMENTS

Select the best term from the list below and complete the following statements.

bitewing	long axis of the tooth
contact area	bisection of the angle technique
crestal bone	diagnostic quality
alveolar bone	parallel
interproximal	central ray
paralleling technique	perpendicular
intersecting	right angle

1. The _____ is an intraoral technique of exposing periapical images in which the teeth and the image receptor are spaced equally to each other.

2. The _____ is an intraoral technique of exposing periapical images in which the film and the teeth create a slanted position that is intersected by the beam.

3. A radiographic image is said to have _____ when it shows correct landmarks, optimum density, contrast, definition, and detail.

4. _____ is a term used to describe the space between two adjacent tooth surfaces.

5. A(n) _____ is a radiographic image used to examine interproximal spaces.

6. The bone that supports and encases the roots of the teeth is the _____.

7. The _____ is the coronal portion of alveolar bone found between the teeth.

8. A portion of a tooth that touches an adjacent tooth in the same arch is the _____.

9. An object is _____ if it is in the same plane and is separated by the same distance.

10. _____ means cutting across or through.

11. Two things are _____ if they intersect at or form a right angle.

12. A 90-degree angle formed by two lines perpendicular to each other is a _____.

13. The _____ is an imaginary line used to divide a tooth longitudinally into two equal halves.

14. The _____ is the central portion of the primary beam of radiation.

MULTIPLE-CHOICE QUESTIONS

Complete each question by circling the best answer.

1. What technique is used for exposing dental images?
   a. Digressive
   b. Parallel
   c. Bisection of angle
   d. b and c

2. Which exposure technique does the American Academy of Oral and Maxillofacial Radiology and the American Dental Education Association recommend?
   a. Bisection of angle
   b. Parallel
   c. Intersection
   d. Dissection

3. Why is the sequencing of exposure important?
   a. So all areas of the mouth are included and images would not have to be retaken
   b. To follow guidelines
   c. For proper mounting of film
   d. So that the operator will know how many films have been exposed

4. When you are exposing images, in which area of the mouth should you begin?
   a. Maxillary right
   b. Mandibular anterior
   c. Mandibular left
   d. Maxillary anterior

5. Which exposure should be the first for the posterior regions?
   a. Maxillary molar
   b. Mandibular premolar
   c. Maxillary premolar
   d. Mandibular molar

6. Why is it not recommended to have the patient hold the image receptor during exposure?
   a. The patient's finger will get in the way of the image.
   b. The dental assistant must position the film or sensor properly.
   c. The patient receives unnecessary radiation.
   d. It does not meet with infection control standards.

7. What type of film holder can be used in the bisecting angle technique?
   a. BAI
   b. EeZee Grip
   c. Stabe
   d. All of the above

8. What error occurs when the horizontal angulation is incorrect?
   a. Elongation
   b. Overlapping
   c. Blurring
   d. Herringbone pattern

9. Which of the following can occur when the vertical angulation is incorrect?
   a. Elongation
   b. Overlapping
   c. Foreshortening
   d. a and c

10. In the bisecting angle technique, how is the image receptor placed in relation to the teeth?
    a. Parallel
    b. Far from the teeth
    c. Close to the teeth
    d. On the opposite side of the arch

11. What is the purpose of bitewing images?
    a. To view the occlusal third of the teeth
    b. To view the gingival third of the teeth
    c. To view the apices of the teeth
    d. To view the interproximal surfaces

12. What vertical angulation should be used for bitewing images?
    a. −10 degrees
    b. −15 degrees
    c. + 10 degrees
    d. + 15 degrees

13. What film size is used in the occlusal technique for an adult?
    a. 1
    b. 2
    c. 3
    d. 4

14. When are occlusal radiographs indicated?
    a. To show a wide view of the arch
    b. To view the sinus
    c. To detect interproximal decay
    d. To view the apex

15. For partially edentulous patients, how can you modify the technique when using a bite-block?
    a. Use a larger film or sensor
    b. Use a cotton roll
    c. Use the patient's partial denture
    d. Use a custom tray

16. When exposing films on a pediatric patient, what analogy can you use to describe the tubehead?
    a. Space gun
    b. Alien machine
    c. Camera
    d. Tubehead

17. What changes are made in the exposure factors of a pediatric patient?
    a. No changes are made.
    b. Exposure factors must be reduced.
    c. Exposure factors must be increased.
    d. It depends on whether the patient is male or female.

18. What film size is recommended for a pediatric patient with all primary dentition?
    a. 0
    b. 1
    c. 2
    d. 3

19. Where would you begin exposures for a patient with a severe gag reflex?
    a. Maxillary posterior
    b. Mandibular molar
    c. Maxillary molar
    d. Mandibular anterior

20. What is a good diagnostic quality image for endodontics?
    a. One that allows you to see an impaction
    b. One that allows you to see interproximally
    c. One that allows you to see 5 mm beyond the apex
    d. One that allows you to see the incisal edge

21. When radiographs are mounted using the labial mounting method, where is the dot placed?
    a. It does not matter.
    b. Facing away from you
    c. Facing down
    d. Facing up

22. Why is it important for the dental assistant to recognize normal anatomic landmarks?
    a. For diagnostic purposes
    b. For mounting of x-ray films
    c. For quality control
    d. For identification of the patient

23. Why is it important to avoid retakes?
    a. The dentist will deduct it from your pay.
    b. To avoid unnecessary radiation exposure.
    c. To avoid wasting film.
    d. Insurance will not pay for retakes.

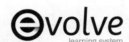

MULTIMEDIA PROCEDURES RECOMMENDED REVIEW

- Assembling XCP Instruments
- Bisecting Technique (8 videos)
- Bitewing Technique (2 videos)
- Mounting Dental Radiographs
- Occlusal Technique
- Paralleling Technique (8 videos)
- Positioning the Patient for Dental Imaging

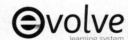

INTERACTIVE DENTAL OFFICE PATIENT CASE EXERCISES

Access the *Interactive Dental Office* on the *Evolve* website and click on the patient case file for Christopher Brooks.
- Review Christopher's file.
- Mount his radiographs.
- Answer the following questions.

1. What types of projections were used for his radiographic survey?

2. What sizes of film were used for each projection?

Access the *Interactive Dental Office* on the Evolve website and click on the patient case file for Antonio DeAngelis.

- Review Mr. DeAngelis's file.
- Mount his radiographs.
- Answer the following questions.

1. What technique error occurred on the mandibular left premolar exposure?

2. What is wrong with the maxillary left molar projection?

3. What is wrong with the right premolar bitewing and what would be the correction?

With the first patient, allow yourself 5 minutes. Time yourself and note how many errors you make when you are placing the radiographs on the mount. Continue this practice until you have your mounting skills down to 2 minutes with no errors.

COMPETENCY 41.1: PREPARING THE PATIENT FOR DENTAL IMAGING

Performance Objective

By following a routine procedure that meets stated protocols, the student will demonstrate the proper technique for preparing a patient for intraoral x-ray imaging procedures.

Evaluation and Grading Criteria

3	Student competently met the stated criteria without assistance.
2	Student required assistance in order to meet the stated criteria.
1	Student showed uncertainty when performing the stated criteria.
0	Student was not prepared and needs to repeat the step.
N/A	No evaluation of this step.

Instructor shall define grades for each point range earned on completion of each performance-evaluated task.

Performance Standards

The minimum number of satisfactory performances required before final evaluation is _____.

Instructor shall identify by * those steps considered critical. If a step is missed or minimum competency is not met, the evaluated procedure fails and must be repeated.

PERFORMANCE CRITERIA	*	SELF	PEER	INSTRUCTOR	COMMENT
1. Explained the procedure to the patient and asked if they have any questions.					
2. Adjusted the chair with the patient positioned upright. Adjusted the level of the chair to a comfortable working height for the operator.					
3. Adjusted the headrest to support and position the patient's head so that the upper arch was parallel to the floor and the midsagittal (midline) plane was perpendicular to the floor.					
4. Placed and secured the lead apron with thyroid collar on the patient. If needed, asked the patient to remove eyeglasses or bulky earrings.					
5. Asked the patient to remove all objects from the mouth, including dentures, retainers, chewing gum, and pierced tongue or pierced lip objects. Placed any objects into the plastic container.					

ADDITIONAL COMMENTS

Total number of points earned _____

Grade _____ Instructor's initials _____

COMPETENCY 41.2: PRODUCING FULL-MOUTH RADIOGRAPHIC SURVEY USING PARALLELING TECHNIQUE

Performance Objective

By following a routine procedure that meets stated protocols, the student will produce a full-mouth radiographic survey using the proper paralleling technique.

Evaluation and Grading Criteria

3   Student competently met the stated criteria without assistance.

2   Student required assistance in order to meet the stated criteria.

1   Student showed uncertainty when performing the stated criteria.

0   Student was not prepared and needs to repeat the step.

N/A   No evaluation of this step.

Instructor shall define grades for each point range earned on completion of each performance-evaluated task.

Performance Standards

The minimum number of satisfactory performances required before final evaluation is _____.

Instructor shall identify by * those steps considered critical. If a step is missed or minimum competency is not met, the evaluated procedure fails and must be repeated.

PERFORMANCE CRITERIA	*	SELF	PEER	INSTRUCTOR	COMMENT
Preparation					
1. Placed personal protective equipment according to the procedure.					
2. Determined the numbers and types of images to be exposed.					
3. Labeled a paper cup, plastic bag, or transfer box, and placed it outside the room where the x-ray machine was used.					
4. Turned on the x-ray machine and checked the basic settings.					
5. Washed hands.					
6. If using conventional film or PSPs, dispensed the desired number of films and stored them outside the room where the x-ray machine was used.					
7. Placed all necessary barriers.					
8. Adjusted the chair with the patient positioned upright. Adjusted the level of the chair to a comfortable working height for the operator.					
9. Adjusted the headrest to support and position the patient's head so that the upper arch was parallel to the floor and the midsagittal (midline) plane was perpendicular to the floor.					

Continued

10. Asked the patient to remove eyeglasses or bulky earrings.				
11. Draped the patient with a lead apron and thyroid collar.				
12. Washed the hands and put on clean examination gloves.				
13. Asked the patient to remove any removable prosthetic appliances from his or her mouth; placed objects in a plastic container.				
14. Opened the package and assembled the sterile film or sensor-holding instruments.				
15. Used a mouth mirror to inspect the oral cavity.				
Maxillary Central or Lateral Incisor Region				
16. Inserted the film packet or sensor vertically into the anterior block.				
17. Positioned the film or sensor.				
18. Instructed the patient to close the mouth slowly but firmly.				
19. Positioned the localizing ring and the position indicator device (PID), and then exposed the film or sensor.				
Maxillary Canine Region				
20. Inserted the film packet or sensor vertically into the anterior bite-block.				
21. Positioned the film packet or sensor with the canine and first premolar centered.				
22. Instructed the patient to close the mouth slowly but firmly.				
23. Positioned the localizing ring and the PID, and then exposed the film or sensor.				
Maxillary Premolar Region				
24. Inserted the film packet or sensor horizontally into the posterior bite-block.				
25. Centered the film packet or sensor on the second premolar.				
26. With the instrument and film or sensor in place, instructed the patient to close the mouth slowly but firmly.				

27. Positioned the localizing ring and PID, and then exposed the film or sensor.					
Maxillary Molar Region					
28. Inserted the film packet or sensor horizontally into the posterior bite-block.					
29. Centered the film packet or sensor on the second molar.					
30. With the instrument and film or sensor in place, instructed the patient to close the mouth slowly but firmly.					
31. Positioned the localizing ring and PID and then exposed the film or sensor.					
Mandibular Incisor Region					
32. Inserted the film packet or sensor vertically into the anterior bite-block.					
33. Centered the film packet or sensor between the central incisors.					
34. With the instrument and film or sensor in place, instructed the patient to close the mouth slowly but firmly.					
35. Positioned the localizing ring and PID and then exposed the film or sensor.					
Mandibular Canine Region					
36. Inserted the film packet or sensor vertically into the anterior bite-block.					
37. Centered the film or sensor on the canine.					
38. Used a cotton roll between the maxillary teeth and the bite-block, if necessary.					
39. With the instrument and film or sensor in place, instructed the patient to close the mouth slowly but firmly.					
40. Positioned the localizing ring and PID and then exposed the film or sensor.					

Continued

Mandibular Premolar Region					
41. Inserted the film or sensor horizontally into the posterior bite-block.					
42. Centered the film or sensor on the contact point between the second premolar and the first molar.					
43. With the instrument and film or sensor in place, instructed the patient to close the mouth slowly but firmly.					
44. Positioned the localizing ring and PID and then exposed the film or sensor.					
Mandibular Molar Region					
45. Inserted the film or sensor horizontally into the posterior bite-block.					
46. Centered the film or sensor on the second molar.					
47. With the instrument and film in place, instructed the patient to close slowly but firmly.					
48. Positioned the localizing ring and PID and then exposed the film or sensor.					
49. Accurately documented the procedure in the patient record.					

ADDITIONAL COMMENTS

Total number of points earned _____

Grade _____ Instructor's initials _____

COMPETENCY 41.3 PRODUCING FULL-MOUTH RADIOGRAPHIC SURVEY USING BISECTING TECHNIQUE

Performance Objective

By following a routine procedure that meets stated protocols, the student will produce a full-mouth radiographic survey using the proper bisecting technique.

Evaluation and Grading Criteria

_3_   Student competently met the stated criteria without assistance.

_2_   Student required assistance in order to meet the stated criteria.

_1_   Student showed uncertainty when performing the stated criteria.

_0_   Student was not prepared and needs to repeat the step.

_N/A_   No evaluation of this step.

Instructor shall define grades for each point range earned on completion of each performance-evaluated task.

Performance Standards

The minimum number of satisfactory performances required before final evaluation is _____.

Instructor shall identify by * those steps considered critical. If a step is missed or minimum competency is not met, the evaluated procedure fails and must be repeated.

PERFORMANCE CRITERIA	*	SELF	PEER	INSTRUCTOR	COMMENT
1. Placed personal protective equipment according to the procedure.					
2. Prepared the operatory with all infection control barriers.					
3. Determined the numbers and types of films to be exposed through a review of the patient's chart, directions from the dentist, or both.					
4. Labeled a paper cup or transfer box with the patient's name and the date and placed it outside the room where the radiograph machine was used.					
5. Turned on the x-ray machine, and checked the basic settings (kilovoltage, milliamperage, exposure time).					
6. Washed and dried hands.					
7. Dispensed the desired number of films or PSPs and stored them outside the room where the x-ray machine was used.					
Maxillary Canine Exposure					
8. Positioned the patient so that the occlusal plane was positioned parallel to the floor and the sagittal plane of the patient's face was perpendicular to the floor.					

Continued

9. Centered the film packet or sensor on the canine.				
10. Positioned the lower edge of the holder to the occlusal plane so that $\frac{1}{8}$ inch extended below the incisal edge of the canine.				
11. Instructed the patient to exert light but firm pressure on the lower edge of the holder.				
12. Established the correct vertical angulation by bisecting the angle and directing the central ray perpendicular to the imaginary bisector.				
13. Established the correct horizontal angulation by directing the central ray between the contacts of the canine and the first premolar.				
14. Centered the PID over the film packet or sensor to avoid cone cutting.				
15. Exposed the film or sensor.				
Maxillary Incisor Exposure				
16. Centered the film packet or sensor on the contact between the two central incisors.				
17. Positioned the lower edge of the film or sensor holder to the occlusal plane so that $\frac{1}{8}$ inch extended below the incisal edge of the canine.				
18. Instructed the patient to exert light but firm pressure on the lower edge of the holder.				
19. Established the correct vertical angulation by bisecting the angle and directing the central ray perpendicular to the imaginary bisector.				
20. Established the correct horizontal angulation by directing the central ray between the contacts of central incisors.				
21. Centered the PID over the film or sensor to avoid cone cutting.				
22. Exposed the film or sensor.				

Mandibular Canine Exposure					
23. Centered the film packet or sensor on the canine.					
24. Positioned the lower edge of the film or sensor holder to the occlusal plane so that $\frac{1}{8}$ inch extended above the incisal edge of the canine.					
25. Instructed the patient to exert light but firm pressure on the lower edge of the holder.					
26. Established the correct vertical angulation by bisecting the angle and directing the central ray perpendicular to the imaginary bisector.					
27. Established the correct horizontal angulation by directing the central ray between the contacts of the canine and the first premolar.					
28. Centered the PID over the film or sensor to avoid cone cutting.					
29. Exposed the film or sensor.					
Mandibular Incisor Exposure					
30. Centered the film packet or sensor on the contact between the two central incisors.					
31. Positioned the upper edge of the holder to the occlusal plane so that $\frac{1}{8}$ inch extended above the incisal edges of the teeth.					
32. Instructed the patient to exert light but firm pressure on the lower edge of the holder.					
33. Established the correct vertical angulation by bisecting the angle and directing the central ray perpendicular to the imaginary bisector.					
34. Established the correct horizontal angulation by directing the central ray between the contacts of the central incisors.					
35. Centered the PID over the film or sensor to avoid cone cutting.					
36. Exposed the film or sensor.					

Continued

Maxillary Premolar Exposure					
37. Centered the film packet or sensor on the second premolar, with the front edge of the film or sensor aligned with the midline of the canine.					
38. Positioned the lower edge of the film or sensor parallel to the occlusal plane so that $\frac{1}{8}$ inch extended below the occlusal edges of the teeth.					
39. Instructed the patient to close gently but firmly on the holder.					
40. Established the correct vertical angulation by bisecting the angle and directing the central ray perpendicular to the imaginary bisector.					
41. Established the correct horizontal angulation by directing the central ray between the contacts of the premolars.					
42. Centered the PID over the film or sensor to avoid cone cutting.					
43. Exposed the film or sensor.					
Maxillary Molar Exposure					
44. Centered the film or sensor holder and film packet or sensor on the second molar, with the front edge of the film or sensor aligned with the midline of the second premolar.					
45. Positioned the lower edge of the holder parallel to the occlusal plane so that $\frac{1}{8}$ inch extended below the occlusal surfaces of the teeth.					
46. Instructed the patient to bite gently but firmly on the holder. *Note:* You may have to ask the patient to lower the chin so that the occlusal surfaces are parallel with the floor.					
47. Established the correct vertical angulation by bisecting the angle and directing the central ray perpendicular to the imaginary bisector.					

48. Established the correct horizontal angulation by directing the central ray between the contacts of the molars.					
49. Centered the PID over the film or sensor to avoid cone cutting.					
50. Exposed the film or sensor.					
Mandibular Premolar Exposure					
51. Centered the film packet or sensor on the second premolar, with the front edge of the film or sensor aligned with the mesial aspect of the canine.					
52. Positioned the upper edge of the film or sensor parallel to the occlusal plane so that $\frac{1}{8}$ inch extended above the occlusal edges of the teeth.					
53. Instructed the patient to close the mouth gently but firmly on the holder.					
54. Established the correct vertical angulation by bisecting the angle and directing the central ray perpendicular to the imaginary bisector.					
55. Established the correct horizontal angulation by directing the central ray between the contacts of the premolars.					
56. Centered the PID over the film or sensor to avoid cone cutting.					
57. Exposed the film or sensor.					
Mandibular Molar Exposure					
58. Centered the film or sensor holder and film packet on the second molar, with the front edge of the film or sensor aligned with the midline of the second premolar.					
59. Positioned the upper edge of the holder parallel to the occlusal plane so that $\frac{1}{8}$ inch extended above the occlusal surfaces of the teeth.					
60. Instructed the patient to bite gently but firmly on the holder.					

Continued

61. Established the correct vertical angulation by bisecting the angle and directing the central ray perpendicular to the imaginary bisector.				
62. Established the correct horizontal angulation by directing the central ray between the contacts of the molars.				
63. Centered the PID over the film or sensor to avoid cone cutting.				
64. Exposed the film or sensor.				
65. Accurately documented the procedure in the patient record.				

ADDITIONAL COMMENTS

Total number of points earned _____

Grade _____ Instructor's initials _____

COMPETENCY 41.4: PRODUCING A FOUR-VIEW RADIOGRAPHIC SURVEY USING THE BITEWING TECHNIQUE

Performance Objective

By following a routine procedure that meets stated protocols, the student will produce a full-mouth radiographic survey using the proper bitewing technique.

Evaluation and Grading Criteria

 3 Student competently met the stated criteria without assistance.

 2 Student required assistance in order to meet the stated criteria.

 1 Student showed uncertainty when performing the stated criteria.

 0 Student was not prepared and needs to repeat the step.

 N/A No evaluation of this step.

Instructor shall define grades for each point range earned on completion of each performance-evaluated task.

Performance Standards

The minimum number of satisfactory performances required before final evaluation is _____.

Instructor shall identify by * those steps considered critical. If a step is missed or minimum competency is not met, the evaluated procedure fails and must be repeated.

PERFORMANCE CRITERIA	*	SELF	PEER	INSTRUCTOR	COMMENT
1. Placed personal protective equipment according to the procedure.					
2. Placed the film or sensor in the patient's mouth for a premolar film.					
3. Put the film or sensor in a proper position.					
4. Set the vertical angulation.					
5. Positioned horizontal angulation.					
6. Placed the position indicator device.					
7. Directed the central ray through the contact areas.					
8. Pressed the exposure button.					
9. Accurately documented the procedure in the patient record.					
ADDITIONAL COMMENTS					

Total number of points earned _____

Grade _____ Instructor's initials _____

COMPETENCY 41.5: PRODUCING MAXILLARY AND MANDIBULAR RADIOGRAPHS USING THE OCCLUSAL TECHNIQUE

Performance Objective

By following a routine procedure that meets stated protocols, the student will produce maxillary and mandibular occlusal radiographs using the proper occlusal technique.

Evaluation and Grading Criteria

3	Student competently met the stated criteria without assistance.
2	Student required assistance in order to meet the stated criteria.
1	Student showed uncertainty when performing the stated criteria.
0	Student was not prepared and needs to repeat the step.
N/A	No evaluation of this step.

Instructor shall define grades for each point range earned on completion of each performance-evaluated task.

Performance Standards

The minimum number of satisfactory performances required before final evaluation is _____.

Instructor shall identify by * those steps considered critical. If a step is missed or minimum competency is not met, the evaluated procedure fails and must be repeated.

PERFORMANCE CRITERIA	*	SELF	PEER	INSTRUCTOR	COMMENT
Maxillary Occlusal Technique					
1. Placed personal protective equipment according to the procedure.					
2. Asked the patient to remove prosthetic appliances or objects from the mouth.					
3. Placed the lead apron and thyroid collar.					
4. Positioned the patient's head so the film plane was parallel to the floor.					
5. Placed the film packet in the patient's mouth with the white side of the film on the occlusal surfaces of the maxillary teeth.					
6. Placed the film as far posterior as possible.					
7. Positioned the position PID so that the central ray was directed at a 65-degree angle through the bridge of the nose to the center of the film packet.					
8. Pressed the x-ray machine-activating button and made the exposure.					
9. Accurately documented the procedure in the patient record.					

Continued

Mandibular Occlusal Technique				
10. Tilted the patient's head back to a comfortable position, ensuring that the midsagittal plane was vertical.				
11. Placed the film packet in the patient's mouth with the white side of the film on the occlusal surfaces of the mandibular teeth.				
12. Positioned the film as far posterior as possible.				
13. Positioned the PID so that the central ray was directed at 90 degrees (a right angle) to the center of the film packet.				
14. Pressed the x-ray machine-activating button and made the exposure.				
15. Accurately documented the procedure in the patient record.				

ADDITIONAL COMMENTS

Total number of points earned _____

Grade _____ Instructor's initials _____

COMPETENCY 41.6: MOUNTING DENTAL RADIOGRAPHS

Performance Objective

By following a routine procedure that meets stated protocols, the student will demonstrate the proper technique for mounting a full-mouth series of radiographs.

Evaluation and Grading Criteria

 3   Student competently met the stated criteria without assistance.

 2   Student required assistance in order to meet the stated criteria.

 1   Student showed uncertainty when performing the stated criteria.

 0   Student was not prepared and needs to repeat the step.

 N/A   No evaluation of this step.

Instructor shall define grades for each point range earned on completion of each performance-evaluated task.

Performance Standards

The minimum number of satisfactory performances required before final evaluation is _____.

Instructor shall identify by * those steps considered critical. If a step is missed or minimum competency is not met, the evaluated procedure fails and must be repeated.

PERFORMANCE CRITERIA	*	SELF	PEER	INSTRUCTOR	COMMENT
1. Ensured that the hands were clean and dry before handling radiographs. Grasped the films only at the edges, not on the front or back.					
2. Selected the appropriately sized mount, and labeled it with the patient's name and the date the radiographs were exposed.					
3. Arranged the dried radiographs in the anatomic order on a piece of clean white paper or on a flat view box.					
4. Once the films were arranged properly, placed them neatly in the mount.					
ADDITIONAL COMMENTS					

Total number of points earned _____

Grade _____ Instructor's initials _____

42 Extraoral Imaging

SHORT-ANSWER QUESTIONS

1. Describe the purposes and uses of extraoral imaging.

2. List the equipment used in panoramic imaging.

3. List the steps for patient preparation and positioning in panoramic imaging.

4. Discuss the advantages and disadvantages of panoramic imaging.

5. Describe the errors that can occur during patient preparation and positioning during panoramic imaging.

6. Describe the equipment used in extraoral imaging.

7. Give the specific purpose of each of the extraoral film projections.

8. Discuss the advantages of 3D imaging.

Select the best term from the list below and complete the following statements.

tomography
extraoral images
Frankfort plane
cone beam computed tomography

midsagittal plane
focal trough
temporomandibular

1. An imaginary three-dimensional curved zone that is horseshoe shaped and used to focus panoramic radiographs is the

   _____.

2. The _____ is the imaginary plane that passes through the top of the ear canal and the bottom of the eye

   socket.

3. The imaginary line that divides the patient's face into right and left sides is the _____.

4. _____ is a radiographic technique that allows imaging of one layer or section of the body while blurring

   images from structures in other planes.

5. _____ is a three-dimensional digital imaging method that uses a cone-shaped beam of radiation that ro-

   tates around the patient.

6. _____ are taken when large areas of the skull or jaw must be examined.

7. _____ is the joint on each side of the head that allows movement of the mandible.

MULTIPLE-CHOICE QUESTIONS

Complete each question by circling the best answer.

1. What types of additional intraoral images are no longer necessary to supplement a panoramic radiograph when using the full-featured digital panoramic units?
   a. Periapical
   b. Bitewing
   c. Occlusal
   d. All of the above

2. A focal trough is _____.
   a. the area where the patient bites down
   b. an imaginary horseshoe-shaped area used for jaw placement
   c. where the patient looks during the process
   d. an earpiece used for positioning

3. Which of the following is NOT an advantage of extra-oral radiographs?
   a. They show a close-up image of something.
   b. They minimize radiation exposure for the patient.
   c. They provide an overview of the skull and jaws.
   d. They prevent the patient from gagging.

4. What type of device is included on a panoramic unit?
   a. Cephalostat
   b. Hemostat
   c. Periapical film holder
   d. Bitewing holder

5. The purpose of a grid is to _____.
   a. increase the size of the image
   b. reduce the amount of scatter radiation
   c. hold the patient's head still
   d. hold the film in place

6. What type of imaging is best for soft tissues of the temporomandibular joint?
   a. Panorex
   b. Digital x-ray examination
   c. Cephalometric
   d. Cone beam computed tomography

7. On new full-featured digital panoramic units, which of the following can now be detected on a panoramic radiograph?
   a. Location of impacted teeth
   b. Lesions in the mandible
   c. Interproximal caries
   d. All of the above

8. What type of technology is used in panoramic units?
   a. Conventional film-based technology
   b. Digital technology
   c. Both a and b

9. Which of the following is a component of a panoramic unit?
   a. Chin rest
   b. Notched bite-block
   c. Forehead rest
   d. All of the above

10. Which of the following can cause "ghost images" on a panoramic image?
    a. Eyeglasses
    b. Earrings
    c. Necklaces
    d. All of the above

CASE STUDY

Sixteen-year-old Jeremy Davis is scheduled for an examination and consultation today. Some of the problems that Jeremy exhibits are class III occlusion, crowding, recurrent decay, and slight gingivitis. For the dentist to proceed with treatment, a more detailed evaluation using radiographs is required.

1. What type of image would reveal a class III occlusion?

2. What type of image would reveal crowding?

3. To what specialist should Jeremy be referred for the class III occlusion and crowding?

4. What type of image would reveal recurrent decay?

5. What type of image would reveal gingivitis?

MULTIMEDIA PROCEDURES RECOMMENDED REVIEW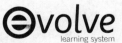

- Preparing Equipment and Positioning the Patient for Panoramic Imaging

INTERACTIVE DENTAL OFFICE PATIENT CASE EXERCISES

Access the *Interactive Dental Office* on the *Evolve* website and click on the patient case file for Cindy Valladares.
- Review the patient's panoramic radiograph.
- Answer the following questions.

1. Are the dark areas over the roots of the mandibular teeth most likely caused by a processing error or by a positioning error?

2. Is this radiograph diagnostically acceptable? Why or why not?

Access the *Interactive Dental Office* on the *Evolve* website and click on the patient case file for Ingrid Pedersen.
- Review the patient's panoramic radiograph.
- Answer the following question.

3. Why are the images of the posterior teeth overlapped? Is this a positioning error?

Access the *Interactive Dental Office* on the *Evolve* website and click on the patient case file for Tiffany Cole.
- Review the patient's panoramic radiograph.
- Answer the following question.

4. On the basis of the development of Tiffany's teeth, how old do you think she is?

COMPETENCY 42.1: PREPARING EQUIPMENT FOR PANORAMIC IMAGING

Performance Objective

By following a routine procedure that meets stated protocols, the student will demonstrate the proper technique for preparing equipment for a panoramic radiograph.

Evaluation and Grading Criteria

3	Student competently met the stated criteria without assistance.
2	Student required assistance in order to meet the stated criteria.
1	Student showed uncertainty when performing the stated criteria.
0	Student was not prepared and needs to repeat the step.
N/A	No evaluation of this step.

Instructor shall define grades for each point range earned on completion of each performance-evaluated task.

Performance Standards

The minimum number of satisfactory performances required before final evaluation is _____.

Instructor shall identify by * those steps considered critical. If a step is missed or minimum competency is not met, the evaluated procedure fails and must be repeated.

PERFORMANCE CRITERIA	*	SELF	PEER	INSTRUCTOR	COMMENT
1. Placed personal protective equipment according to the procedure.					
2. Loaded the panoramic cassette in the darkroom under safelight conditions. Handled the film only by its edges to avoid fingerprints.					
3. Placed all infection control barriers and containers.					
4. Covered the bite-block with a disposable plastic barrier. If the bite-block was not covered, sterilized it before using it on the next patient.					
5. Covered or disinfected (or both) any part of the machine that came in contact with the patient.					
6. Set the exposure factors (kilovoltage, milliamperage) according to the manufacturer's recommendations.					

Continued

353

7. Adjusted the machine to accommodate the height of the patient and aligned all movable parts properly.					
8. Loaded the cassette into the carrier of the panoramic unit.					

ADDITIONAL COMMENTS

Total number of points earned _____

Grade _____ Instructor's initials _____

COMPETENCY 42.2: PREPARING THE PATIENT FOR PANORAMIC IMAGING

Performance Objective

By following a routine procedure that meets stated protocols, the student will demonstrate the proper technique for preparing a patient for panoramic imaging.

Evaluation and Grading Criteria

<u>3</u> Student competently met the stated criteria without assistance.

<u>2</u> Student required assistance in order to meet the stated criteria.

<u>1</u> Student showed uncertainty when performing the stated criteria.

<u>0</u> Student was not prepared and needs to repeat the step.

<u>N/A</u> No evaluation of this step.

Instructor shall define grades for each point range earned on completion of each performance-evaluated task.

Performance Standards

The minimum number of satisfactory performances required before final evaluation is _____.

Instructor shall identify by * those steps considered critical. If a step is missed or minimum competency is not met, the evaluated procedure fails and must be repeated.

PERFORMANCE CRITERIA	*	SELF	PEER	INSTRUCTOR	COMMENT
1. Explained the procedure to the patient. Gave the patient the opportunity to ask questions.					
2. Placed personal protective equipment according to the procedure.					
3. Asked the patient to remove all objects from the head and neck area, including eyeglasses, earrings, lip piercing and tongue piercing objects, necklaces, napkin chains, hearing aids, hairpins, and complete and partial dentures. Placed the objects in separate containers.					
4. Placed a double-sided (for protecting the front and back of the patient) lead apron on the patient, or used the style of lead apron recommended by the manufacturer.					
ADDITIONAL COMMENTS					

Total number of points earned _____

Grade _____ Instructor's initials _____

COMPETENCY 42.3: POSITIONING THE PATIENT FOR PANORAMIC IMAGING

Performance Objective

By following a routine procedure that meets stated protocols, the student will demonstrate the proper technique for positioning a patient for panoramic imaging.

Evaluation and Grading Criteria

3	Student competently met the stated criteria without assistance.
2	Student required assistance in order to meet the stated criteria.
1	Student showed uncertainty when performing the stated criteria.
0	Student was not prepared and needs to repeat the step.
N/A	No evaluation of this step.

Instructor shall define grades for each point range earned on completion of each performance-evaluated task.

Performance Standards

The minimum number of satisfactory performances required before final evaluation is _____.

Instructor shall identify by * those steps considered critical. If a step is missed or minimum competency is not met, the evaluated procedure fails and must be repeated.

PERFORMANCE CRITERIA	*	SELF	PEER	INSTRUCTOR	COMMENT
1. Placed personal protective equipment according to the procedure.					
2. Instructed the patient to sit or stand "as tall as possible" with the back straight and erect.					
3. Instructed the patient to bite on the plastic bite-block and slide the upper and lower teeth into the notch (groove) on the end of the bite-block.					
4. Positioned the midsagittal plane perpendicular to the floor.					
5. Positioned the Frankfort plane parallel to the floor.					
6. Instructed the patient to position the tongue on the roof of the mouth and then to close the lips around the bite-block.					
7. After the patient was positioned, instructed him or her to remain still while the machine rotated during exposure.					

Continued

8. Exposed the film and proceeded with film processing.				
9. Accurately documented the procedure in the patient record.				

ADDITIONAL COMMENTS

Total number of points earned _____

Grade _____ Instructor's initials _____

43 Restorative and Esthetic Dental Materials

SHORT-ANSWER QUESTIONS

1. Describe how a dental material is evaluated before it is marketed to the dental profession.

2. List the properties a dental material must have in the application and to withstand the oral environment.

3. Differentiate between direct and indirect restorative materials.

4. List the standards a dental material must meet.

5. Provide the makeup of amalgam and its use in the restoration of teeth.

6. Provide the makeup of composite resin and its use in the restoration of teeth.

7. Provide the makeup of glass ionomers and its use in the restoration of teeth.

8. Provide the makeup of a temporary restorative material and its use in the restoration of teeth.

9. Discuss the composition and variety of tooth-whitening products.

10. Describe the properties of gold alloys and their application in the restoration of teeth.

11. Describe the properties of porcelain and its application in the restoration of teeth.

359

FILL-IN-THE-BLANK STATEMENTS

Select the best term from the list below and complete the following statements.

adhere	microleakage
alloy	palladium
amalgam	pestle
auto-cure	porcelain
ceramic	restorative
cured	retention
esthetic	spherical
filler	strain
galvanic	stress
gold	viscosity

1. A(n) _____ reaction is the effect of an electrical shock that results when two metals come into contact.

2. A type of dental restorative material that is nonmetallic, is resistant to heat and corrosion, and resembles clay is _____.

3. For a material to become hardened or set, it is said to be _____.

4. To bond or attach two items together is to _____.

5. _____ is a soft, silvery white metallic chemical element that resembles platinum.

6. _____ is a term used to bring a tooth or teeth back to their natural appearance.

7. An object within the amalgam capsule used for pounding or pulverizing is a _____.

8. _____ is a solid white, translucent ceramic material made by firing pure clay and then glazing it.

9. An artistically pleasing and attractive appearance is said to be _____.

10. _____ is a soft, yellow, corrosion-resistant metal used in the making of indirect restorations.

11. The property of a liquid that prevents it from flowing easily is the _____.

12. _____ is a mixture of alloys triturated with mercury to produce a restorative material.

13. _____ refers to how a dental material hardens or sets by means of a chemical reaction.

14. A(n) _____ is a microscopic area where moisture and contaminants can enter.

15. A(n) _____ is a combination of two or more metals.

16. _____ is the means of preparing a tooth surface for retaining or holding something in place.

17. Something that is round is said to be _____.

18. _____ is the distortion or change produced by stress.

19. An internal resistance to an externally applied force is referred to as _____.

20. _____ is an inorganic material that adds strength and other characteristics to composite resins.

MULTIPLE-CHOICE QUESTIONS

Complete each question by circling the best answer.

1. Which professional organization evaluates a new dental material?
   a. FDA
   b. DDS
   c. ADA
   d. MDA

2. What type of reaction does a dental material undergo when a person is chewing?
   a. Thermal change
   b. Compressive stress
   c. Galvanic reaction
   d. Corrosion

3. What happens to a dental material when it is exposed to extreme temperatures of hot and then cold?
   a. Contraction and expansion
   b. Melting and hardening
   c. Galvanic reaction
   d. Strain and stress

4. Which is an example of how galvanic action can occur?
   a. Salt within saliva
   b. Leakage of a material
   c. Touching of two metals
   d. a and c

5. How does an auto-cured material harden or set?
   a. It air-dries
   b. By chemical reaction
   c. With light
   d. With heat

6. Select the correct makeup of the alloy powder in amalgam.
   a. Porcelain, glass, zinc, and composite
   b. Gold, tin, silver, and aluminum
   c. Mercury, silver, zinc, and tin
   d. Silver, tin, copper, and zinc

7. Why would dental amalgam not be placed in anterior teeth?
   a. Esthetics
   b. It is not strong enough.
   c. It is difficult to finish.
   d. Retention

8. Most amalgams have a high copper content. What does copper provide to amalgam restorations?
   a. Strength
   b. Malleability
   c. Corrosion resistance
   d. a and c

9. Where are amalgam scraps disposed of?
   a. In the garbage
   b. Down the sink
   c. In an airtight container
   d. In a biohazard bag

10. What is used to triturate capsulated dental materials?
    a. Mortar and pestle
    b. Amalgamator
    c. Paper pad and spatula
    d. Bowl and spatula

11. The term commonly used to refer to dimethacrylate is _____.
    a. alloy
    b. composite resin
    c. mercury
    d. BIS-GMA

12. Which filler type of composite resin has the strongest makeup and is used most commonly for posterior restorations?
    a. Macrofilled
    b. Microfilled
    c. Monofilled
    d. Autofilled

13. In light-curing of composite resins, which factor can affect curing time of the material?
    a. Type of tooth
    b. Depth or extent of restoration
    c. Surface that is being restored
    d. Type of composite

14. What is used to determine the color of composite resin material for a procedure?
    a. Color palate
    b. Picture
    c. Shade guide
    d. Radiograph

15. The final step in finishing a composite resin is _____.
    a. Use of a diamond bur
    b. Use of a sandpaper strip
    c. Use of a rubber cup and polishing paste
    d. Use of a white stone

16. The acronym *IRM* stands for _____.
    a. inside the restorative matrix
    b. intermediate restorative material
    c. interdental resin material
    d. international restorative material

17. What temporary restorative material would be selected for a class II cavity preparation?
    a. Acrylic resin
    b. Amalgam
    c. Glass ionomer
    d. IRM

18. Which material would be selected for the fabrication of provisional coverage?
    a. IRM
    b. Acrylic resin
    c. Amalgam
    d. Glass ionomer

19. The three noble metals used in making indirect restorations are _____.
    a. gold, palladium, and platinum
    b. silver, tin, and zinc
    c. mercury, copper, and tin
    d. glass, porcelain, and fillers

20. What type of restoration is always made in a dental laboratory setting?
    a. Direct restoration
    b. Provisional coverage
    c. Indirect restoration
    d. Temporary restoration

CASE STUDY

You are assisting in a restorative procedure. The patient record indicates the decay is located on the gingival third of the facial surfaces of teeth #10 and #11. The dentist informs you that you will be using the dental dam for this procedure.

1. What cavity classification would this type of decay represent?

2. What type of restorative material would most likely be selected for this procedure?

3. Why do you think the dentist has requested the use of the dental dam for this procedure?

4. What instrument is in the setup for the placement of the restorative dental material?

5. What additional piece of equipment will be used for the hardening or setting of the restorative material?

6. How will the dentist finish or carve this material?

7. How would this procedure be charted on a patient record?

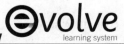

MULTIMEDIA PROCEDURES RECOMMENDED REVIEW

- Mixing and Transferring Amalgam

COMPETENCY 43.1: MIXING AND TRANSFERRING DENTAL AMALGAM

Performance Objective

By following a routine procedure that meets stated protocols, the student will demonstrate the proper skills for mixing and transferring amalgam.

Evaluation and Grading Criteria

3   Student competently met the stated criteria without assistance.

2   Student required assistance in order to meet the stated criteria.

1   Student showed uncertainty when performing the stated criteria.

0   Student was not prepared and needs to repeat the step.

N/A   No evaluation of this step.

Instructor shall define grades for each point range earned on completion of each performance-evaluated task.

Performance Standards

The minimum number of satisfactory performances required before final evaluation is _____.

Instructor shall identify by * those steps considered critical. If a step is missed or minimum competency is not met, the evaluated procedure fails and must be repeated.

PERFORMANCE CRITERIA	*	SELF	PEER	INSTRUCTOR	COMMENTS
1. Selected the proper equipment and supplies.					
2. Placed personal protective equipment according to the procedure.					
3. Activated the capsule for trituration.					
4. Placed the capsule in the amalgamator.					
5. Adjusted the settings for the specific type of amalgam.					
6. Closed the cover on the amalgamator and began trituration.					
7. Removed the capsule and dispensed amalgam in the well.					
8. Filled the small end of the carrier and transferred it to the dentist.					
9. Ensured that the carrier was directed toward the preparation.					
10. Continued delivery until the preparation was overfilled.					
ADDITIONAL COMMENTS					

Total number of points earned _____

Grade _____ Instructor's initials _____

COMPETENCY 43.2: PREPARING COMPOSITE RESIN MATERIALS

Performance Objective

By following a routine procedure that meets stated protocols, the student will assemble the necessary supplies and then prepare composite resin for a restorative procedure.

Evaluation and Grading Criteria

<u>3</u>   Student competently met the stated criteria without assistance.

<u>2</u>   Student required assistance in order to meet the stated criteria.

<u>1</u>   Student showed uncertainty when performing the stated criteria.

<u>0</u>   Student was not prepared and needs to repeat the step.

<u>N/A</u>   No evaluation of this step.

Instructor shall define grades for each point range earned on completion of each performance-evaluated task.

Performance Standards

The minimum number of satisfactory performances required before final evaluation is _____.

Instructor shall identify by * those steps considered critical. If a step is missed or minimum competency is not met, the evaluated procedure fails and must be repeated.

PERFORMANCE CRITERIA	*	SELF	PEER	INSTRUCTOR	COMMENTS
1. Selected the proper equipment and supplies.					
2. Placed personal protective equipment according to the procedure.					
3. Shade selected with the use of a shade guide and natural light at the beginning of the procedure.					
4. Readied the composite material either from syringe, treatment pad or light protected well.					
5. Transferred the composite instrument and material to the dentist in the transfer zone.					
6. Made gauze available for the dentist to clean the composite instrument.					
7. Readied curing light or positioned light correctly on the tooth.					
8. When finished, cared for the supplies and materials appropriately.					

ADDITIONAL COMMENTS

Total number of points earned _____

Grade _____ Instructor's initials _____

COMPETENCY 43.3: MIXING INTERMEDIATE RESTORATIVE MATERIALS

Performance Objective

By following a routine procedure that meets stated protocols, the student will assemble the necessary supplies and then correctly manipulate the intermediate restorative material for placement into a class I cavity preparation.

Evaluation and Grading Criteria

 3   Student competently met the stated criteria without assistance.

 2   Student required assistance in order to meet the stated criteria.

 1   Student showed uncertainty when performing the stated criteria.

 0   Student was not prepared and needs to repeat the step.

 N/A   No evaluation of this step.

Note: In states where it is legal, the assistant may place the temporary restoration in a prepared tooth.

Instructor shall define grades for each point range earned on completion of each performance-evaluated task.

Performance Standards

The minimum number of satisfactory performances required before final evaluation is _____.

Instructor shall identify by * those steps considered critical. If a step is missed or minimum competency is not met, the evaluated procedure fails and must be repeated.

PERFORMANCE CRITERIA	*	SELF	PEER	INSTRUCTOR	COMMENTS
1. Selected the proper material and assembled the appropriate supplies.					
2. Placed personal protective equipment according to the procedure.					
3. Dispensed materials in the proper sequence and quantity; recapped the containers.					
4. Incorporated the powder and liquid according to the manufacturer's instructions.					
5. Completed the mix within the appropriate working time.					
6. Ensured that the completed mix was of the appropriate consistency for a temporary restoration.					
7. When finished, cared for the supplies and materials appropriately.					

ADDITIONAL COMMENTS

Total number of points earned _____

Grade _____ Instructor's initials _____

44 Dental Liners, Bases, and Bonding Systems

SHORT-ANSWER QUESTIONS

1. Explain how the sensitivity of a tooth will determine the types of supplemental dental materials selected for the restoration of a tooth.

2. Explain why and how a cavity liner is used in the restoration process.

3. Explain why and how a varnish is used in the restoration process.

4. Explain why and how a dentin sealer is used in the restoration process.

5. Explain why and how a dental base is used in the restoration process.

6. Describe the etching process of a tooth and its importance in the bonding procedure.

7. Describe the bonding system and how this procedure provides better adaptation of a dental material to the tooth structure.

FILL-IN-THE-BLANK STATEMENTS

Select the best term from the list below and complete the following statements.

desiccate
etching
eugenol
hybrid layer
insulating
micromechanical

obliterating
polymerization
sedative
smear layer
thermal

1. The _____ is a very thin film of debris on newly prepared dentin.

2. _____ refers to using, producing, or caused by heat.

3. A _____ is a thin layer created between dentin and the adhesive resin to seal the space.

4. A dental material is _____ if it prevents the passage of heat or electricity.

5. _____ is the process of opening or removing enamel rods with the use of an acid product.

6. The process of bonding two or more monomers is _____.

7. A liquid made from clove oil and selected for its soothing effect is _____.

8. To _____ means to remove all moisture from an item.

9. _____ refers to minute cuttings of a preparation that lock a dental material and tooth structure together.

10. _____ is the process of complete removal.

11. Some dental materials are designed to have a _____ effect, which is soothing.

MULTIPLE-CHOICE QUESTIONS

Complete each question by circling the best answer.

1. The purpose of a dental liner is to _____.
   a. make the restorative material look natural
   b. protect the pulp from any type of irritation
   c. create a mechanical lock of the dental material
   d. cover the smear layer

2. What tooth structure is calcium hydroxide placed in a prepared tooth?
   a. Enamel
   b. Cementum
   c. Dentin
   d. Pulp

3. Which statement is not a characteristic of calcium hydroxide?
   a. Protects the tooth from chemical irritation
   b. Produces reparative dentin
   c. Is compatible with all restorative materials
   d. Replaces the need for a dentin sealer

4. The key ingredient in varnish is _____.
   a. resin
   b. acid
   c. eugenol
   d. sealant

5. Which supplemental material is contraindicated under composite resins and glass ionomer restorations?
   a. Etchant
   b. Calcium hydroxide
   c. Dentin sealer
   d. Varnish

6. Another name for dentin sealer is _____.
   a. cement
   b. desensitizer
   c. etchant
   d. base

7. What does a cavity sealer seal?
   a. Enamel rods
   b. Etched tags
   c. Dentin tubules
   d. Pulpal chambers

8. An insulating base is placed to _____.
   a. protect the pulp from thermal shock
   b. protect the pulp from moisture
   c. help soothe the pulp
   d. protect the pulp from the restoration

9. What effect does eugenol have on the pulp?
   a. Regenerative
   b. Soothing
   c. Irritant
   d. Restorative

10. A base is placed in or on the _____ of a cavity preparation.
    a. proximal box
    b. cavity walls
    c. enamel margin
    d. pulpal floor

11. What dental instrument is selected to press a base into the cavity preparation?
    a. Explorer
    b. Hollenback
    c. Condenser
    d. Burnisher

12. The purpose of a dental bonding material is to _____.
    a. seal the dentinal tubules
    b. bond the restorative material to the tooth structure
    c. etch the tooth structure
    d. act as a permanent restorative material

13. _____ is/are (an) example(s) of an enamel bonding procedure.
    a. orthodontic brackets
    b. sealants
    c. amalgam
    d. a and b

14. What is removed from the tooth structure before a bonding material is placed?
    a. Enamel
    b. Decay
    c. Smear layer
    d. Dentin tubules

15. Which sequence is recommended for the application of supplementary materials for a deep restoration?
    a. Liner, base, dentin sealer, bonding system
    b. Base, liner, dentin sealer, bonding system
    c. Bonding system, base, liner, dentin sealer
    d. Dentin sealer, base, bonding system, liner

CASE STUDY

Dr. Clark has completed the preparation of a class III restoration on the distal surface of tooth #7. She has asked you to prepare and ready the supplemental materials for placement. You inquire about the depth of the preparation and Dr. Clark indicates that it is moderately deep.

1. What type of direct restorative material would be selected for a class III restoration on tooth #7?

2. What supplemental materials should be set up for this procedure?

3. What types of instruments and mixing pad or slab will be set out?

4. How many steps will be required to complete the application of these supplemental materials?

5. What type of moisture control is commonly placed for this type of restoration and for the application of these materials?

6. Is it legal in your state for the expanded-functions assistant to apply any of these materials? If so, which ones?

MULTIMEDIA PROCEDURES RECOMMENDED REVIEW ⊖volve
learning system

- Mixing and Applying Calcium Hydroxide
- Mixing and Applying Zinc Oxide-Eugenol Cement as a Base
- Mixing Polycarboxylate Cement as a Base

COMPETENCY 44.1: APPLYING CALCIUM HYDROXIDE (EXPANDED FUNCTION)

Performance Objective

By following a routine procedure that meets stated protocols, the student will assemble the necessary supplies and then will correctly manipulate and place the cavity liner in a prepared tooth.

Evaluation and Grading Criteria

_3_	Student competently met the stated criteria without assistance.
_2_	Student required assistance in order to meet the stated criteria.
_1_	Student showed uncertainty when performing the stated criteria.
_0_	Student was not prepared and needs to repeat the step.
_N/A_	No evaluation of this step.

Instructor shall define grades for each point range earned on completion of each performance-evaluated task.

Performance Standards

The minimum number of satisfactory performances required before final evaluation is _____.

Instructor shall identify by * those steps considered critical. If a step is missed or minimum competency is not met, the evaluated procedure fails and must be repeated.

PERFORMANCE CRITERIA	*	SELF	PEER	INSTRUCTOR	COMMENTS
1. Selected the proper material and assembled the appropriate supplies.					
2. Placed personal protective equipment according to the procedure.					
3. Identified the preparation and where the material is to be placed.					
4. Dispensed small, equal quantities of the catalyst and the base pastes onto the paper mixing pad.					
5. Used a circular motion to mix the material over a small area of the paper pad with the spatula.					
6. Immediately used gauze to clean the spatula before setting.					
7. With the tip of the applicator, picked up a small amount of the material and applied a thin layer at the deepest area of the preparation.					
8. Used an explorer to remove any excess material from the enamel before drying.					

Continued

373

9. Cleaned and disinfected the equipment.				
10. Accurately documented the procedure in the patient record.				

ADDITIONAL COMMENTS

Total number of points earned _____

Grade _____ Instructor's initials _____

COMPETENCY 44.2: APPLYING DENTAL VARNISH (EXPANDED FUNCTION)

Performance Objective

By following a routine procedure that meets stated protocols, the student will assemble the necessary supplies and then will correctly apply dental varnish to a prepared tooth surface.

Evaluation and Grading Criteria

<u>3</u>   Student competently met the stated criteria without assistance.

<u>2</u>   Student required assistance in order to meet the stated criteria.

<u>1</u>   Student showed uncertainty when performing the stated criteria.

<u>0</u>   Student was not prepared and needs to repeat the step.

<u>N/A</u>   No evaluation of this step.

Instructor shall define grades for each point range earned on completion of each performance-evaluated task.

Performance Standards

The minimum number of satisfactory performances required before final evaluation is _____.

Instructor shall identify by * those steps considered critical. If a step is missed or minimum competency is not met, the evaluated procedure fails and must be repeated.

PERFORMANCE CRITERIA	*	SELF	PEER	INSTRUCTOR	COMMENTS
1. Selected the proper material and assembled the appropriate supplies.					
2. Placed personal protective equipment according to the procedure.					
3. Identified the cavity preparation and where the material is to be placed.					
4. Retrieved the applicator or sterile cotton pellets in cotton pliers.					
5. Opened the bottle of varnish and placed the tip of the applicator or cotton pellet into the liquid, making sure not to wet the cotton pliers.					
6. Replaced the cap on the bottle immediately.					
7. Placed a coating of the varnish on the walls, floor, and margin of the cavity preparation.					
8. Applied a second coat.					

Continued

9. Cleaned and disinfected the equipment.				
10. Accurately documented the procedure in the patient record.				

ADDITIONAL COMMENTS

Total number of points earned _____

Grade _____ Instructor's initials _____

COMPETENCY 44.3: APPLYING A DESENSITIZER (EXPANDED FUNCTION)

Performance Objective

By following a routine procedure that meets stated protocols, the student will assemble the necessary supplies and then will correctly apply a dentin sealer to a prepared tooth surface.

Evaluation and Grading Criteria

_3_   Student competently met the stated criteria without assistance.

_2_   Student required assistance in order to meet the stated criteria.

_1_   Student showed uncertainty when performing the stated criteria.

_0_   Student was not prepared and needs to repeat the step.

_N/A_   No evaluation of this step.

Instructor shall define grades for each point range earned on completion of each performance-evaluated task.

Performance Standards

The minimum number of satisfactory performances required before final evaluation is _____.

Instructor shall identify by * those steps considered critical. If a step is missed or minimum competency is not met, the evaluated procedure fails and must be repeated.

PERFORMANCE CRITERIA	*	SELF	PEER	INSTRUCTOR	COMMENTS
1. Selected the proper material and assembled the appropriate supplies.					
2. Placed personal protective equipment according to the procedure.					
3. Identified the cavity outline and where the material was to be placed.					
4. Rinsed the area with water, not overdrying the preparation.					
5. Applied the dentin sealer with the applicator over all surfaces of the dentin.					
6. Waited 30 seconds and dried the area thoroughly.					
7. Repeated application of the sealer if sensitivity was a problem for the patient.					
8. Cleaned and disinfected the equipment.					
9. Accurately documented the procedure in the patient record.					

ADDITIONAL COMMENTS

Total number of points earned _____

Grade _____ Instructor's initials _____

COMPETENCIES 44.4 TO 44.6: MIXING A SELECTED TYPE OF CEMENT AS A BASE (EXPANDED FUNCTION)

Performance Objective

By following a routine procedure that meets stated protocols, the student will select the appropriate cement, assemble the necessary supplies, and correctly manipulate the material for use as a base.

Evaluation and Grading Criteria

__3__   Student competently met the stated criteria without assistance.

__2__   Student required assistance in order to meet the stated criteria.

__1__   Student showed uncertainty when performing the stated criteria.

__0__   Student was not prepared and needs to repeat the step.

__N/A__   No evaluation of this step.

Instructor shall define grades for each point range earned on completion of each performance-evaluated task.

Performance Standards

The minimum number of satisfactory performances required before final evaluation is _____.

Instructor shall identify by * those steps considered critical. If a step is missed or minimum competency is not met, the evaluated procedure fails and must be repeated.

PERFORMANCE CRITERIA	*	SELF	PEER	INSTRUCTOR	COMMENTS
Name of Material					
1. Selected the proper material for the procedure and assembled the appropriate supplies.					
2. Placed personal protective equipment according to the procedure.					
3. Dispensed the materials in the proper sequence and quantity and then immediately recapped the containers.					
4. Incorporated the powder and liquid according to the manufacturer's instructions.					
5. Completed the mix within the appropriate working time.					
6. Ensured that the completed mix was the appropriate consistency for use as a base.					

Continued

7. When finished, cared for supplies and materials appropriately.					
8. Accurately documented the procedure in the patient record.					

ADDITIONAL COMMENTS

Total number of points earned _____

Grade _____ Instructor's initials _____

COMPETENCY 44.7: APPLYING AN ETCHANT MATERIAL (EXPANDED FUNCTION)

Performance Objective

By following a routine procedure that meets stated protocols, the student will assemble the necessary supplies and then will correctly apply an etchant to a prepared tooth surface.

Evaluation and Grading Criteria

_3_	Student competently met the stated criteria without assistance.
_2_	Student required assistance in order to meet the stated criteria.
_1_	Student showed uncertainty when performing the stated criteria.
_0_	Student was not prepared and needs to repeat the step.
_N/A_	No evaluation of this step.

Instructor shall define grades for each point range earned on completion of each performance-evaluated task.

Performance Standards

The minimum number of satisfactory performances required before final evaluation is _____.

Instructor shall identify by * those steps considered critical. If a step is missed or minimum competency is not met, the evaluated procedure fails and must be repeated.

PERFORMANCE CRITERIA	*	SELF	PEER	INSTRUCTOR	COMMENT
1. Selected the proper material and assembled the appropriate supplies.					
2. Placed personal protective equipment according to the procedure.					
3. Identified the cavity outline and where material is to be placed.					
4. Uses a dental dam or cotton rolls to isolate the prepared tooth.					
5. Ensured that the surface of the tooth structure was clean and free of any debris, plaque, and calculus before etching.					
6. Carefully dried (but did not desiccate) the surface.					
7. Applied the etchant to the enamel or dentin.					
8. Etched the tooth structure for the time recommended by the manufacturer.					
9. After etching, thoroughly rinsed and dried the surface for 15 to 30 seconds.					

Continued

10. Ensured that the etched surface had a frosty-white appearance.					
11. When finished, cared for supplies and materials appropriately.					
12. Accurately documented the procedure in the patient record.					

ADDITIONAL COMMENTS

Total number of points earned _____

Grade _____ Instructor's initials _____

COMPETENCY 44.8: APPLYING A BONDING SYSTEM (EXPANDED FUNCTION)

Performance Objective

By following a routine procedure that meets stated protocols, the student will assemble the necessary supplies and then will correctly apply a bonding system to a prepared tooth surface.

Evaluation and Grading Criteria

3 Student competently met the stated criteria without assistance.

2 Student required assistance in order to meet the stated criteria.

1 Student showed uncertainty when performing the stated criteria.

0 Student was not prepared and needs to repeat the step.

N/A No evaluation of this step.

Instructor shall define grades for each point range earned on completion of each performance-evaluated task.

Performance Standards

The minimum number of satisfactory performances required before final evaluation is _____.

Instructor shall identify by * those steps considered critical. If a step is missed or minimum competency is not met, the evaluated procedure fails and must be repeated.

PERFORMANCE CRITERIA	*	SELF	PEER	INSTRUCTOR	COMMENT
1. Selected the proper material and assembled the appropriate supplies.					
2. Placed personal protective equipment according to the procedure.					
3. Identified the cavity outline and placement of the material.					
4. If a metal matrix band was required, prepared the band with cavity varnish or wax before placing it around the tooth.					
5. Etched the cavity preparation and the enamel margins according to the manufacturer's instructions.					
6. If a primer was part of the system, applied a primer to the entire preparation, using the number of applications specified by the manufacturer's instructions.					
7. Placed the dual-cured bonding resin in the entire cavity preparation and lightly air-thinned the material. The resin should have appeared unset or semi-set.					

Continued

383

8. When finished, cared for supplies and materials appropriately.					
9. Accurately documented the procedure in the patient record.					

ADDITIONAL COMMENTS

Total number of points earned _____

Grade _____ Instructor's initials _____

45 Dental Cements

SHORT-ANSWER QUESTIONS

1. Describe luting cements and the difference between permanent and temporary cements.

2. Discuss the factors that influence luting cements.

3. List the six cements discussed in the chapter and describe their similarities and differences.

FILL-IN-THE-BLANK STATEMENTS

Select the best term from the list below and complete the following statements.

cement	provisional
exothermic	retard
luting agent	spatulate

1. _____ is the method of mixing a cement by using a flat flexible metal or plastic instrument.

2. _____ is a type of reaction or process in the release of heat.

3. A(n) _____ refers to a temporary type of tooth coverage used for a short time.

4. _____ is a type of dental material that is designed to temporarily or permanently hold an indirect restoration in place.

5. To _____ is to slow down the process of something.

6. Another name for a type I dental cement is _____.

MULTIPLE-CHOICE QUESTIONS

Complete each question by circling the best answer.

1. Another name used to describe a permanent cement is _____.
   a. liner
   b. luting agent
   c. resin
   d. base

2. Which of the following procedures would you include a temporary cement on the tray setup?
   a. Composite restoration
   b. Sealants
   c. Amalgam restoration
   d. Provisional coverage

3. Which variable can affect the addition or loss of water in a material?
   a. Time
   b. Speed of spatulation
   c. Humidity
   d. Moisture control

4. What type of zinc oxide–eugenol (ZOE) is used for permanent cementation?
   a. Type I
   b. Type II
   c. Type III
   d. Type IV

5. On what type of mixing pad is ZOE mixed?
   a. Treated paper pad
   b. Glass
   c. Plastic
   d. Tile

6. Temp bond is supplied as _____.
   a. powder and liquid
   b. paste and powder
   c. two tubes of paste
   d. two liquids

7. The main ingredient in the liquid of zinc phosphate is

   _____.
   a. hydrogen peroxide
   b. zinc oxide
   c. resin
   d. phosphoric acid

8. How do you dissipate the heat from zinc phosphate in the mixing process?
   a. Cool the spatula
   b. Use a cool glass slab
   c. Decrease the temperature in the room
   d. Chill the material

9. If the powder of a dental material is dispersed in increments, what size increment is commonly brought into the liquid first?
   a. Smallest
   b. Medium
   c. Half of the material
   d. Largest

10. How is the liquid portion of polycarboxylate cement supplied?
    a. Tube
    b. Squeeze bottle
    c. Calibrated syringe
    d. b and c

11. At the completion of the process for mixing polycarboxylate cement, the end product should appear

    _____.
    a. dull
    b. glossy
    c. streaky
    d. clear

12. Can a glass ionomer material be used as a restorative material?
    a. Yes
    b. No

13. What unique ingredient in the powder of glass ionomer cement helps inhibit recurrent decay?
    a. Zinc
    b. Composite resin
    c. Iron
    d. Calcium

14. Can a resin cement be used with a metal casting?
    a. Yes
    b. No

CASE STUDY

Dr. Matthews will be cementing four stainless steel crowns on four primary molars of a 10-year-old patient. He has indicated that Duralon will be the cement of choice.

1. Are stainless steel crowns for this procedure considered permanent or provisional?

2. What type of cement is Duralon?

3. List what is needed for the cementation setup.

4. Describe the mixing technique for this cement.

5. How would the excess cement be removed from around the cemented crown?

MULTIMEDIA PROCEDURES RECOMMENDED REVIEW ☉volve
learning system

- Mixing Glass Ionomer for Permanent Cementation
- Mixing Zinc Oxide–Eugenol for Temporary Cementation
- Mixing Polycarboxylate for Permanent Cementation
- Mixing Zinc Phosphate for Permanent Cementation
- Removing Cement

COMPETENCY 45.1: MIXING GLASS FOR PERMANENT CEMENTATION

Performance Objective

By following a routine procedure that meets stated protocols, the student will assemble the necessary supplies and will correctly manipulate the material for use in the cementation of a cast crown.

Evaluation and Grading Criteria

 3   Student competently met the stated criteria without assistance.

 2   Student required assistance in order to meet the stated criteria.

 1   Student showed uncertainty when performing the stated criteria.

 0   Student was not prepared and needs to repeat the step.

 N/A   No evaluation of this step.

Instructor shall define grades for each point range earned on completion of each performance-evaluated task.

Performance Standards

The minimum number of satisfactory performances required before final evaluation is _____.

Instructor shall identify by * those steps considered critical. If a step is missed or minimum competency is not met, the evaluated procedure fails and must be repeated.

PERFORMANCE CRITERIA	*	SELF	PEER	INSTRUCTOR	COMMENT
1. Selected the proper material and assembled the appropriate supplies.					
2. Placed personal protective equipment according to the procedure.					
3. Dispenses the manufacturer's recommended proportion of the *liquid* on one half of the paper pad.					
4. Dispenses the manufacturer's recommended proportion of the *powder* on the other half of the pad; this usually is divided into two or three increments.					
5. Incorporates the powder into the liquid for the recommended mixing time until the material had a glossy appearance.					
6. Lined the inside of the crown with cement.					
7. Turned the casting over in the palm and transferred it to the dentist.					

Continued

8. Transferred a cotton roll so the patient could bite down, to help seat the crown and displace the excess cement.				
9. When finished, cared for supplies and materials appropriately.				
ADDITIONAL COMMENTS				

Total number of points earned _____

Grade _____ Instructor's initials _____

COMPETENCY 45.2: MIXING COMPOSITE RESIN FOR PERMANENT CEMENTATION

Performance Objective

By following a routine procedure that meets stated protocols, the student will assemble the necessary supplies and will correctly manipulate the material for use in the cementation of a cast crown.

Evaluation and Grading Criteria

<u>3</u>   Student competently met the stated criteria without assistance.

<u>2</u>   Student required assistance in order to meet the stated criteria.

<u>1</u>   Student showed uncertainty when performing the stated criteria.

<u>0</u>   Student was not prepared and needs to repeat the step.

<u>N/A</u>   No evaluation of this step.

Instructor shall define grades for each point range earned on completion of each performance-evaluated task.

Performance Standards

The minimum number of satisfactory performances required before final evaluation is _____.

Instructor shall identify by * those steps considered critical. If a step is missed or minimum competency is not met, the evaluated procedure fails and must be repeated.

PERFORMANCE CRITERIA	*	SELF	PEER	INSTRUCTOR	COMMENT
1. Selected the proper material and assembled the appropriate supplies.					
2. Placed personal protective equipment according to the procedure.					
3. Applied the etchant to the enamel and dentin for 15 seconds and then rinsed. Blotted excess water with a moist cotton pellet, leaving the tooth moist.					
4. Applied a bond adhesive to the enamel and dentin and dried gently. Avoided excess adhesive on all prepared surfaces.					
5. Light-cured each surface for 10 seconds.					
6. Applied primer to the etched porcelain or roughened metal surfaces. Dried for 5 seconds.					
7. Dispensed a 1:1 ratio of powder to liquid onto a mixing pad and mixed for 10 seconds. Applied a thin layer of cement to the bonding surface of the restoration.					

Continued

8. After the crown was seated, light-cured the margins for 40 seconds, or allowed to self-cure for 10 minutes from the start of the mixing.				
9. When finished, cared for supplies and materials appropriately.				

ADDITIONAL COMMENTS

Total number of points earned _____

Grade _____ Instructor's initials _____

COMPETENCY 45.3: MIXING ZINC OXIDE–EUGENOL FOR TEMPORARY CEMENTATION

Performance Objective

By following a routine procedure that meets stated protocols, the student will assemble the necessary supplies and will correctly manipulate ZOE for temporary cementation.

Evaluation and Grading Criteria

 3   Student competently met the stated criteria without assistance.

 2   Student required assistance in order to meet the stated criteria.

 1   Student showed uncertainty when performing the stated criteria.

 0   Student was not prepared and needs to repeat the step.

 N/A   No evaluation of this step.

Instructor shall define grades for each point range earned on completion of each performance-evaluated task.

Performance Standards

The minimum number of satisfactory performances required before final evaluation is _____.

Instructor shall identify by * those steps considered critical. If a step is missed or minimum competency is not met, the evaluated procedure fails and must be repeated.

PERFORMANCE CRITERIA	*	SELF	PEER	INSTRUCTOR	COMMENT
1. Selected the proper material and assembled the appropriate supplies.					
2. Placed personal protective equipment according to the procedure.					
3. Measured the pastes onto the mixing pad at equal lengths, approximately $\frac{1}{2}$ inch per unit of restoration.					
4. Replaced the caps immediately.					
5. Incorporated the two pastes.					
6. Spatulated the material over an area of the mixing pad.					
7. Ensured that the material was smooth and creamy, and that the process was completed within 20 to 30 seconds.					
8. Filled the temporary coverage with the cement immediately.					

Continued

Chapter **45** **Dental Cements**

9. Inverted the crown in the palm and readied for transfer.				
10. When finished, cared for supplies and materials appropriately.				

ADDITIONAL COMMENTS

Total number of points earned _____

Grade _____ Instructor's initials _____

COMPETENCY 45.4: MIXING ZINC OXIDE–EUGENOL FOR PERMANENT CEMENTATION

Performance Objective
By following a routine procedure that meets stated protocols, the student will assemble the necessary supplies and will correctly manipulate ZOE for permanent cementation.

Evaluation and Grading Criteria

 3   Student competently met the stated criteria without assistance.

 2   Student required assistance in order to meet the stated criteria.

 1   Student showed uncertainty when performing the stated criteria.

 0   Student was not prepared and needs to repeat the step.

 N/A   No evaluation of this step.

Instructor shall define grades for each point range earned on completion of each performance-evaluated task.

Performance Standards
The minimum number of satisfactory performances required before final evaluation is _____.

Instructor shall identify by * those steps considered critical. If a step is missed or minimum competency is not met, the evaluated procedure fails and must be repeated.

PERFORMANCE CRITERIA	*	SELF	PEER	INSTRUCTOR	COMMENT
1. Selected the proper material and assembled the appropriate supplies.					
2. Placed personal protective equipment according to the procedure.					
3. Measured the powder and placed it onto the mixing pad. Replaced the cap on the powder immediately.					
4. Dispensed the liquid near the powder on the mixing pad. Replaced the cap on the liquid container immediately.					
5. Incorporated the powder and liquid all at once and mixed them with the spatula for 30 seconds.					
6. After ensuring a putty-like consistency of the initial mix, mixed for an additional 30 seconds until it became more fluid for loading into a casting.					
7. Lined the crown with the permanent cement.					

Continued

8. Inverted the crown in the palm and readied for transfer.				
9. When finished, cared for supplies and materials appropriately.				

ADDITIONAL COMMENTS

Total number of points earned _____

Grade _____ Instructor's initials _____

COMPETENCY 45.5: MIXING POLYCARBOXYLATE FOR PERMANENT CEMENTATION

Performance Objective

By following a routine procedure that meets stated protocols, the student will assemble the necessary supplies and will correctly manipulate the material for use in cementation.

Evaluation and Grading Criteria

 3   Student competently met the stated criteria without assistance.

 2   Student required assistance in order to meet the stated criteria.

 1   Student showed uncertainty when performing the stated criteria.

 0   Student was not prepared and needs to repeat the step.

 N/A   No evaluation of this step.

Instructor shall define grades for each point range earned on completion of each performance-evaluated task.

Performance Standards

The minimum number of satisfactory performances required before final evaluation is _____.

Instructor shall identify by * those steps considered critical. If a step is missed or minimum competency is not met, the evaluated procedure fails and must be repeated.

PERFORMANCE CRITERIA	*	SELF	PEER	INSTRUCTOR	COMMENT
Prepare the Mix					
1. Selected the proper material and assembled the appropriate supplies.					
2. Placed personal protective equipment according to the procedure.					
3. Gently shook the powder to fluff the ingredients.					
4. Measured the powder onto the mixing pad and immediately recapped the container.					
5. Dispensed the liquid and then recapped the container.					
6. Used the flat side of the spatula to incorporate all the powder quickly into the liquid at one time. Completed the mix within 30 seconds.					
7. Ensured that the mix was somewhat thick with a shiny, glossy surface.					
8. Lined the inside of the crown with cement.					
9. Turned the casting over in the palm and transferred it to the dentist.					

Continued

10. Transferred a cotton roll so the patient could bite down on it to help seat the crown and displace the excess cement.				
11. When finished, cared for supplies and materials appropriately.				

ADDITIONAL COMMENTS

Total number of points earned _____

Grade _____ Instructor's initials _____

COMPETENCY 45.6: MIXING ZINC PHOSPHATE FOR PERMANENT CEMENTATION

Performance Objective

By following a routine procedure that meets stated protocols, the student will assemble the necessary supplies and will correctly manipulate zinc phosphate for use in the cementation of a cast crown.

Evaluation and Grading Criteria

3   Student competently met the stated criteria without assistance.

2   Student required assistance in order to meet the stated criteria.

1   Student showed uncertainty when performing the stated criteria.

0   Student was not prepared and needs to repeat the step.

N/A   No evaluation of this step.

Instructor shall define grades for each point range earned on completion of each performance-evaluated task.

Performance Standards

The minimum number of satisfactory performances required before final evaluation is _____.

Instructor shall identify by * those steps considered critical. If a step is missed or minimum competency is not met, the evaluated procedure fails and must be repeated.

PERFORMANCE CRITERIA	*	SELF	PEER	INSTRUCTOR	COMMENT
Preparing the Mix					
1. Selected the proper material and assembled the appropriate supplies.					
2. Placed personal protective equipment according to the procedure.					
3. Cooled and dried a glass slab for mixing.					
4. Dispensed the powder toward one end of the slab and the liquid at the opposite end. Recapped the containers.					
5. Divided the powder into small increments as directed by the manufacturer.					
6. Incorporated each powder increment into the liquid, beginning with smaller increments.					
7. Spatulated the mix thoroughly, using broad strokes or a figure-eight movement over a large area of the slab.					
8. Tested the material for appropriate consistency. (The cement should "string up" and break about 1 inch from the slab.)					

Continued

9. Held the casting with the inner portion facing upward.				
10. Loaded the cement onto the spatula/black spoon. Scraped the edge of instrument along the margin to cause the cement to flow into the casting.				
11. Used the instrument to move the cement around so that it covered all internal walls with a thin lining of cement.				
12. Turned the casting over in the palm and transferred it to the dentist.				
13. Transferred a cotton roll so the patient could bite down on it to help seat the crown and displace the excess cement.				
14. When finished, cared for supplies and materials appropriately.				

ADDITIONAL COMMENTS

Total number of points earned _____

Grade _____ Instructor's initials _____

COMPETENCY 45.7: REMOVING CEMENT FROM PERMANENT OR TEMPORARY CEMENTATION (EXPANDED FUNCTION)

Performance Objective

By following a routine procedure that meets stated protocols, in states where it is legal, the student will remove excess cement from the coronal surfaces of a cast restoration.

Evaluation and Grading Criteria

  3   Student competently met the stated criteria without assistance.

  2   Student required assistance in order to meet the stated criteria.

  1   Student showed uncertainty when performing the stated criteria.

  0   Student was not prepared and needs to repeat the step.

 N/A   No evaluation of this step.

Instructor shall define grades for each point range earned on completion of each performance-evaluated task.

Performance Standards

The minimum number of satisfactory performances required before final evaluation is _____.

Instructor shall identify by * those steps considered critical. If a step is missed or minimum competency is not met, the evaluated procedure fails and must be repeated.

PERFORMANCE CRITERIA	*	SELF	PEER	INSTRUCTOR	COMMENT
Preparing the Mix					
1. Assembled the appropriate setup.					
2. Placed personal protective equipment according to the procedure.					
3. Determined that the cement had set by testing with an explorer. Removed the cotton rolls from the patient's mouth.					
4. Established a firm fulcrum for the use of the explorer.					
5. Placed the tip of the instrument at the gingival edge of the cement and used overlapping horizontal strokes (away from the gingiva) to remove the bulk of the cement.					
6. Applied a slight lateral pressure (toward the tooth surface) to remove the remaining cement.					
7. Passed a length of dental floss, with knot tied in it, through the mesial and distal contact areas to remove the excess cement from the interproximal areas.					
8. Used overlapping strokes with an explorer to examine all tooth surfaces.					

Continued

9. Completed the procedure without scratching the cast restoration.				
10. Removed any remaining cement particles and performed a complete mouth rinse.				
11. Maintained patient comfort and followed appropriate infection-control measures throughout the procedure.				

ADDITIONAL COMMENTS

Total number of points earned _____

Grade _____ Instructor's initials _____

46 Impression Materials

SHORT-ANSWER QUESTIONS

1. List the different types of impressions that are taken in a dental procedure.

2. Describe the types of impression trays and their characteristics of use.

3. Discuss hydrocolloid impression materials, and describe their use, mixing techniques, and application of material.

4. Discuss elastomeric impression materials, and describe their use, mixing techniques, and application of material.

5. Explain the importance of an occlusal registration and its use.

6. List the advantages and disadvantages of digital impressions.

FILL-IN-THE-BLANK STATEMENTS

Select the best term from the list below and complete the following statements.

agar
alginate
base
border molding
catalyst
centric
colloid
elastomeric

hydro-
hysteresis
imbibition
occlusal registration
syneresis
tempering
viscosity

1. A(n) _____ is a gel or sol substance with its particles suspended in a water-based medium.

2. _____ is the process of using the fingers to achieve a closer adaptation of the edges of an impression.

3. A(n) _____ impression material has flexible properties and is made from rubber.

4. A foundation or main ingredient of a material is the _____.

5. To have something _____ is to have it aligned, such as the maxillary teeth centered over the mandibular teeth.

6. _____ is a gelatin-type material derived from seaweed found in a reversible hydrocolloid material.

7. _____ is the loss of water, which causes shrinkage.

8. _____ is a way of bringing a material to a desired temperature and consistency.

9. _____ describes a property of fluids with a high resistance to flow.

10. _____ is the material of choice in dentistry for preliminary impressions.

11. _____ is to transform a material from one physical state to another.

12. _____ means water.

13. A(n) _____ is a reproduction of someone's bite with the use of wax or an elastomeric material.

14. A(n) _____ is a substance that modifies or increases the rate of a chemical reaction.

15. _____ is the absorption of water, which causes an object to swell.

MULTIPLE-CHOICE QUESTIONS

Complete each question by circling the best answer.

1. An impression would be considered a _____.
   a. negative reproduction
   b. mirror image
   c. positive reproduction
   d. duplication

2. Of the three classifications of impressions, which of these could be an expanded function for the certified dental assistant?
   a. Preliminary
   b. Final
   c. Bite registration
   d. a and c

3. Of the three classifications of impressions, which would be used by the dental lab tech for determining occlusal relationship?
   a. Preliminary
   b. Final
   c. Bite registration
   d. a and c

4. Which type of stock tray would be selected and prepared to cover half of an arch?
   a. Anterior
   b. Quadrant
   c. Full
   d. Custom

5. Which type of impression tray allows the impression material to mechanically lock on?
   a. Metal
   b. Plastic
   c. Custom
   d. Perforated

6. Which type of tray is constructed to fit the mouth of a specific patient?
   a. Metal
   b. Plastic
   c. Custom
   d. Perforated

7. _____ would be used to extend the length of a tray to accommodate third molars.
   a. Utility wax
   b. Impression material
   c. Border molding
   d. Boxing wax

8. The organic substance of a hydrocolloid material is _____.
   a. tree bark
   b. volcanic ash
   c. seaweed
   d. mud

9. Why would a fast-set alginate be indicated when taking a preliminary impression?
   a. The patient is late for the appointment.
   b. The patient has a strong gag reflex.
   c. The patient does not like the taste.
   d. To keep the patient from talking.

10. The powder/water ratio for a maxillary preliminary impression is _____.
    a. 1 scoop of powder to 1 measure of water
    b. 2 scoops of powder to 2 measures of water
    c. 3 scoops of powder to 3 measures of water
    d. 4 scoops of powder to 4 measures of water

11. Hydro- means _____.
    a. air
    b. mass
    c. water
    d. temperature

12. Irreversible hydrocolloid material is also referred to as _____.
    a. alginate
    b. elastomeric
    c. polyether
    d. polysulfide

13. Irreversible hydrocolloid material is mixed in/on a/an _____.
    a. Glass slab
    b. Mixing bowl
    c. Paper pad
    d. Automix system

14. Where would a reversible hydrocolloid material be placed prior to taking the impression?
    a. Refrigerator
    b. Autoclave
    c. Patient tray
    d. Conditioning bath

15. Elastomeric materials are intended for what type of impression?
    a. Final
    b. Preliminary
    c. Bite registration
    d. a and c

16. How is an elastomeric material supplied?
    a. Paste
    b. Cartridge
    c. Putty
    d. All of the above

17. Which viscosity of a final impression material is applied first to the prepared tooth or teeth?
    a. Light body
    b. Medium body
    c. Heavy body

18. Another name for polysulfide is _____.
    a. polyether
    b. rubber base
    c. silicone
    d. alginate

19. How is the light-body impression material applied during the final impression procedure?
    a. Extruder with tip
    b. Tray
    c. Spatula
    d. a or c

20. What additional method can be used to mix final impression material instead of using an extruder?
    a. Vibrator
    b. Amalgamator
    c. Triturator
    d. Spatula and pad

21. _____ is the material universally used for taking a bite registration.
    a. Baseplate wax
    b. Alginate
    c. Silicone
    d. Rubber base

22. What type of tray is most commonly selected when zinc oxide-eugenol bite registration material is used?
    a. Perforated
    b. Metal
    c. Gauze
    d. Water-cooled

23. Baseplate wax is _____ before being placed in the patient's mouth for a bite registration.
    a. molded
    b. cooled
    c. placed in a tray
    d. warmed

24. While the dentist is dispensing the syringe material around the prepared tooth, what should the dental assistant be doing during a final impression procedure?
    a. Suctioning
    b. Preparing the provisional coverage
    c. Readying the tray with heavy-body material
    d. Triturating the restorative material

25. A preliminary impression is _____ before being transported to the lab for pouring up.
    a. immersed in a disinfectant solution
    b. rinsed, disinfected, wrapped in a moist paper towel, and placed in a precautionary bag
    c. placed in a rubber mixing bowl and filled with cold water
    d. left on the patient tray to dry completely

405

CASE STUDY

Dr. Clark asks you to take the maxillary and mandibular preliminary impressions on the next patient for the fabrication of tooth whitening trays.

1. What impression material will you select to take preliminary impressions?

2. What type of trays will you select for the impression?

3. How do you know which size tray to use? How are the trays prepared for the impression material?

4. Describe the setup that is required for taking these impressions.

5. Describe the mixing technique used for taking this type of impression.

6. Which impression will you take first, and why?

7. Is there any specific area in the mouth that is most critical while this type of impression is taken?

8. What will you do with these impressions once they are taken?

MULTIMEDIA PROCEDURES RECOMMENDED REVIEW   ⊖volve
                                               learning system

■ Mixing Alginate and Taking Preliminary Impressions

COMPETENCY 46.1: MIXING ALGINATE IMPRESSION MATERIAL

Performance Objective

By following a routine procedure that meets stated protocols, the student will mix alginate impression material.

Evaluation and Grading Criteria

 3   Student competently met the stated criteria without assistance.

 2   Student required assistance in order to meet the stated criteria.

 1   Student showed uncertainty when performing the stated criteria.

 0   Student was not prepared and needs to repeat the step.

 N/A   No evaluation of this step.

Instructor shall define grades for each point range earned on completion of each performance-evaluated task.

Performance Standards

The minimum number of satisfactory performances required before final evaluation is _____.

Instructor shall identify by * those steps considered critical. If a step is missed or minimum competency is not met, the evaluated procedure fails and must be repeated.

PERFORMANCE CRITERIA	*	SELF	PEER	INSTRUCTOR	COMMENT
1. Gathered appropriate supplies.					
2. Placed personal protective equipment according to the procedure.					
3. Placed the appropriate amount of water into the bowl using the calibrated measure.					
4. Shook the can of alginate to "fluff" the contents. After fluffing, carefully lifted the lid to prevent the particles from flying into the air.					
5. Using the correct scoop, sifted the powder into the water.					
6. Used the spatula to mix with a stirring action to wet the powder until it was all moistened.					
7. Firmly spread the alginate between the spatula and the side of the rubber bowl.					

Continued

8. Spatulated the material for the appropriate length of time, until the mixture appeared smooth and creamy.				
9. Wiped the alginate mix into one mass on the inside edge of the bowl.				
10. When finished, cared for supplies and materials appropriately.				

ADDITIONAL COMMENTS

Total number of points earned _____

Grade _____ Instructor's initials _____

COMPETENCIES 46.2 AND 46.3: TAKING A MANDIBULAR AND/OR MAXILLARY PRELIMINARY IMPRESSION (EXPANDED FUNCTION)

Performance Objective

By following a routine procedure that meets stated protocols, the student will take mandibular and maxillary alginate impressions of diagnostic quality.

Evaluation and Grading Criteria

 3   Student competently met the stated criteria without assistance.

 2   Student required assistance in order to meet the stated criteria.

 1   Student showed uncertainty when performing the stated criteria.

 0   Student was not prepared and needs to repeat the step.

 N/A   No evaluation of this step.

Instructor shall define grades for each point range earned on completion of each performance-evaluated task.

Performance Standards

The minimum number of satisfactory performances required before final evaluation is _____.

Instructor shall identify by * those steps considered critical. If a step is missed or minimum competency is not met, the evaluated procedure fails and must be repeated.

PERFORMANCE CRITERIA	*	SELF	PEER	INSTRUCTOR	COMMENT
1. Gathered all necessary supplies.					
2. Placed personal protective equipment according to the procedure.					
3. Seated and prepared the patient.					
4. Explained the procedure to the patient.					
Taking the Mandibular Impression					
1. Selected and prepared the mandibular impression tray.					
2. Obtained 2 measures of room temperature water with 2 scoops of alginate and mixed the material.					
3. Gathered half the alginate in the bowl onto the spatula, and then wiped the alginate into one side of the tray from the lingual side. Quickly pressed the material down to the base of the tray.					
4. Gathered the remaining half of the alginate in the bowl onto the spatula, and then loaded the other side of the tray in the same way.					
5. Smoothed the surface of the alginate by wiping a moistened finger along the surface.					

Continued

6. Placed the additional material over the occlusal surfaces of the mandibular teeth.				
7. Retracted the patient's cheek with the index finger.				
8. Turned the tray slightly sideways when placing it into the mouth.				
9. Centered the tray over the teeth.				
10. Seated the tray from the posterior border first.				
11. Instructed the patient to breathe normally while the material set.				
12. Observed the alginate around the tray to determine when the material had set.				
13. Placed fingers on top of the impression tray, and gently broke the seal between the impression and the peripheral tissues by moving the inside of the patient's cheeks or lips with the finger.				
14. Grasped the handle of the tray with the thumb and index finger, and used a firm lifting motion to break the seal.				
15. Snapped up the tray and impression from the dentition.				
16. Instructed the patient to rinse with water to remove the excess alginate material.				
17. Evaluated the impression for accuracy.				
18. Documented the procedure in the patient record.				
Taking the Maxillary Impression				
1. For a maxillary impression, mixed 3 measures of water and 3 scoops of powder.				
2. Loaded the maxillary tray in one large increment and used a wiping motion to fill the tray from the posterior end.				
3. Placed the bulk of the material toward the anterior palatal area of the tray.				

4. Moistened the fingertips with tap water and smoothed the surface of the alginate.					
5. Used the index finger to retract the patient's cheek.					
6. Turned the tray slightly sideways to position the tray into the mouth.					
7. Centered the tray over the patient's teeth.					
8. Seated the posterior border (back) of the tray up against the posterior border of the hard palate to form a seal.					
9. Directed the anterior portion of the tray upward over the teeth.					
10. Gently lifted the patient's lips out of the way as the tray was seated and instructed the patient to tilt their head forward.					
11. Checked the posterior border of the tray to ensure that no material was flowing into the patient's throat. If necessary, wiped the excess material away with a cotton-tipped applicator.					
12. Held the tray firmly in place while the alginate set.					
13. To avoid injury to the impression and the patient's teeth, placed a finger along the lateral borders of the tray to push down and break the palatal seal.					
14. Used a straight, downward snapping motion to remove the tray from the teeth.					
15. Instructed the patient to rinse with water to remove any excess alginate impression material.					
16. Gently rinsed the impression under cold tap water to remove any blood or saliva.					
17. Sprayed the impression with an approved disinfectant.					

Continued

18. Wrapped the impression in a damp paper towel and stored it in a covered container or a plastic biohazard bag labeled with the patient's name.				
19. Examined the patient's mouth for any remaining fragments of alginate and removed them using an explorer and dental floss.				
20. Used a moist facial tissue to remove any alginate from the patient's face and lips.				
21. Documented the procedure in the patient record.				

ADDITIONAL COMMENTS

Total number of points earned _____

Grade _____ Instructor's initials _____

COMPETENCY 46.4: MIXING A TWO-PASTE FINAL IMPRESSION MATERIAL

Performance Objective

By following a routine procedure that meets stated protocols, the student will prepare and mix a two-paste final impression material.

Evaluation and Grading Criteria

 3   Student competently met the stated criteria without assistance.

 2   Student required assistance in order to meet the stated criteria.

 1   Student showed uncertainty when performing the stated criteria.

 0   Student was not prepared and needs to repeat the step.

 N/A   No evaluation of this step.

Instructor shall define grades for each point range earned on completion of each performance-evaluated task.

Performance Standards

The minimum number of satisfactory performances required before final evaluation is _____.

Instructor shall identify by * those steps considered critical. If a step is missed or minimum competency is not met, the evaluated procedure fails and must be repeated.

PERFORMANCE CRITERIA	*	SELF	PEER	INSTRUCTOR	COMMENT
1. Gathered appropriate supplies.					
2. Placed personal protective equipment according to the procedure.					
Preparing the Light-Bodied Syringe Material					
1. Dispensed equal lengths—approximately 1½ to 2 inches—of the base and catalyst of the light-bodied material onto the top third of the pad, ensuring that the materials were not too close to each other.					
2. Wiped the tube openings clean with gauze and recapped them immediately.					
3. Placed the tip of the spatula blade into the catalyst and base and mixed in a swirling direction for approximately 5 seconds.					
4. Gathered the material onto the flat portion of the spatula and placed it on a clean area of the pad, preferably the center.					
5. Spatulated smoothly, wiping back and forth using only one side of the spatula during the mixing process.					

Continued

6. To obtain a more homogeneous mix, picked the material up by the spatula blade and wiped it onto the pad.					
7. Gathered the material together, took the syringe tube, and began "cookie cutting" the material into the syringe. Inserted the plunger and expressed a small amount of the material to ensure that the syringe was in working order.					
8. Transferred the syringe to the dentist, ensuring that the tip of the syringe was directed toward the tooth.					
Preparing the Heavy-Bodied Tray Material					
1. Dispensed equal lengths of the base and catalyst of the heavy-bodied material on the top third of the pad for a quadrant tray.					
2. Placed the tip of the spatula blade into the catalyst and base, and mixed in a swirling direction for approximately 5 seconds.					
3. Gathered the material onto the flat portion of the spatula and placed it onto a clean area of the pad.					
4. Spatulated smoothly, wiping back and forth, using only one side of the spatula during the mixing process.					
5. To get a more homogeneous mix, picked the material up with the spatula blade and wiped it onto the pad.					
6. Gathered the bulk of the material with the spatula and loaded the material into the tray.					
7. Using the tip of the spatula, spread the material evenly from one end of the tray to the other without picking up the material.					
8. Retrieved the syringe from the dentist and transferred the tray, ensuring that the dentist could grasp the handle of the tray properly.					

9. When finished, cared for supplies and materials appropriately.					
10. Documented the procedure in the patient record.					

ADDITIONAL COMMENTS

Total number of points earned _____

Grade _____ Instructor's initials _____

COMPETENCY 46.5: PREPARING AN AUTOMIX FINAL IMPRESSION MATERIAL

Performance Objective

By following a routine procedure that meets stated protocols, the student will prepare an automix final impression material.

Evaluation and Grading Criteria

<u>3</u> ·   Student competently met the stated criteria without assistance.

<u>2</u>   Student required assistance in order to meet the stated criteria.

<u>1</u>   Student showed uncertainty when performing the stated criteria.

<u>0</u>   Student was not prepared and needs to repeat the step.

<u>N/A</u>   No evaluation of this step.

Instructor shall define grades for each point range earned on completion of each performance-evaluated task.

Performance Standards

The minimum number of satisfactory performances required before final evaluation is _____.

Instructor shall identify by * those steps considered critical. If a step is missed or minimum competency is not met, the evaluated procedure fails and must be repeated.

PERFORMANCE CRITERIA	*	SELF	PEER	INSTRUCTOR	COMMENT
1. Gathered appropriate supplies.					
2. Placed personal protective equipment according to the procedure.					
3. Loaded the extruder with dual cartridges of the base and the catalyst of a light-bodied material.					
4. Removed the caps from the tube and extruded a small amount of the unmixed material onto the gauze pad.					
5. Attached a mixing tip to the extruder, along with a syringe tip for light-bodied application by the dentist.					
6. When the dentist signaled, began squeezing the trigger until the material reached the tip.					
7. Transferred the extruder to the dentist, directing the tip toward the area of the impression.					
8. Placed the heavy-bodied cartridges in the extruder, expressing a small amount as before with the light-bodied material. Attached the mixing tip to the cartridge.					
9. When the dentist signaled, began squeezing the trigger, mixing the heavy-bodied material.					

Continued

417

10. Loaded the impression tray with the heavy-bodied material, making sure not to trap air in the material.				
11. Transferred the tray, ensuring that the dentist could grasp the handle of the tray.				
12. Disinfected the impression, placed it in a biohazard bag, labeled it with the patient's name, and readied it for the laboratory.				
13. Documented the procedure in the patient record.				

ADDITIONAL COMMENTS

Total number of points earned _____

Grade _____ Instructor's initials _____

COMPETENCY 46.6: MIXING POLYSILOXANE MATERIAL FOR A BITE REGISTRATION

Performance Objective

By following a routine procedure that meets stated protocols, the student will mix and prepare a polysiloxane material for a bite registration.

Evaluation and Grading Criteria

_3_	Student competently met the stated criteria without assistance.
_2_	Student required assistance in order to meet the stated criteria.
_1_	Student showed uncertainty when performing the stated criteria.
_0_	Student was not prepared and needs to repeat the step.
_N/A_	No evaluation of this step.

Note: Mandibular and maxillary impressions have already been taken for this patient.

Instructor shall define grades for each point range earned on completion of each performance-evaluated task.

Performance Standards

The minimum number of satisfactory performances required before final evaluation is _____.

Instructor shall identify by * those steps considered critical. If a step is missed or minimum competency is not met, the evaluated procedure fails and must be repeated.

PERFORMANCE CRITERIA	*	SELF	PEER	INSTRUCTOR	COMMENT
1. Gathered appropriate supplies.					
2. Placed personal protective equipment according to the procedure.					
3. Mixed the material and dispensed it using an extruder.					
4. Extruded the material directly onto the tray, making sure to fill both sides of the tray.					
5. Instructed the patient to close in proper occlusion.					
6. After the material was set (about 1 minute), removed the impression and had dentist check it for accuracy.					
7. Rinsed, disinfected, and dried the impression and sent it to the laboratory with the written prescription and other impressions.					

Continued

8. When finished, cared for supplies and materials appropriately.				
9. Documented the procedure in the patient record.				

ADDITIONAL COMMENTS

Total number of points earned _____

Grade _____ Instructor's initials _____

47 Laboratory Materials and Procedures

SHORT-ANSWER QUESTIONS

1. Discuss the types of safety precautions followed when working in the dental laboratory.

2. List the types of equipment commonly found in a dental laboratory and describe their use.

3. Define the dental model/cast and explain its use in dentistry.

4. List the advantages of using digital models.

5. Discuss gypsum products and their use in fabricating dental models.

6. Describe the three types of custom impression trays and their use in dentistry.

7. List the types of dental waxes and describe their use in dentistry.

FILL-IN-THE-BLANK STATEMENTS

Select the best term from the list below and complete the following statements.

anatomic portion	lathe
articulator	dental model
dihydrate	monomer
dimensionally stable	nuclei crystallization
facebow	polymer
gypsum	slurry
hemihydrate	volatile
homogeneous	

1. A dental material that is uniform in mixture and consistent throughout is said to be _____.

2. A(n) _____ is a dental lab machine used for cutting, grinding and polishing dental appliances.

3. _____ is a type of mineral used in the formation of plaster of paris and stone.

4. A substance is said to be _____ if it has an explosive property.

421

5. A _____ is a compound of a gypsum product with two parts water to one part calcium sulfate.

6. If an object is resistant to change in width, height, and length, it is said to be _____.

7. The _____ is the portion of an articulator used to transfer the relationship of the upper teeth and the temporomandibular joint to a cast.

8. A(n) _____ is a compound of many molecules.

9. _____ is a chemical process in which crystals form into a structure.

10. _____ is the removal of one-half part water to one-part calcium sulfate to form the powder product of gypsum.

11. A(n) _____ is a replica of the maxillary and mandibular arches fabricated from an impression.

12. _____ refers to the structural portion of a dental model/cast.

13. A(n) _____ is a dental laboratory device that simulates the movement of the mandible and the temporomandibular joint when models of the dental arches are attached.

14. A(n) _____ is a molecule that when combined with others forms a polymer.

15. _____ is a mixture of gypsum and water to be used in the finishing of models.

MULTIPLE-CHOICE QUESTIONS

Complete each question by circling the best answer.

1. Where would you commonly find the lab in a dental office?
   a. In proximity to the business area
   b. In proximity the reception area
   c. In proximity to the clinical operatory
   d. In proximity to the dentist's private office

2. Which specialty practice would have a more extensive laboratory setup?
   a. Oral surgery
   b. Fixed prosthodontics
   c. Orthodontics
   d. b and c

3. An example of a contaminated item that could be found in the dental lab would be a(n)_____.
   a. explorer
   b. x-ray
   c. impression
   d. high-speed handpiece

4. Which piece of lab equipment would be used to grind away plaster or stone?
   a. Model trimmer
   b. Lathe
   c. Bunsen burner
   d. Laboratory handpiece

5. Which piece of lab equipment would the dentist use to determine centric relation from a diagnostic model?
   a. Vibrator
   b. Model trimmer
   c. Face bow
   d. Bunsen burner

6. The size of the wax spatula most commonly used in the laboratory is a _____.
   a. #1
   b. #3
   c. #5
   d. #7

7. Another name for a dental model is _____.
   a. dental die
   b. dental impression
   c. dental cast
   d. dental wax-up

8. What dental material is used in creating a dental model?
   a. Hydrocolloid
   b. Gypsum
   c. Elastomeric
   d. Wax

9. Which type of gypsum is used to fabricate a replica for an inlay or crown?
   a. Plaster
   b. Dental stone
   c. Die stone
   d. High-strength stone

10. The powder (g)/water (ml) ratio of model plaster for pouring a dental model is _____.
    a. 75/100
    b. 100/50
    c. 30/100
    d. 150/30

11. When a gypsum material is mixed, how is the powder and water incorporated?
    a. Add water and powder at the same time.
    b. Add water to the powder.
    c. Add powder to the water.
    d. It does not matter.

12. Gypsum materials are mixed using a(n) _____.
    a. spatula and rubber bowl
    b. spatula and paper pad
    c. automix syringe
    d. amalgamator

13. Which of the following terms are the description of the portions of a dental model?
    a. Anatomic / Art
    b. Gingiva / Teeth
    c. Base / Teeth
    d. a and c

14. When pouring up an impression, where would you begin placing the gypsum material in a mandibular impression?
    a. Anterior teeth
    b. Palatal area
    c. Most posterior tooth
    d. Premolar teeth

15. How long should you wait before you separate a model from its impression?
    a. 15 to 20 minutes
    b. 30 to 45 minutes
    c. 45 to 60 minutes
    d. 24 hours

16. Which model (maxillary or mandibular) should you begin trimming first?
    a. Maxillary
    b. Smallest model
    c. Mandibular
    d. Does not matter

17. What is the one specific area of a dental model where the maxillary and mandibular models are trimmed differently?
    a. Heels
    b. Buccal surfaces
    c. Base
    d. Anterior portion

18. What should be placed between the two models during trimming?
    a. Tongue depressor
    b. Wax bite
    c. Hydrocolloid material
    d. Cotton rolls

19. Digital models and traditional plaster models have the same advantages listed below except:
    a. Diagnosing and treatment planning
    b. Accuracy
    c. Unbreakable
    d. Shows a 3-D image

20. Of the three types of custom trays discussed in the chapter, which technique uses a volatile hazardous material?
    a. Acrylic resin
    b. Light-cured resin
    c. Thermoplastic resin
    d. Composite resin

21. What type of custom tray would be made for a vital bleaching procedure?
    a. Acrylic resin
    b. Light-cured resin
    c. Thermoplastic resin
    d. Composite resin

22. What type of wax is used to form a barrier around a preliminary impression when it is poured up?
    a. Rope wax
    b. Boxing wax
    c. Inlay wax
    d. Baseplate wax

23. To extend an impression tray, what type of wax is used?
    a. Utility wax
    b. Boxing wax
    c. Inlay wax
    d. Baseplate wax

24. What type of wax is used to obtain a patient's bite?
    a. Rope wax
    b. Boxing wax
    c. Inlay wax
    d. Registration wax

25. What is placed to prevent a tray from seating too deeply onto the arch or quadrant?
    a. Undercut
    b. Separating medium
    c. Spacer stops
    d. Finisher

CASE STUDY

It is 4:30 PM and Dr. Campbell has asked you to take preliminary impressions on the patient in Room 3. The conventional study models from these impressions will be used for a case presentation at a scheduled appointment.

1. What type of impression material will be used for this impression?

2. What type of tray is commonly selected for this procedure?

3. Is this a procedure that the dental assistant can complete independently? If so, how and why?

4. How are preliminary impressions cared for before they are taken to the dental laboratory?

5. Because of the time of day, can you wait until tomorrow morning to pour them up?

6. Because these models will be used for a case presentation, which gypsum material would provide a more professional presentation?

7. How will you prepare the models for a more professional appearance?

8. How will you polish the finished model?

MULTIMEDIA PROCEDURES RECOMMENDED REVIEW

- Constructing a Vacuum-Formed Tray
- Pouring Dental Models Using the Inverted-Pour Method

COMPETENCY 47.1: TAKING A FACE-BOW REGISTRATION (EXPANDED FUNCTION)

Performance Objective

By following a routine procedure that meets stated protocols, the student will take a face-bow registration that will be used by the dentist or dental laboratory technician in the mounting of the study cast.

Evaluation and Grading Criteria

<u>3</u>   Student competently met the stated criteria without assistance.

<u>2</u>   Student required assistance in order to meet the stated criteria.

<u>1</u>   Student showed uncertainty when performing the stated criteria.

<u>0</u>   Student was not prepared and needs to repeat the step.

<u>N/A</u>   No evaluation of this step.

Instructor shall define grades for each point range earned on completion of each performance-evaluated task.

Performance Standards

The minimum number of satisfactory performances required before final evaluation is _____.

Instructor shall identify by * those steps considered critical. If a step is missed or minimum competency is not met, the evaluated procedure fails and must be repeated.

PERFORMANCE CRITERIA	*	SELF	PEER	INSTRUCTOR	COMMENT
1. Gathered appropriate supplies and materials.					
2. Placed personal protective equipment according to the procedure.					
3. Attached the vertical indicator rod to the analyzer bow.					
4. Attached either a disposable index tray or a bite-fork to the analyzer bow.					
5. Prepared the bite-fork with either a disposable index tray or compound bite tabs.					
6. Made sure the patient bit slowly when the bite-fork was positioned in the mouth.					
7. Aligned the vertical indicator rod with the patient's facial midline.					
8. Positioned the analyzer bow so that the lateral wings were level.					

Continued

425

9. Removed the tray or bite-fork from the bow.				
10. Documented the procedure in the patient record.				

ADDITIONAL COMMENTS

Total number of points earned _____

Grade _____ Instructor's initials _____

COMPETENCY 47.2: MIXING DENTAL PLASTER

Performance Objective

By following a routine procedure that meets stated protocols, the student will mix dental plaster in preparation for pouring a dental model.

Evaluation and Grading Criteria

 3 Student competently met the stated criteria without assistance.

 2 Student required assistance in order to meet the stated criteria.

 1 Student showed uncertainty when performing the stated criteria.

 0 Student was not prepared and needs to repeat the step.

 N/A No evaluation of this step.

Note: Mandibular and maxillary impressions have already been taken.

Instructor shall define grades for each point range earned on completion of each performance-evaluated task.

Performance Standards

The minimum number of satisfactory performances required before final evaluation is _____.

Instructor shall identify by * those steps considered critical. If a step is missed or minimum competency is not met, the evaluated procedure fails and must be repeated.

PERFORMANCE CRITERIA	*	SELF	PEER	INSTRUCTOR	COMMENT
1. Gathered appropriate supplies.					
2. Placed personal protective equipment according to the procedure.					
3. Measured 50 ml of room temperature water into a clean rubber mixing bowl.					
4. Weighed out 100 g of dental plaster.					
5. Added the powder to the water in steady increments. Allowed the powder to settle into the water for about 30 seconds.					
6. Used the spatula to incorporate the powder slowly into the water.					
7. Achieved a smooth and creamy mix in about 20 seconds.					
8. Turned the vibrator to a low or medium speed and placed the bowl of plaster mix on the vibrator platform.					
9. Lightly pressed and rotated the bowl on the vibrator until air bubbles rose to the surface.					

Continued

10. Completed mixing and vibration of the plaster in 2 minutes or less.				
11. When finished, cared for supplies and materials appropriately.				

ADDITIONAL COMMENTS

Total number of points earned _____

Grade _____ Instructor's initials _____

COMPETENCY 47.3: POURING DENTAL MODELS USING THE INVERTED-POUR METHOD

Performance Objective

By following a routine procedure that meets stated protocols, the student will pour a maxillary and mandibular dental model using the inverted-pour method.

Evaluation and Grading Criteria

3   Student competently met the stated criteria without assistance.

2   Student required assistance in order to meet the stated criteria.

1   Student showed uncertainty when performing the stated criteria.

0   Student was not prepared and needs to repeat the step.

N/A   No evaluation of this step.

Instructor shall define grades for each point range earned on completion of each performance-evaluated task.

Performance Standards

The minimum number of satisfactory performances required before final evaluation is _____.

Instructor shall identify by * those steps considered critical. If a step is missed or minimum competency is not met, the evaluated procedure fails and must be repeated.

PERFORMANCE CRITERIA	*	SELF	PEER	INSTRUCTOR	COMMENT
1. Gathered the appropriate supplies.					
2. Placed personal protective equipment according to the procedure.					
3. Used air to remove excess moisture from the impression.					
4. Used a laboratory knife or laboratory cutters to remove any excess impression material that would interfere with pouring of the model.					
5. Mixed the plaster, and then set the vibrator at a low to medium speed.					
Pouring the Mandibular Cast					
1. Held the impression tray by the handle and placed the edge of the tray onto the vibrator.					
2. Placed small increments of plaster in the impression near the most posterior tooth.					
3. Continued to place small increments in the same area as the first increment and allowed the plaster to flow toward the anterior teeth.					
4. Turned the tray on its side to provide a continuous flow of the material forward into each tooth impression.					

Continued

5. When all teeth in the impression were covered, added larger increments until the entire impression was filled.				
6. Placed the additional material onto a glass slab (or tile) and shaped the base to approximately 2×2 inches and 1 inch thick.				
7. Inverted the impression onto the new mix without pushing the impression into the base.				
8. Used a spatula to smooth the plaster base mix up onto the margins of the initial pour.				
Pouring the Maxillary Cast				
1. Repeated steps 3 to 5 above, using clean equipment for the fresh mix of plaster.				
2. Placed a small increment of plaster at the posterior area of the impression. Guided the material as it flowed down into the impression of the most posterior tooth.				
3. Continued to place small increments in the same area as the first increment and allowed the plaster to flow toward the anterior teeth.				
4. Turned the tray on its side to provide a continuous flow of the material into each tooth impression.				
5. When all teeth in the impression were covered, added larger increments until the entire impression was filled.				
6. Placed the mix onto a glass slab (or tile) and shaped the base to approximately 2×2 inches and 1 inch thick.				
7. Inverted the impression onto the new mix.				
8. Used a spatula to smooth the stone base mix up onto the margins of the initial pour.				
9. Placed the impression tray on the base so the handle and the occlusal plane of the teeth on the cast were parallel with the surface of the glass slab (or tile).				

Separating the Casts from the Impression					
1. Waited 45 to 60 minutes after the base was poured before separating the impression from the model.					
2. Used the laboratory knife to gently separate the margins of the tray.					
3. Applied firm, straight, upward pressure on the handle of the tray to remove the impression.					
4. Pulled the tray handle straight up from the model.					
5. The models were ready for trimming and polishing.					
6. When finished, cared for supplies and materials appropriately.					

ADDITIONAL COMMENTS

Total number of points earned _____

Grade _____ Instructor's initials _____

COMPETENCY 47.4: TRIMMING AND FINISHING DENTAL MODELS

Performance Objective

By following a routine procedure that meets stated protocols, the student will trim and finish a set of dental models to be used for diagnostic purposes.

Evaluation and Grading Criteria

3	Student competently met the stated criteria without assistance.
2	Student required assistance in order to meet the stated criteria.
1	Student showed uncertainty when performing the stated criteria.
0	Student was not prepared and needs to repeat the step.
N/A	No evaluation of this step.

Instructor shall define grades for each point range earned on completion of each performance-evaluated task.

Performance Standards

The minimum number of satisfactory performances required before final evaluation is _____.

Instructor shall identify by * those steps considered critical. If a step is missed or minimum competency is not met, the evaluated procedure fails and must be repeated.

PERFORMANCE CRITERIA	*	SELF	PEER	INSTRUCTOR	COMMENT
1. Gathered appropriate supplies.					
2. Placed personal protective equipment according to the procedure.					
3. Soaked the art portion of the model in a bowl of water for at least 5 minutes.					
4. Placed the maxillary model on a flat countertop with the teeth resting on the table.					
5. Measured up 1¼ inches from the counter and drew a line around the model.					
6. Turned on the trimmer, held the model firmly against the trimmer, and trimmed the bottom of the base to the line drawn.					
7. Drew a line ¼ inch behind the maxillary tuberosities. With the base flat on the trimmer, removed excess plaster in the posterior area of the model to the marked line.					
8. Drew a line through the center of the occlusal ridges on one side of the model. Measured out ¼ inch from the line and drew a line parallel to the line drawn.					
9. Repeated these measurements on the other side of the model.					

Continued

433

10. Trimmed the sides of the cast to the lines drawn.				
11. Trimmed the maxillary heel cuts by drawing a line behind the tuberosity that was perpendicular to the opposite canine.				
12. Made the final cut by drawing a line from the canine to the midline at an angle (completed this step on both sides) and trimmed to the line.				
13. Occluded the mandibular model with the maxillary model using the wax bite.				
14. With the mandibular base on the trimmer, trimmed the posterior portion of the mandibular model until it was even with the maxillary model.				
15. Placed the models upside down (maxillary base on the table), measured 3 inches from the surface up, and marked a line around the base of the mandibular model.				
16. Trimmed the mandibular model base to the line drawn.				
17. With the models in occlusion with the wax bite, placed the mandibular model on the trimmer and trimmed the lateral cuts to match the maxillary lateral cuts.				
18. Trimmed the back and heel cuts to match the maxillary heel cuts.				
19. Checked that the mandibular anterior cut was a rounded circle from mandibular canine to mandibular canine.				
20. Mixed a slurry of gypsum and filled any voids.				

21. Used a laboratory knife to remove any extra gypsum that appeared as beads on the occlusion or model.					
22. When finished, cared for supplies and materials appropriately.					

ADDITIONAL COMMENTS

Total number of points earned _____

Grade _____ Instructor's initials _____

COMPETENCY 47.5: CONSTRUCTING AN ACRYLIC RESIN CUSTOM TRAY

Performance Objective

By following a routine procedure that meets stated protocols, the student will construct an acrylic resin custom tray.

Evaluation and Grading Criteria

3	Student competently met the stated criteria without assistance.
2	Student required assistance in order to meet the stated criteria.
1	Student showed uncertainty when performing the stated criteria.
0	Student was not prepared and needs to repeat the step.
N/A	No evaluation of this step.

Instructor shall define grades for each point range earned on completion of each performance-evaluated task.

Performance Standards

The minimum number of satisfactory performances required before final evaluation is _____.

Instructor shall identify by * those steps considered critical. If a step is missed or minimum competency is not met, the evaluated procedure fails and must be repeated.

PERFORMANCE CRITERIA	*	SELF	PEER	INSTRUCTOR	COMMENT
1. Gathered appropriate supplies.					
2. Placed personal protective equipment according to the procedure.					
Preparing the Model					
1. Filled the undercuts on the diagnostic model.					
2. Outlined the tray in pencil.					
3. Placed the baseplate wax spacer, trimmed the wax, and luted it to the cast.					
4. Cut the appropriate stops in the spacer.					
5. Painted the spacer and surrounding area with the separating medium.					
Mixing the Acrylic Resin					
1. Used the manufacturer's measuring devices to measure the powder into the mixing container, then added an equal part of liquid and recapped the container immediately.					
2. Used the tongue blade to mix the powder and liquid until the mix appeared thin and sticky.					
3. Set the mix aside for 2 to 3 minutes to allow polymerization.					

Continued

437

Forming the Tray					
1. When the mix reached a "doughy" stage, removed it from the container with the spatula or tongue blade.					
2. Lubricated the palms of the hands with petroleum jelly and kneaded the resin to form a flat patty approximately the size of the wax spacer.					
3. Placed the material on the cast to cover the wax spacer. Adapted it to extend 1 to 1.5 mm beyond the edges of the wax spacer.					
4. Used an instrument or laboratory knife to trim away the excess tray material quickly while it was still soft.					
Creating the Handle					
1. Used the excess material to shape the handle.					
2. Placed a drop of monomer on the handle and on the tray, where they join.					
3. Attached the handle so it extended out of the mouth and was parallel with the occlusal surfaces of the teeth.					
4. Held the handle in place until it was firm.					
Finishing the Tray					
1. After the initial set (7 to 10 minutes), removed the spacer and returned the tray to the cast.					
2. Cleaned the wax completely from the inside of the tray after the tray resin had reached final cure.					

3. Finished the edges and then cleaned and disinfected the tray.					
4. When finished, cared for supplies and materials appropriately.					

ADDITIONAL COMMENTS

Total number of points earned _____

Grade _____ Instructor's initials _____

COMPETENCY 47.6: CREATING A LIGHT-CURED CUSTOM TRAY

Performance Objective

By following a routine procedure that meets stated protocols, the student will construct a light-cured custom tray.

Evaluation and Grading Criteria

 3 Student competently met the stated criteria without assistance.

 2 Student required assistance in order to meet the stated criteria.

 1 Student showed uncertainty when performing the stated criteria.

 0 Student was not prepared and needs to repeat the step.

 N/A No evaluation of this step.

Instructor shall define grades for each point range earned on completion of each performance-evaluated task.

Performance Standards

The minimum number of satisfactory performances required before final evaluation is _____.

Instructor shall identify by * those steps considered critical. If a step is missed or minimum competency is not met, the evaluated procedure fails and must be repeated.

PERFORMANCE CRITERIA	*	SELF	PEER	INSTRUCTOR	COMMENT
1. Gathered appropriate supplies.					
2. Placed personal protective equipment according to the procedure.					
3. Completed a model before tray construction.					
4. Used a pencil to outline the vestibular area and posterior tray border on the stone model.					
5. Painted the separating medium on the model before placement of the material.					
6. Adapted precut sections of the custom tray material for use on the maxillary model with full palatal coverage, and on the mandibular model without full palatal coverage.					
7. Molded the sheet of tray material to conform to the study model using the thumb and forefinger with a minimal pressure.					
8. Trimmed away the excess tray material with a laboratory knife. *Note:* If desired, the excess material can be used to form a handle on the tray.					
9. Placed the model and tray in a light-curing unit. Cured the tray for 2 minutes.					

Continued

10. After curing, placed the model and tray in cool water to solidify the wax spacer and facilitate separation of the tray from the model.				
11. Used the acrylic extruded through the holes in the spacer to create occlusal stops on the inside of the tray.				
12. Removed the wax spacer from the tray using a #7 wax spatula.				
13. Placed the tray in hot water to remove any remnants of wax from the inside.				
14. Trimmed the borders of the tray using an acrylic laboratory bur.				
15. Used a thin acrylic bur to perforate the custom tray.				
16. Using a laboratory acrylic bur, trimmed the borders of the edentulous tray to 2 mm short of the vestibule to allow for the border molding material.				
17. When finished, cared for supplies and materials appropriately.				

ADDITIONAL COMMENTS

Total number of points earned _____

Grade _____ Instructor's initials _____

COMPETENCY 47.7: CONSTRUCTING A VACUUM-FORMED CUSTOM TRAY

Performance Objective

By following a routine procedure that meets stated protocols, the student will construct a vacuum-formed custom tray.

Evaluation and Grading Criteria

 3   Student competently met the stated criteria without assistance.

 2   Student required assistance in order to meet the stated criteria.

 1   Student showed uncertainty when performing the stated criteria.

 0   Student was not prepared and needs to repeat the step.

 N/A   No evaluation of this step.

Instructor shall define grades for each point range earned on completion of each performance-evaluated task.

Performance Standards

The minimum number of satisfactory performances required before final evaluation is _____.

Instructor shall identify by * those steps considered critical. If a step is missed or minimum competency is not met, the evaluated procedure fails and must be repeated.

PERFORMANCE CRITERIA	*	SELF	PEER	INSTRUCTOR	COMMENT
1. Gathered appropriate supplies.					
2. Placed personal protective equipment according to the procedure.					
3. Readied a set of completed models.					
4. Trimmed the model so it extended 3 to 4 mm past the gingival border.					
5. To extend the tray from the teeth for the purpose of holding the bleaching solution, placed a spacer material on the facial surfaces of the teeth on the model.					
6. Using a vacuum former, heated a tray sheet until it sagged ½ to 1 inch.					
7. Lowered the sheet over the model and turned on the vacuum for 10 seconds.					
8. Removed the sheet after allowing it to cool completely.					
9. Using scissors, cut the excess material from the tray.					
10. Used small, sharp scissors to trim the tray approximately 0.5 mm away from the gingival margin.					

Continued

11. Placed the tray onto the original model and checked gingival extensions.				
12. If necessary, applied a thin coat of petroleum jelly to the facial surface. Using a low flame, gently heated and readapted the margins on the model so that all of the teeth were covered, taking care to avoid overlapping onto the gingiva.				
13. After re-adapting the margins, retrimmed the excess material.				
14. Left the tray on the model until the delivery appointment, at which time it was washed in cold, soapy water and then cold-sterilized.				
15. When finished, cared for supplies and materials appropriately.				

ADDITIONAL COMMENTS

Total number of points earned _____

Grade _____ Instructor's initials _____

48 General Dentistry

SHORT-ANSWER QUESTIONS

1. Describe the process and principles of cavity preparation.

2. Besides the restorative material itself, what is the most unique difference of an amalgam and composite procedure?

3. Why is the use of retention pins included in a complex restoration?

4. Discuss the rationales for placing an intermediate restoration.

5. How would you describe a composite veneer to your patient?

6. Describe the role of the dental assistant in a tooth whitening in-office procedure.

FILL-IN-THE-BLANK STATEMENTS

Select the best term from the list below and complete the following statements.

axial wall
cavity
cavity wall
convenience form
diastema
line angle

operative dentistry
outline form
pulpal floor
restoration
retention form
resin veneer

1. The dentist will place a direct _____ to replace a decayed tooth structure.

2. The _____ _____ is an internal surface of a cavity preparation.

3. A _____ _____ is placed within a cavity preparation to help retain and support the restorative material.

4. An open space between teeth #8 and #9 is termed a(n) _____.

5. A(n) _____ _____ is a thin layer of tooth-colored material used to correct the facial surface of a tooth.

6. Another term for decay is _____.

7. _____ _____ is the cavity preparation step that allows the dentist easier access when restoring a tooth.

8. The _____ _____ is an internal surface of the cavity preparation that is perpendicular to the long axis of the tooth.

9. The _____ _____ is the design and specific shape of the cavity preparation used by the dentist to restore a tooth.

10. A common term used to describe restorative and esthetic procedures is _____ _____.

11. The junction of two walls in a cavity preparation forms a(n) _____ _____.

12. A(n) _____ _____ is an internal wall of a cavity preparation that runs parallel to the long axis of the tooth.

MULTIPLE-CHOICE QUESTIONS

Complete each question by circling the best answer.

1. Restorative dentistry is often referred to as _____.
   a. fillings
   b. operative dentistry
   c. prosthetic dentistry
   d. surgical dentistry

2. Another term for decay is _____.
   a. abscess
   b. hole
   c. preparation
   d. cavity

3. The process of removing decay is known as _____.
   a. cavity preparation
   b. drill and fill
   c. extraction
   d. restoration

4. Which wall of the cavity preparation is perpendicular to the long axis of the tooth?
   a. Proximal wall
   b. Pulpal floor
   c. External wall
   d. Marginal wall

5. Where would a class I restoration be located throughout the dentition?
   a. Occlusal surface
   b. Buccal pit of posterior teeth
   c. Lingual pit of anterior teeth
   d. All the above

6. What is the minimum number of surfaces a class II restoration could involve?
   a. One
   b. Two
   c. Three
   d. b and c

7. Which tooth would receive a class II restoration?
   a. Tooth #8
   b. Tooth #13
   c. Tooth #22
   d. Tooth #26

8. What restorative material is indicated for a class IV restoration?
   a. Composite resin
   b. Amalgam
   c. Veneer
   d. Bleaching

9. The type of moisture control recommended for class III and IV procedures is _____?
   a. cotton rolls
   b. 2 × 2-inch gauze
   c. dental dam
   d. saliva ejector

10. The population with a higher incidence of class V lesion includes _____?
   a. children
   b. teenagers
   c. adults
   d. older adults

11. An intermediate restoration is placed for which of the following reasons?
    a. Determine the health of a tooth
    b. Interim period for a permanent restoration
    c. Financial reasons
    d. All the above

12. What tooth surface would receive a resin veneer?
    a. Lingual
    b. Facial
    c. Distal
    d. Incisal

13. The types of veneers placed are _____.
    a. direct composite resin
    b. indirect porcelain
    c. whitening
    d. a and b

14. Indications for tooth whitening are _____.
    a. extrinsic stains
    b. aged teeth
    c. intrinsic stains
    d. all the above

15. _____ is utilized to keep the tooth-whitening gel against the teeth.
    a. A custom fitted tray
    b. A toothbrush
    c. A gauze tray
    d. Molded wax

16. The main ingredient of a tooth-whitening strip is _____.
    a. carbamide peroxide
    b. phosphoric acid
    c. hydrogen peroxide
    d. toothpaste

17. What adverse effect may a patient experience during tooth whitening?
    a. Nausea
    b. Fever
    c. Sensitivity
    d. Decay

18. What classification of tooth preparation is a MOD on tooth #14?
    a. Class I
    b. Class II
    c. Class III
    d. Class IV

19. What classification of a tooth preparation is a lingual pit on tooth #8?
    a. Class I
    b. Class II
    c. Class III
    d. Class IV

20. Which classification would require the use of a matrix system?
    a. Class I
    b. Class II
    c. Class III
    d. b and c

CASE STUDY

Your next patient is scheduled to have an MO restoration on tooth #19.

1. What surfaces of the tooth are M and O?

2. What type of restorative material is indicated for this specific tooth?

3. Are there expanded functions that could be delegated to you in this procedure? If so, what are they?

447

4. You will be preparing the dental dam for this procedure. Dr. Campbell prefers to isolate one tooth distal to the opposite canine. Which teeth are included in the isolation?

5. Will a matrix system be used for the procedure? If so, how many wedges will be placed?

6. The preparation is moderately deep. What supplemental materials besides the restorative material will you set out for this procedure? (Remember, this list depends on the restorative material chosen.)

7. After the procedure has been completed, how is this charted in the patient record?

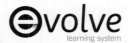

MULTIMEDIA PROCEDURES RECOMMENDED REVIEW

- Assisting in a Class II Amalgam Restoration
- Placing an Intermediate Restoration

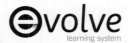

INTERACTIVE DENTAL OFFICE PATIENT CASE EXERCISE

Access the *Interactive Dental Office* on the *Evolve* website and click on the patient case file for Crystal Malone.
- Review Ms. Malone's file.
- Complete all exercises on the website for Ms. Malone's case.
- Answer the following questions.

1. How many teeth have undergone restorations in each of the following classifications: classes I, II, III, and IV?

2. Does Ms. Malone have any composite restorations in place at this time?

3. For what restorative procedure should Ms. Malone be scheduled?

4. Ms. Malone discovers that her insurance does not cover whitening and she cannot afford to have the procedure completed at this time. What would be an alternative that the dental team could educate Ms. Malone about?

5. Ms. Malone underwent restoration of tooth #19 with a root canal and porcelain-fused-to-metal crown. What dental specialists might have been involved in this restoration process?

COMPETENCIES 48.1 AND 48.2: ASSISTING IN AN AMALGAM RESTORATION

Performance Objective

By following a routine procedure that meets stated protocols, the student will demonstrate the proper techniques when assisting with the preparation, placement, and finishing of an amalgam restoration.

Evaluation and Grading Criteria

3   Student competently met the stated criteria without assistance.

2   Student required assistance in order to meet the stated criteria.

1   Student showed uncertainty when performing the stated criteria.

0   Student was not prepared and needs to repeat the step.

N/A   No evaluation of this step.

Instructor shall define grades for each point range earned on completion of each performance-evaluated task.

Performance Standards

The minimum number of satisfactory performances required before final evaluation is _____.

Instructor shall identify by * those steps considered critical. If a step is missed or minimum competency is not met, the evaluated procedure fails and must be repeated.

PERFORMANCE CRITERIA	*	SELF	PEER	INSTRUCTOR	COMMENTS
1. Gathered the appropriate setup.					
2. Placed personal protective equipment according to the procedure.					
3. Ensured that the dental materials were placed and readied.					
4. Assisted during administration of topical and local anesthetic solutions.					
5. Assisted in the placement of the dental dam or other moisture control devices.					
Preparing the Tooth					
1. Transferred the mirror and explorer.					
2. During cavity preparation, used the HVE and air-water syringe, adjusted the light, and retracted as necessary to maintain a clear field.					
3. Transferred the explorer, excavators, and hand cutting instruments as needed throughout cavity preparation.					

Continued

Placing the Matrix Band and Wedge (If Required)					
1. Prepared the universal retainer and matrix band according to the preparation.					
2. Assisted in the placement or performed complete placement of the matrix band.					
3. Assisted in the insertion or performed complete insertion of wedges using #110 pliers.					
Placing Dental Materials					
1. Rinsed and dried the preparation for evaluation.					
2. Mixed and transferred the base, liner, sealer, etchant, and bonding materials in the proper sequence.					
Mixing the Amalgam					
1. Activated the capsule, placed it in the amalgamator, and set the correct time for trituration.					
2. Placed mixed amalgam in the well.					
3. Reassembled the capsule and discarded it properly.					
Placing, Condensing, and Carving the Amalgam					
1. Filled the amalgam carrier and transferred it to the dentist in its correct position.					
2. Transferred restorative instruments to the dentist as needed.					
3. Transferred the carving instruments.					
4. Assisted with removal of the wedge, retainer, matrix band, and dental dam.					
5. Assisted during final carving and occlusal adjustment.					
6. Gave postoperative instructions to the patient.					
7. Maintained patient comfort and followed appropriate infection control measures throughout the procedure.					

8. When finished, cared for supplies and materials appropriately.					
9. Documented the procedure in the patient record.					

ADDITIONAL COMMENTS

Total number of points earned _____

Grade _____ Instructor's initials _____

COMPETENCIES 48.3 AND 48.4: ASSISTING IN A COMPOSITE RESTORATION

Performance Objective

By following a routine procedure that meets stated protocols, the student will demonstrate the proper techniques when assisting with the preparation, placement, and finishing of a composite restoration.

Evaluation and Grading Criteria

3   Student competently met the stated criteria without assistance.

2   Student required assistance in order to meet the stated criteria.

1   Student showed uncertainty when performing the stated criteria.

0   Student was not prepared and needs to repeat the step.

N/A   No evaluation of this step.

Instructor shall define grades for each point range earned on completion of each performance-evaluated task.

Performance Standards

The minimum number of satisfactory performances required before final evaluation is _____.

Instructor shall identify by * those steps considered critical. If a step is missed or minimum competency is not met, the evaluated procedure fails and must be repeated.

PERFORMANCE CRITERIA	*	SELF	PEER	INSTRUCTOR	COMMENTS
1. Gathered the appropriate setup.					
2. Placed personal protective equipment according to the procedure.					
3. Ensured that the dental materials were placed and readied.					
4. Assisted during administration of the topical and local anesthetic solutions.					
5. Assisted in selection of the shade of the composite material.					
6. Assisted in the placement of the dental dam or other moisture control devices.					
Preparing the Tooth					
1. Transferred the mirror and explorer.					
2. During cavity preparation, used the HVE and air-water syringe, adjusted the light, and retracted as necessary to maintain a clear field.					
3. Transferred the explorer, excavators, and hand cutting instruments as needed throughout cavity preparation.					

Continued

Placing the Matrix Band and Wedge (If Required)					
1. Prepared a clear strip and wedge according to the preparation.					
2. Assisted in the placement or performed complete placement of the matrix band.					
3. Assisted in the insertion or performed complete insertion of the wedges using #110 pliers.					
Placing Dental Materials					
1. Rinsed and dried the preparation for evaluation.					
2. Mixed and transferred the base, liner, sealer, etchant, and bonding materials in proper sequence.					
Preparing the Composite					
1. Dispensed the composite material on the paper pad and transferred it to the dentist.					
2. Transferred the restorative instruments to the dentist as needed.					
3. Assisted in light-curing of the material.					
Finishing the Restoration					
1. Assisted with the transfer of burs or diamonds for the high-speed handpiece.					
2. Transferred the finishing strips.					
3. Assisted with removal of the wedge, matrix band, and dental dam.					
4. Assisted during final polishing and occlusal adjustment.					
5. Gave postoperative instructions to the patient.					

6. Maintained patient comfort and followed appropriate infection control measures throughout the procedure.				
7. When finished, cared for supplies and materials appropriately.				
8. Documented the procedure in the patient record.				

ADDITIONAL COMMENTS

Total number of points earned _____

Grade _____ Instructor's initials _____

COMPETENCY 48.5: PLACING AND CARVING AN INTERMEDIATE RESTORATION (EXPANDED FUNCTION)

Performance Objective

By following a routine procedure that meets stated protocols, the student will demonstrate the proper technique for placing and carving an intermediate restoration.

Evaluation and Grading Criteria

<u>3</u>   Student competently met the stated criteria without assistance.

<u>2</u>   Student required assistance in order to meet the stated criteria.

<u>1</u>   Student showed uncertainty when performing the stated criteria.

<u>0</u>   Student was not prepared and needs to repeat the step.

<u>N/A</u>   No evaluation of this step.

Instructor shall define grades for each point range earned on completion of each performance-evaluated task.

Performance Standards

The minimum number of satisfactory performances required before final evaluation is _____.

Instructor shall identify by * those steps considered critical. If a step is missed or minimum competency is not met, the evaluated procedure fails and must be repeated.

PERFORMANCE CRITERIA	*	SELF	PEER	INSTRUCTOR	COMMENTS
1. Gathered the appropriate setup.					
2. Placed personal protective equipment according to the procedure.					
3. Cleaned, dried, and isolated the site with cotton rolls or a dental dam.					
4. Examined the tooth and preparation.					
5. If the preparation included a proximal wall, assembled and placed a matrix band and wedge.					
6. Mixed the IRM to the appropriate consistency.					
7. Used a plastic instrument or FP1 and took increments of the materials to the preparation. If there was an interproximal box, began filling this area first.					
8. After each increment, condensed the material using the small end of the condenser or nib first.					
9. Continued filling the preparation until it was overfilled.					

Continued

10. While the material was still in putty form, used an explorer to remove the excess material from the marginal ridge and the proximal box.				
11. Removed any excess material from the occlusal surface using the discoid-cleoid carver.				
12. If a matrix system was used, removed it at this time, leaving the wedge in place.				
13. Completed the final carving of the occlusal surface with the discoid-cleoid carver, making sure to carve back to the tooth's normal anatomy.				
14. If the interproximal surface was involved, used the Hollenback carver to remove excess material from the interproximal area, making sure not to create an overhang or indentation in the material.				
15. Removed the wedge when carving was completed.				
16. Instructed the patient to bite down gently on articulating paper to check the occlusion.				
17. After the final carving, used a wet cotton pellet to wipe over the restoration.				
18. Informed the patient that the restoration was "short term" and instructed him or her not to chew sticky foods on that side.				
19. When finished, cared for supplies and materials appropriately.				
20. Documented the procedure in the patient record.				

ADDITIONAL COMMENTS

Total number of points earned _____

Grade _____ Instructor's initials _____

COMPETENCY 48.6: ASSISTING IN THE PLACEMENT OF A DIRECT VENEER

Performance Objective

By following a routine procedure that meets stated protocols, the student will demonstrate the proper techniques when assisting in the placement of a veneer.

Evaluation and Grading Criteria

_3_   Student competently met the stated criteria without assistance.

_2_   Student required assistance in order to meet the stated criteria.

_1_   Student showed uncertainty when performing the stated criteria.

_0_   Student was not prepared and needs to repeat the step.

_N/A_   No evaluation of this step.

Instructor shall define grades for each point range earned on completion of each performance-evaluated task.

Performance Standards

The minimum number of satisfactory performances required before final evaluation is _____.

Instructor shall identify by * those steps considered critical. If a step is missed or minimum competency is not met, the evaluated procedure fails and must be repeated.

PERFORMANCE CRITERIA	*	SELF	PEER	INSTRUCTOR	COMMENTS
1. Gathered the appropriate setup.					
2. Placed personal protective equipment according to the procedure.					
3. Assisted in the administration of topical and local anesthetic solutions.					
4. Assisted with shade selection of the composite material.					
5. Assisted in the placement of cotton rolls or of the dental dam.					
6. Assisted in the measurement of the appropriate crown form size.					
7. Assisted in the tooth preparation by maintaining moisture control and retraction for better visibility.					
8. Assisted in the the placement of liners, etchant, and matrix.					
9. If veneers were being placed to cover dark stains, prepared an opaque material.					
10. Transferred the restorative instruments throughout the procedure.					

Continued

11. Assisted with light-curing for the time recommended by the manufacturer.				
12. Assisted with sandpaper discs, strips, and finishing burs to trim and smooth the veneer.				
13. Assisted as needed for each tooth to receive a veneer.				
14. When finished, cared for supplies and materials appropriately.				
15. Documented the procedure in the patient record.				

ADDITIONAL COMMENTS

Total number of points earned _____

Grade _____ Instructor's initials _____

49 Matrix Systems for Restorative Dentistry

SHORT-ANSWER QUESTIONS

1. Describe why a matrix system is an essential component of a class II, III, and IV restoration.

2. Give two types of matrix systems used for posterior restorations.

3. Describe the types of matrix system used for anterior composite restorations.

4. Discuss the purpose and use of a wedge in the matrix procedure.

5. Discuss alternative methods of matrix systems used in restorative dentistry.

FILL-IN-THE-BLANK STATEMENTS

Select the best term from the list below and complete the following statements.

Retainerless Matrix	overhang
celluloid strip	sectional matrix
cupping	Tofflemire retainer
matrix band	wedge
Mylar	

1. _____ and _____ are names for a clear plastic strip that is used to provide a temporary wall for the restoration of an anterior tooth.

2. Improper placement of the wedge can cause the excess restorative material to extend beyond the cavity margin, resulting in a/an _____.

3. _____ is a term used when a restorative material becomes concave from improper wedge placement and not being contoured properly.

4. A(n) _____ is placed in the embrasure of a class II, III, or IV preparation to provide the contour needed when being restored.

5. A(n) _____ acts as a temporary wall for a tooth structure during restoration of the proximal contours and contacts to their normal shape and function.

461

6. A(n) _____ is matrix system made with sectional bands and a tension ring that can be used for posterior amalgam and composite materials.

7. The _____ is a matrix system designed to establish a temporary wall on a primary tooth

8. The _____ is a matrix system that hold a matrix band in place during a class II restoration.

MULTIPLE-CHOICE QUESTIONS

Complete each question by circling the best answer.

1. Which classification would require the use of a matrix system?
   a. I
   b. II
   c. V
   d. VI

2. The plural word for matrix is _____.
   a. matrixes
   b. martinis
   c. matrices
   d. martins

3. Which item would be used to hold a posterior matrix band in position?
   a. Cotton pliers
   b. #110 pliers
   c. Wedge
   d. Tofflemire retainer

4. In what direction is the smaller circumference of the Tofflemire matrix band positioned when placed properly?
   a. Gingival
   b. Occlusal
   c. Facial
   d. Lingual

5. Which instrument would be selected to thin and contour a matrix band for placement?
   a. Carver
   b. Explorer
   c. #110 pliers
   d. Burnisher

6. What additional item is placed in a posterior matrix system to reestablish proper interproximal contact of the newly placed material?
   a. Retraction cord
   b. Wedge
   c. Cotton roll
   d. Articulating paper

7. Improper wedge placement can result in _____.
   a. overfilling
   b. cupping
   c. overhang
   d. b and c

8. Which would be an alternative to the Tofflemire retainer/matrix system for a permanent tooth?
   a. Celluloid strip
   b. Dental dam
   c. T-band
   d. Retainerless matrix

9. Another term for a clear matrix is _____.
   a. celluloid
   b. sandpaper strip
   c. Mylar strip
   d. a and c

CASE STUDY

You are assisting in a MOD amalgam restoration on tooth #29. During the preparation of the tooth, the dentist removes an extensive amount of the tooth structure, which includes the mesial facial cusp. The cavity preparation is now below the gingival margin, creating a large preparation.

1. Have the surfaces of the restoration changed from what was noted in the patient record because of the final preparation? If so, what surfaces are now involved?

2. You have been asked to place the matrix system. What type of matrix system would you select for this preparation?

3. Because the preparation has changed, do any adaptations to the matrix need to be made? If so, what are they?

4. How will the matrix band be adapted for the preparation just described?

5. Which surfaces of the preparation are most critical for stabilizing the newly placed amalgam before carving?

6. How many wedges will be used and from what direction will they be inserted?

7. Could any other matrix system have been used for this procedure? If so, what would it be?

MULTIMEDIA PROCEDURES RECOMMENDED REVIEW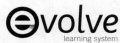

- Assembling a Matrix Band and Tofflemire Retainer
- Placing a Matrix Band and Wedge for a class II Restoration

INTERACTIVE DENTAL OFFICE PATIENT CASE EXERCISE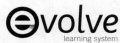

Access the *Interactive Dental Office* on the *Evolve* website and click on the patient case file for Miguel Ricardo.
- Review Mr. Ricardo's record.
- Complete all exercises on the website for Mr. Ricardo's case.
- Answer the following questions:

1. Which teeth received a matrix in the restoration process?

2. Does Mr. Ricardo have any composite restorations in place at this time?

3. For what restorative procedure should Mr. Ricardo be scheduled?

4. Which tooth will be restored?

5. What type of matrix system will be prepared for the procedure?

COMPETENCY 49.1: ASSEMBLING A MATRIX BAND AND TOFFLEMIRE RETAINER

Performance Objective

By following a routine procedure that meets stated protocols, the student will demonstrate the proper technique for assembling a matrix band and Tofflemire retainer for each quadrant of the dental arch.

Evaluation and Grading Criteria

 3   Student competently met the stated criteria without assistance.

 2   Student required assistance in order to meet the stated criteria.

 1   Student showed uncertainty when performing the stated criteria.

 0   Student was not prepared and needs to repeat the step.

 N/A   No evaluation of this step.

Instructor shall define grades for each point range earned on completion of each performance-evaluated task.

Performance Standards

The minimum number of satisfactory performances required before final evaluation is _____.

Instructor shall identify by * those steps considered critical. If a step is missed or minimum competency is not met, the evaluated procedure fails and must be repeated.

PERFORMANCE CRITERIA	*	SELF	PEER	INSTRUCTOR	COMMENTS
1. Gathered the appropriate supplies.					
2. Placed personal protective equipment according to the procedure.					
3. Stated which guide slot would be used for each quadrant.					
4. Determined the tooth to be treated and selected the appropriate band.					
5. Placed the middle of the band on the paper pad and burnished the band with a ball burnisher.					
6. Held the retainer so that the diagonal slot was visible and turned the outer knob clockwise until the end of the spindle was visible in the diagonal slot in the vise.					
7. Turned the inner knob counterclockwise until the vise moved next to the guide slots and the retainer was ready to receive the matrix band.					
8. Identified the occlusal and gingival aspects of the matrix band and brought the ends of the band together to form a loop.					

Continued

9. Placed the occlusal edge of the band into the retainer first, and then guided the band between the correct guide slots.				
10. Locked the band in the vise.				
11. Used the handle end of the mouth mirror to open and round the loop of the band.				
12. Adjusted the size of the loop to fit the selected tooth.				

ADDITIONAL COMMENTS

Total number of points earned _____

Grade _____ Instructor's initials _____

COMPETENCY 49.2: PLACING AND REMOVING A MATRIX BAND AND WEDGE FOR A CLASS II RESTORATION (EXPANDED FUNCTION)

Performance Objective

By following a routine procedure that meets stated protocols, the student will demonstrate the proper technique for placing a Tofflemire retainer, matrix band, and wedge on a tooth with a class II amalgam preparation. The student will then remove the matrix band, retainer, and wedge.

Evaluation and Grading Criteria

 3   Student competently met the stated criteria without assistance.

 2   Student required assistance in order to meet the stated criteria.

 1   Student showed uncertainty when performing the stated criteria.

 0   Student was not prepared and needs to repeat the step.

 N/A   No evaluation of this step.

Instructor shall define grades for each point range earned on completion of each performance-evaluated task.

Performance Standards

The minimum number of satisfactory performances required before final evaluation is _____.

Instructor shall identify by * those steps considered critical. If a step is missed or minimum competency is not met, the evaluated procedure fails and must be repeated.

PERFORMANCE CRITERIA	*	SELF	PEER	INSTRUCTOR	COMMENTS
1. Placed personal protective equipment according to the procedure.					
2. Used mirror and explorer to evaluate the tooth for matrix.					
3. Assembled the matrix band correctly in the retainer for the procedure.					
4. Positioned and seated the band's loop over the occlusal surface.					
5. Held the band securely while tightening it by turning the inner knob clockwise.					
6. Used an explorer to check adaptation of the band to determine that it was firm and extended no farther than 1 to 1.5 mm beyond the gingival margin of the cavity preparation.					
7. Selected the correct size and number of wedges.					
8. Used cotton pliers or #110 pliers to insert the wedge from the lingual embrasure so that the flat side of the wedge was toward the gingiva.					
9. Verified the proximal contact and sealed the gingival margin.					

Continued

Band Removal					
1. Held the band securely while slowly turning the outer knob of the retainer in a counterclockwise direction.					
2. Carefully slid the retainer toward the occlusal surface.					
3. Used cotton pliers to gently spread open the ends of the matrix band and gently lift the matrix band in an occlusal direction using a seesaw motion.					
4. Removed the wedge using #110 pliers or cotton pliers.					
5. Discarded the used matrix band in the sharps container.					
6. Maintained patient comfort and followed appropriate infection control measures throughout the procedure.					

ADDITIONAL COMMENTS

Total number of points earned _____

Grade _____ Instructor's initials _____

COMPETENCY 49.3: PLACING A PLASTIC MATRIX FOR A CLASS III OR CLASS IV RESTORATION

Performance Objective

By following a routine procedure that meets stated protocols, the student will demonstrate the proper technique for placing and removing a plastic matrix band.

Evaluation and Grading Criteria

_3_   Student competently met the stated criteria without assistance.

_2_   Student required assistance in order to meet the stated criteria.

_1_   Student showed uncertainty when performing the stated criteria.

_0_   Student was not prepared and needs to repeat the step.

_N/A_   No evaluation of this step.

Instructor shall define grades for each point range earned on completion of each performance-evaluated task.

Performance Standards

The minimum number of satisfactory performances required before final evaluation is _____.

Instructor shall identify by * those steps considered critical. If a step is missed or minimum competency is not met, the evaluated procedure fails and must be repeated.

PERFORMANCE CRITERIA	*	SELF	PEER	INSTRUCTOR	COMMENTS
1. Gathered the appropriate setup.					
2. Placed personal protective equipment according to the procedure.					
3. Examined the contour of the tooth and preparation site, paying special attention to the outline of the preparation.					
4. Contoured the matrix strip.					
5. Slid the matrix interproximally, ensuring that the gingival edge of the matrix extended beyond the preparation.					
6. Using the thumb and forefinger, pulled the band over the prepared tooth on the facial and lingual surfaces.					
7. Using cotton pliers, positioned the wedge into the gingival embrasure.					

Continued

8. Removed the matrix after the preparation was filled and light-cured.					
9. Maintained patient comfort and followed appropriate infection control measures throughout the procedure.					

ADDITIONAL COMMENTS

Total number of points earned _____

Grade _____ Instructor's initials _____

50 Fixed Prosthodontics

SHORT-ANSWER QUESTIONS

1. List the indications and contraindications to a fixed prosthetic.

2. Identify the steps of a diagnostic treatment plan for someone receiving a fixed prosthetic.

3. Describe the role of the laboratory technician for this specialty of dentistry.

4. Describe the following indirect restorations: inlay, onlay, full crown, and veneer.

5. List the components of a fixed bridge.

6. Describe the preparation and placement of a fixed restoration

7. Discuss why the use of a core buildup, pin, or post may be required for retention.

8. Describe the rationale for use of a retraction cord when a final impression is taken.

9. Describe why provisional coverage is used for a crown or fixed bridge procedure.

10. Describe the home care instructions given to a patient following a fixed prosthetic procedure.

FILL-IN-THE-BLANK STATEMENTS

Select the best term from the list below and complete the following statements.

abutment
articulator
cast post
core
die
fixed bridge
full crown
gingival retraction cord
hypertrophied
inlay

investment material
master cast
onlay
opaquer
pontic
porcelain fused to metal
resin-bonded bridge
three-quarter crown
unit
veneer

1. A(n) _____ is a preformed component fitted into the canal of an endodontically treated tooth to improve the retention of a cast restoration.

2. The _____ is a buildup of a restorative material that provides a larger area of retention for the permanent crown or abutment of a bridge.

3. A positive reproduction of the prepared tooth used in a laboratory for the making of a cast restoration is a _____.

4. A(n) _____ is either a tooth or an implant that supports a fixed bridge.

5. A dental laboratory device that simulates the relation of the mandible to the maxilla is the _____.

6. A _____ is a type of permanent prosthetic that includes both natural teeth and artificial teeth.

7. _____ is placed prior to taking the final impression to displace gingival tissues away from the tooth.

8. A cast restoration that covers the entire anatomic portion of a single tooth is a _____.

9. A cast restoration designed to restore a conservative class II preparation is a(n) _____.

10. _____ means overgrown tissue.

11. A(n) _____ is a type of dental model created from a final impression and is used in the construction of baseplates, bite rims, wax setups, and the finished prosthesis.

12. _____ is a type of gypsum material used during the casting process

13. The _____ is an artificial tooth in a bridge that replaces a natural missing tooth.

14. A type of indirect restoration in which a thin porcelain material is fused to the facial portion of a metal crown is called a _____.

15. A(n) _____ is a layer of tooth-colored material that is bonded or cemented to the prepared facial surface of a tooth.

16. The _____ is a cast restoration designed to cover occlusal, one or more cusps, and proximal surfaces of a posterior tooth.

Chapter **50** **Fixed Prosthodontics**

17. A(n) _____, also referred to as a *Maryland bridge,* has wing-like projections that are bonded to the lingual surfaces of adjacent teeth.

18. A(n) _____ is a resin material that is placed under a porcelain restoration to prevent discoloration of the tooth from showing.

19. A(n) _____ is a cast restoration that covers the anatomic crown of a tooth and either a facial or buccal portion.

20. Each single component of a fixed bridge is considered a _____.

MULTIPLE-CHOICE QUESTIONS

Complete each question by circling the best answer.

1. Fixed prosthodontics is commonly referred to as _____.
   a. operative
   b. crown and bridge
   c. dentures
   d. prosthetics

2. What feature of a patient could be a contraindication to his or her receiving a fixed prosthesis?
   a. Diagnosed with diabetes
   b. Over 60 years old
   c. Poor oral hygiene
   d. Arthritis

3. What would be readied for the dentist to use to reduce the height and contour of a tooth for a casting?
   a. Hand cutting instrument
   b. Sandpaper disc
   c. Model trimmer
   d. Rotary instruments

4. If a tooth is nonvital, what is fabricated and placed into the pulp for better retention of a crown?
   a. Post and core
   b. Root canal filling
   c. Abutment
   d. Pontic

5. A(n) _____ is used during a crown and bridge preparation to displace gingival tissue.
   a. Cotton roll
   b. Dental dam
   c. Gingival retraction cord
   d. Explorer

6. _____ is a type of astringent that can be applied to a retraction cord to control bleeding.
   a. Hydrogen peroxide
   b. Hemodent agent
   c. Disinfectant
   d. Coumadin

7. A term for overgrown gingival tissue is
   a. hyperthyroid
   b. hypertension
   c. hypertrophied
   d. b and c

8. The type of impression to be sent to the dental laboratory for the preparation of a crown is the _____ impression.
   a. preliminary
   b. final
   c. wax bite
   d. b and c

9. How does the dentist convey to the laboratory technician what type of crown is to be fabricated?
   a. Conference call
   b. Fax
   c. Laboratory prescription
   d. Copy of the patient record

10. The laboratory technician prepares an exact replica of the prepared tooth to make a crown. What is this replica called?
    a. Model
    b. Die
    c. Temporary
    d. Impression

11. What is placed on a prepared tooth while the laboratory is fabricating a permanent crown or bridge?
    a. Amalgam
    b. Provisional
    c. Wax
    d. Intermediate restorative material

12. Who in the dental office can legally cement a provisional crown or bridge?
    a. Dentist
    b. EFDA Assistant
    c. Laboratory Technician
    d. a and b

13. Which of the following is the minimum number of appointments needed to fabricate a crown or fixed bridge?
    a. One
    b. Two
    c. Three
    d. Four

14. What accessory would be recommened to the patient to help in flossing a bridge?
    a. Waterpik
    b. Rubber tip
    c. Bridge threader
    d. Electric toothbrush

15. An advantage of a computer-assisted (CAD/CAM) restoration is _____.
    a. fewer appointments
    b. no impressions
    c. reduced tooth sensitivity
    d. all of the above

CASE STUDY

Treatment has been planned for Mandy Moore to receive a three-unit bridge on teeth #11, #12, and #13. Because of prolonged neglect of her dental needs, Mandy must go through a series of dental appointments to correct oral hygiene and restorative needs before bridge preparation can begin.

1. What hygiene problems might interfere with Mandy's having a bridge placed?

2. What type of bridge might be recommended for the charted teeth?

3. Which teeth are the abutment(s) and which are the pontic(s) for the bridge?

4. What type(s) of impression(s) would be taken through the series of procedures?

5. Chart the procedure for the type of bridge described in question 2.

6. What expanded functions may be possible for you to complete throughout this procedure?

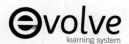

- Placing and Removing a Retraction Cord

INTERACTIVE DENTAL OFFICE PATIENT CASE EXERCISE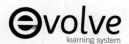

Access the *Interactive Dental Office* on the *Evolve* website and click on the patient case file for Jessica Brooks.
- Review Ms. Brooks's record.
- Complete all exercises on the website for Ms. Brooks's case.
- Answer the following questions:

1. Does Ms. Brooks have any existing crown and bridge work?

2. If she was charted to have an amalgam, why did the procedure change to that for a crown?

3. Why did Ms. Brooks require a core buildup?

4. What type of crown was prescribed for the preparation?

5. Should any specific oral hygiene procedures be given to Ms. Brooks for the care of a crown?

COMPETENCY 50.1: PLACING AND REMOVING A GINGIVAL RETRACTION CORD (EXPANDED FUNCTION)

Performance Objective

By following a routine procedure that meets stated protocols, the student will demonstrate the proper technique for placing, packing, and removing a gingival retraction cord.

Evaluation and Grading Criteria

3	Student competently met the stated criteria without assistance.
2	Student required assistance in order to meet the stated criteria.
1	Student showed uncertainty when performing the stated criteria.
0	Student was not prepared and needs to repeat the step.
N/A	No evaluation of this step.

Instructor shall define grades for each point range earned on completion of each performance-evaluated task.

Performance Standards

The minimum number of satisfactory performances required before final evaluation is _____.

Instructor shall identify by * those steps considered critical. If a step is missed or minimum competency is not met, the evaluated procedure fails and must be repeated.

PERFORMANCE CRITERIA	*	SELF	PEER	INSTRUCTOR	COMMENT
1. Gathered the appropriate setup.					
2. Placed personal protective equipment according to the procedure.					
3. Rinsed and gently dried the prepared tooth and isolated the quadrant with cotton rolls.					
4. Cut a piece of the retraction cord 1 to 1½ inches in length, depending on the size and type of the tooth under preparation.					
5. Formed a loose loop of the cord and placed the cord in the cotton pliers.					
6. Slipped the loop of the retraction cord over the tooth so that the overlapping ends were on the facial or buccal surface.					
7. Laid the cord into the sulcus, then used the packing instrument and, working in a clockwise direction, packed the cord gently but firmly into the sulcus.					

Continued

Chapter **50** **Fixed Prosthodontics**

8. Used a gentle rocking movement of the instrument as it moved forward to the next loose section of the retraction cord. Repeated this action until the length of the cord was packed in place.				
9. Overlapped the working end of the cord where it met the other end. Tucked the ends into the sulcus on the facial aspect.				
10. Left the cord in place for no longer than 5 to 7 minutes. During this time, advised the patient to remain still, and kept the area dry.				
Removing the Cord				
1. Grasped the end of the retraction cord with cotton pliers and removed the cord in a counterclockwise direction.				
2. If instructed by the operator, gently dried the area and placed fresh cotton rolls.				
3. Documented the procedure in the patient record.				

ADDITIONAL COMMENTS

Total number of points earned _____

Grade _____ Instructor's initials _____

COMPETENCY 50.2: ASSISTING IN A CROWN OR BRIDGE PREPARATION

Performance Objective

By following a routine procedure that meets stated protocols, the student will demonstrate the proper technique when assisting with the preparation for a crown and bridge restoration.

Evaluation and Grading Criteria

_3_   Student competently met the stated criteria without assistance.

_2_   Student required assistance in order to meet the stated criteria.

_1_   Student showed uncertainty when performing the stated criteria.

_0_   Student was not prepared and needs to repeat the step.

_N/A_   No evaluation of this step.

Instructor shall define grades for each point range earned on completion of each performance-evaluated task.

Performance Standards

The minimum number of satisfactory performances required before final evaluation is _____.

Instructor shall identify by * those steps considered critical. If a step is missed or minimum competency is not met, the evaluated procedure fails and must be repeated.

PERFORMANCE CRITERIA	*	SELF	PEER	INSTRUCTOR	COMMENT
1. Gathered the appropriate setup.					
2. Placed personal protective equipment according to the procedure.					
3. Assisted during administration of topical and local anesthetic solutions.					
4. Took a preliminary impression for making the provisional coverage.					
5. Throughout the preparation, maintained a clear, well-lighted operating field.					
6. Anticipated the dentist's needs. Transferred instruments and changed burs as necessary.					
7. Assisted in the placement of or placed the gingival retraction cord.					
8. Assisted in mixing the impression material and taking the final impression.					
9. Assisted in the fabrication of or fabricated the provisional coverage.					

Continued

10. Temporarily cemented the provisional coverage.				
11. Provided full mouth rinse.				
12. Documented the procedure in the patient record.				
13. Prepared the laboratory prescription to be sent with impression.				
14. Maintained patient comfort and followed appropriate infection control measures throughout the procedure.				

ADDITIONAL COMMENTS

Total number of points earned _____

Grade _____ Instructor's initials _____

COMPETENCY 50.3: ASSISTING IN THE DELIVERY AND CEMENTATION OF A CAST RESTORATION

Performance Objective

By following a routine procedure that meets stated protocols, the student will demonstrate the proper technique when assisting during the cementation of a crown and bridge restoration.

Evaluation and Grading Criteria

 3 Student competently met the stated criteria without assistance.

 2 Student required assistance in order to meet the stated criteria.

 1 Student showed uncertainty when performing the stated criteria.

 0 Student was not prepared and needs to repeat the step.

 N/A No evaluation of this step.

Instructor shall define grades for each point range earned on completion of each performance-evaluated task.

Performance Standards

The minimum number of satisfactory performances required before final evaluation is _____.

Instructor shall identify by * those steps considered critical. If a step is missed or minimum competency is not met, the evaluated procedure fails and must be repeated.

PERFORMANCE CRITERIA	*	SELF	PEER	INSTRUCTOR	COMMENT
1. Determined in advance that the cast had been returned from the laboratory.					
2. Gathered the appropriate setup.					
3. Placed personal protective equipment according to the procedure.					
4. Assisted during administration of topical and local anesthetic solutions.					
5. Assisted during the removal of provisional coverage. (In a state where it is legal, removed the provisional coverage.)					
6. Anticipated the dentist's needs while the casting was tried and adjusted.					
7. Assisted with the placement of or placed cotton rolls to isolate the quadrant and keep the area dry.					
8. Assisted during the placement of cavity varnish or desensitizer.					
9. At a signal from the dentist, mixed the cement, lined the internal surface of the casting with a thin coating of cement, and transferred the prepared crown to the dentist.					

Continued

10. Instructed the patient to bite down on the cotton rolls while the cement hardened.				
11. Removed the excess cement using an explorer, floss, and air/water to clean around the crown.				
12. Provided home care instructions to the patient.				
13. Maintained patient comfort and followed appropriate infection control measures throughout the procedure.				
14. Documented the procedure in the patient record.				

ADDITIONAL COMMENTS

Total number of points earned _____

Grade _____ Instructor's initials _____

COMPETENCY 50.4: ASSISTING IN A CAD/CAM PROCEDURE (EXPANDED FUNCTION)

Performance Objective

By following a routine procedure that meets stated protocols, the student will demonstrate the proper procedures when assisting during a CAD/CAM restoration.

Evaluation and Grading Criteria

<u>3</u>   Student competently met the stated criteria without assistance.

<u>2</u>   Student required assistance in order to meet the stated criteria.

<u>1</u>   Student showed uncertainty when performing the stated criteria.

<u>0</u>   Student was not prepared and needs to repeat the step.

<u>N/A</u>   No evaluation of this step.

Instructor shall define grades for each point range earned on completion of each performance-evaluated task.

Performance Standards

The minimum number of satisfactory performances required before final evaluation is _____.

Instructor shall identify by * those steps considered critical. If a step is missed or minimum competency is not met, the evaluated procedure fails and must be repeated.

PERFORMANCE CRITERIA	*	SELF	PEER	INSTRUCTOR	COMMENT
1. Gathered the appropriate setup.					
2. Placed personal protective equipment according to the procedure.					
3. Selected the shade of ceramic to be used.					
4. Assisted during administration of topical and local anesthetic solutions.					
5. Placed cotton rolls, Dri-Angle, or dental dam to control moisture.					
6. Prepared the surrounding teeth with Optispray to obtain photos of the occlusal registration before the removal of tooth structure or restorative material.					
7. Assisted in the removal of the tooth structure, exchanging the handpiece and hand cutting instruments.					
8. Completed moisture control throughout the procedure. Rinsed and dried the tooth.					
9. Assisted in the placement of the gingival retraction cord if needed.					

Continued

10. Prepared the surrounding soft tissue with the Optispray for the taking of an optical impression.				
11. Took a digital impression using the system camera.				
12. Using the images taken, outlined the new restoration.				
13. Transferred the images to the screen using the toggle switch to view all sides of the restoration to examine the margins.				
14. Viewed the contacts and anatomy and made changes on the computer screen.				
15. Initiated the computer to mill the restoration from the ceramic block.				
16. Tried in the restoration and readied the finishing burs and discs for adjustment.				
17. Assisted in use of the etching and bonding agents.				
18. Readied the cement and placed a thin film in the restoration.				
19. Following the cementation, readied the articulating paper and floss to check the occlusal bite and contacts for accuracy.				
20. Maintained patient comfort and followed appropriate infection control measures throughout the procedure.				
21. Documented the procedure in the patient record.				

ADDITIONAL COMMENTS

Total number of points earned _____

Grade _____ Instructor's initials _____

51 Provisional Coverage

SHORT-ANSWER QUESTIONS

1. Discuss the indications for the placement of provisional coverage.

2. Give the types of provisional coverage.

3. Identify home care instructions for provisional coverage.

4. Identify the criteria used to determine an acceptable temporary restoration.

FILL-IN-THE-BLANK STATEMENTS

Select the best term from the list below and complete the following statements.

custom provisional
polycarbonate crown
preformed

provisional
stainless steel crown

1. A(n) _____ is a type of temporary coverage designed from a preliminary impression or a thermoplastic tray that replicates the tooth being prepared.

2. A(n) _____ is the term used for temporary coverage that is to be worn during cast preparation.

3. An item that is already shaped in the appearance required is termed _____.

4. The _____ is a thin metal material used for provisional coverage of primary molars.

5. A(n) _____ is a preformed provisional that is tooth-colored and used commonly for anterior teeth.

MULTIPLE-CHOICE QUESTIONS

Complete each question by circling the best answer.

1. A temporary covering for a single crown or a bridge is referred to as a(n) _____.
   a. interim
   b. provisional
   c. crown
   d. tray

2. In most cases, what is the length of time a patient will normally wear a provisional?
   a. 2 to 4 weeks
   b. 2 to 4 months
   c. 6 months
   d. 1 year

3. Who can legally fabricate and temporarily cement a provisional in the dental office?
   a. Dentist
   b. Expanded-functions dental assistant
   c. Laboratory technician
   d. a and b

4. What type of provisional is the most natural looking?
   a. Polycarbonate
   b. Aluminum
   c. Preformed acrylic
   d. Custom

5. What type of provisional is fabricated for anterior teeth?
   a. Stainless steel
   b. Aluminum
   c. Preformed polycarbonate
   d. a and c

6. What step of the procedure is required before the dentist prepares a tooth for a custom provisional?
   a. Preliminary impression
   b. Placement of a gingival retraction cord
   c. Post and core
   d. Final impression

7. _____ is the type of dental material used when making a custom provisional.
   a. Hydrocolloid
   b. Silicone
   c. Acrylic resin
   d. Amalgam

8. When a polycarbonate crown is selected for provisional coverage, the crown _____.
   a. remains on the prepared tooth
   b. acts as a mold for the material
   c. polycarbonate crowns are not used as provisional coverage
   d. either a or b

9. The acrylic resin material is placed in the _____ _____ during construction of a provisional crown.
   a. gingival sulcus
   b. preliminary impression
   c. thermoplastic tray
   d. b or c

CASE STUDY

You have been asked to fabricate a custom provisional for tooth #30.

1. Is there a provisional other than a custom that could be used for this procedure? If so, what kind?

2. Describe two techniques to fabricate a custom provisional.

3. What specific areas of the provisional are the most critical when fitting and when trimming?

4. List the specific instruments you would use in trimming and finishing the provisional.

5. After placing the provisional on the prepared tooth, you notice there is a 1 mm marginal discrepancy. What is your plan of action to improve the provisional so that it fits properly?

6. When the provisional is fitting properly, what is the next step before it is cemented?

7. Describe the setup for cementation of the provisional. List the steps for removal of the excess cement around the provisional.

MULTIMEDIA PROCEDURES RECOMMENDED REVIEW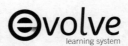

■ Fabricating a Custom Acrylic Provisional Crown

INTERACTIVE DENTAL OFFICE PATIENT CASE EXERCISE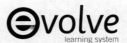

Access the *Interactive Dental Office* on the *Evolve* website and click on the patient case file for Chester Higgins.
■ Review Mr. Higgins's record.
■ Complete all exercises on the website for Mr. Higgins's case.
■ Answer the following questions.

1. What teeth are involved in the three-unit bridge?

2. What type of provisional was selected to fabricate for this case?

3. Besides an alginate impression, what can be used in making a custom provisional?

4. What cement should be used for the cementation of the provisional?

5. What type of home care instructions should be given for provisional coverage?

COMPETENCIES 51.1 AND 51.2: FABRICATING AND CEMENTING A CUSTOM ACRYLIC PROVISIONAL CROWN OR BRIDGE

Performance Objective

By following a routine procedure that meets stated protocols, the student will demonstrate the proper technique for preparing and placing temporary coverage for a tooth prepared to receive a crown.

Evaluation and Grading Criteria

- 3   Student competently met the stated criteria without assistance.
- 2   Student required assistance in order to meet the stated criteria.
- 1   Student showed uncertainty when performing the stated criteria.
- 0   Student was not prepared and needs to repeat the step.
- N/A   No evaluation of this step.

Instructor shall define grades for each point range earned on completion of each performance-evaluated task.

Performance Standards

The minimum number of satisfactory performances required before final evaluation is _____.

Instructor shall identify by * those steps considered critical. If a step is missed or minimum competency is not met, the evaluated procedure fails and must be repeated.

PERFORMANCE CRITERIA	*	SELF	PEER	INSTRUCTOR	COMMENT
Preliminary Impression					
1. Gathered the appropriate setup.					
2. Placed personal protective equipment according to the procedure.					
3. Obtained the preliminary impression.					
4. Isolated and dried the prepared tooth.					
5. If using a separating medium, placed a thin layer on the tooth.					
6. Prepared provisional material according to the manufacturer's directions.					
7. Placed the material in the impression in the area of the tooth. Returned the impression to the mouth and allowed it to set for a minimum of 3 minutes.					
8. Removed the impression from the patient's mouth and removed the provisional from the impression.					
9. Located the interproximal contact point and margin of the provisional, and marked these areas with a pencil.					
10. After the setting or curing of the material, trimmed the provisional with an acrylic bur outside of the mouth.					

Continued

11. Replaced the provisional and checked the occlusion with articulating paper.				
12. Made adjustment on the occlusion using the laboratory burs and discs on the provisional outside the mouth.				
13. Completed final polishing using rubber discs and polishing lathe and pumice.				
Cementation				
1. Cleaned and dried the prepared tooth, making sure isolation is maintained.				
2. Mixed the temporary cement and filled the crown.				
3. Seated the provisional coverage and instructed the patient to bite down on cotton roll and allowed the cement to set.				
4. Using an explorer, tested the material for setting, and removed the excess cement using a horizontal movement with the explorer. Passed floss through both contacts, making sure to slide the floss out from the facial side.				
5. Checked the occlusion with articulating paper.				
6. Had the dentist check and evaluate the procedure.				
7. Provided the patient with home care instructions.				
8. Maintained patient comfort and followed appropriate infection control measures throughout the procedure.				
9. Documented the procedure in the patient record.				

ADDITIONAL COMMENTS

Total number of points earned _____

Grade _____ Instructor's initials _____

COMPETENCY 51.3: FABRICATING AND CEMENTING A PREFORMED PROVISIONAL CROWN

Performance Objective

By following a routine procedure that meets stated protocols, the student will prepare and temporarily cement a preformed provisional crown.

Grading Criteria

_3_	Student competently met the stated criteria without assistance.
_2_	Student required assistance in order to meet the stated criteria.
_1_	Student showed uncertainty when performing the stated criteria.
_0_	Student was not prepared and needs to repeat the step.
_N/A_	No evaluation of this step.

Instructor shall define grades for each point range earned on completion of each performance-evaluated task.

Performance Standards

The minimum number of satisfactory performances required before final evaluation is _____.

Instructor shall identify by * those steps considered critical. If a step is missed or minimum competency is not met, the evaluated procedure fails and must be repeated.

PERFORMANCE CRITERIA	*	SELF	PEER	INSTRUCTOR	COMMENT
Preparation					
1. Gathered the appropriate setup.					
2. Placed personal protective equipment according to the procedure.					
3. Selected a crown of appropriate shape and size, and checked for width, length, and adaptation at the margins.					
4. Used crown and bridge scissors to reduce the height of the crown by trimming the cervical margin.					
5. Smoothed the rough edges with an acrylic trimming stone or an acrylic bur.					
6. Polished the edges with a Burlew wheel or on a lathe with pumice.					
Cementation					
1. Mixed the temporary cement and filled the crown.					
2. Seated the provisional coverage and allowed the cement to set.					
3. Removed the excess cement with explorer and floss.					
4. Readied articulating paper to check occlusion.					

Continued

5. Provided the patient with home care instructions.				
6. Maintained patient comfort and followed appropriate infection control measures throughout the procedure.				
7. Documented the procedure in the patient record.				
ADDITIONAL COMMENTS				

Total number of points earned _____

Grade _____ Instructor's initials _____

52 Removable Prosthodontics

SHORT-ANSWER QUESTIONS

1. Differentiate between a partial denture and a full denture.

2. Give indications and contraindications for a removable partial denture and a full denture.

3. List the components of a partial denture.

4. List the components of a full denture.

5. Describe the steps in the construction of a removable partial denture.

6. Describe the steps in the construction of a full denture.

7. Discuss the differences of an overdenture and an immediate denture.

8. What type of home care instructions are provided for a prosthesis removal?

9. Identify the process of relining or repairing a partial or full denture.

FILL-IN-THE-BLANK STATEMENTS

Select the best term from the list below and complete the following statements.

border molding
centric relation
connectors
coping
edentulous
festooning
flange

framework
full denture
immediate denture
lateral excursion
mastication
occlusal rim
partial denture

post dam
pressure points
protrusion

relining
retainer
retrusion

1. _____ is a position of the maxillary and mandibular arches that produces a proper occlusion.

2. A metal bar that joins various parts of the partial denture together is the _____.

3. In _____, the fingers are used to contour a closer adaptation of the margins of an impression while it is still in the mouth.

4. Tooth structure is protected with a thin metal covering called _____ in the placement of an overdenture.

5. _____ means without teeth.

6. The process of carving or trimming the base material of a denture to simulate normal tissue contours is _____.

7. The parts of a full or partial denture that extend from the teeth to the border of the denture are the _____.

8. The _____ is the metal skeleton of the removable partial denture.

9. _____ is the term for chewing.

10. A(n) _____ is a prosthesis that replaces all teeth in one arch.

11. A temporary denture placed after the extraction of anterior teeth is a(n) _____.

12. _____ is the sliding position of the mandible to the left or right of the centric position.

13. The _____ is positioned on the baseplate to register vertical dimension and occlusal relationship of the mandibular and maxillary arches.

14. The _____ is a seal at the posterior of a full denture that holds it in place.

15. Specific areas in the mouth where a removable prosthesis may rub or apply more force are the _____.

16. _____ is the position of the mandible placed forward in relation to the maxilla.

17. A(n) _____ is a removable prosthesis that replaces several teeth within the same arch.

18. _____ is the process of coating the tissue side of a partial or full denture so that it fits more accurately.

19. The _____ is a device used to hold something in place, such as the attachments or abutments of a removable prosthesis.

20. _____ is the position of the mandible posterior from the centric position in relation to the maxilla.

MULTIPLE-CHOICE QUESTIONS

Complete each question by circling the best answer.

1. What single type of prosthesis would be indicated for replacing teeth #18 through #21 and #28 through #31

   is a(n) _____.
   a. bridge
   b. full denture
   c. partial denture
   d. onlay

2. What can affect a person's decision when choosing a removable prosthesis?
   a. Cost
   b. Appearance
   c. Confidence
   d. All the above

3. The presence of a new remoavalable prosthesis will

   generally _____ saliva.
   a. increase the flow of
   b. decrease the flow of
   c. change the consistency of
   d. cause no change in

4. Why is it important for the alveolar ridge to be evenly contoured for the fitting of a removable prosthesis?
   a. For mastication
   b. For a natural smile
   c. For a better fit
   d. a and c

5. What oral habits could affect the choice in having a removable prosthesis?
   a. Clenching
   b. Grinding
   c. Mouth breathing
   d. All the above

6. The metal skeleton of a partial is referred to as the

   _____.
   a. internal partial
   b. framework
   c. clasp
   d. retainer

7. The retainer of a partial is also referred to as the

   _____.
   a. connector
   b. base
   c. rest
   d. clasp

8. What component of a partial affects the way it is seated in the mouth?
   a. Connectors
   b. Base
   c. Rests
   d. Clasp

9. A type of final impression material used for the fabri-

   cation of a partial is _____.
   a. reversible hydrocolloid
   b. elastomeric
   c. alginate
   d. a and b

10. A dental material the laboratory technician uses to set the teeth for the try-in appointment for a denture is

    _____.
    a. alginate
    b. plaster
    c. stone
    d. wax

11. The suction seal that is created between the maxillary

    denture and the palate is the _____.
    a. post dam
    b. base
    c. border molding
    d. reline

12. How many teeth are in a full set of dentures?
    a. 8
    b. 16
    c. 28
    d. 32

13. What technique does the dentist use to modify the margins of an impression?
    a. Relining
    b. Tissue conditioning
    c. Articulating
    d. Border molding

14. What is a "smile line"?
    a. Space between the maxillary and mandibular teeth
    b. The teeth shown when a patient smiles
    c. Shape of the teeth
    d. Level of the patient's happiness with the dentures

495

15. Which position of the jaw does the dentist measure when articulating a denture?
    a. Centric relation
    b. Protrusion
    c. Retrusion
    d. All the above

16. An immediate denture would most commonly be a treatment planned after _____.
    a. root canal
    b. extraction of multiple teeth
    c. extraction of one tooth
    d. periodontal surgery

17. An immediate denture is commonly worn for _____.
    a. a few days
    b. a few weeks
    c. a few months
    d. a year

18. How is an overdenture supported in the mouth?
    a. Teeth
    b. Implant
    c. Oral mucosa
    d. All the above

19. The term for adding a new layer of resin over the tissue surface of a prosthesis is _____.
    a. border molding
    b. relining
    c. waxing
    d. polishing

20. A denture repair that involves the replacement of teeth or repair of a fracture in the framework would be completed by the _____.
    a. dentist
    b. dental assistant
    c. dental laboratory technician
    d. prosthodontist

CASE STUDY

A friend of the family comes to you for advice. Her dentist has recommended that she have a partial made to replace teeth #19 through #21 and #28 through #30. She is confused as to the options that her dentist discussed with her and she wants your advice.

1. What is your position in giving family and friends advice about their dental needs?

2. What are the reasons a dentist would recommend a partial rather than two separate bridges?

3. What are the reasons a dentist would recommend a partial rather than extraction of the remaining teeth and fabrication of a denture?

4. What are the motives a dentist would recommend a partial rather than implants?

5. What is the role of the dental laboratory technician in making a partial?

INTERACTIVE DENTAL OFFICE PATIENT CASE EXERCISE

Access the *Interactive Dental Office* on the *Evolve* website and click on the patient case file for Jose Escobar.
- Review Mr. Escobar's record.
- Complete all exercises on the website for Mr. Escobar's case.
- Answer the following questions.

1. How many of Mr. Escobar's teeth are already missing?

2. What other specialists might have been involved in the development of the treatment plan?

3. Is Mr. Escobar receiving a full or a partial denture?

4. Why were implants not discussed as a possible treatment?

5. Is it probable that Mr. Escobar will need to have his denture relined? Why or why not?

COMPETENCIES 52.1 TO 52.3: ASSISTING IN THE DELIVERY OF A PARTIAL AND/OR COMPLETE DENTURE

Performance Objective

By following a routine procedure that meets stated protocols, the student will demonstrate the proper technique when assisting with the preparation and placement of a complete and/or partial denture.

Evaluation and Grading Criteria

  3   Student competently met the stated criteria without assistance.

  2   Student required assistance in order to meet the stated criteria.

  1   Student showed uncertainty when performing the stated criteria.

  0   Student was not prepared and needs to repeat the step.

 N/A No evaluation of this step.

Instructor shall define grades for each point range earned on completion of each performance-evaluated task.

Performance Standards

The minimum number of satisfactory performances required before final evaluation is _____.

Instructor shall identify by * those steps considered critical. If a step is missed or minimum competency is not met, the evaluated procedure fails and must be repeated.

PERFORMANCE CRITERIA	*	SELF	PEER	INSTRUCTOR	COMMENT
Preliminary Visits					
1. Exposed radiographs as requested.					
2. Prepared diagnostic cast.					
3. Prepared custom tray.					
Preparation Visit					
1. Gathered the appropriate setup.					
2. Placed personal protective equipment according to the procedure.					
3. Assisted during preparation of the teeth.					
4. Assisted in obtaining the final impression, opposing arch impression, and intraoral occlusal registration.					
5. Disinfected the completed impressions.					
6. Recorded the shade and type of artificial teeth in the patient's record.					
7. Prepared the case for shipment to the commercial laboratory.					

Continued

Try-in Visit(s)					
1. Before the patient's appointment, determined that the case had been returned from the laboratory.					
2. Assisted the dentist during try-in and adjustment of the appliance.					
3. When the appliance was removed, disinfected it and prepared the case to be returned to the laboratory for completion.					
Delivery Visit					
1. Before the patient's appointment, determined that the completed case had been returned from the laboratory.					
2. Gathered the appropriate setup.					
3. Assisted in making any necessary adjustments.					
4. Provided the patient with home care instructions.					
5. Documented the procedure in the patient record.					

ADDITIONAL COMMENTS

Total number of points earned _____

Grade _____ Instructor's initials _____

COMPETENCY 52.4: REPAIRING A FRACTURED DENTURE

Performance Objective

By following a routine procedure that meets stated protocols, the student will demonstrate the proper technique for repairing an upper or lower partial or full denture. Infection control protocol must be followed during the procedure.

Evaluation and Grading Criteria

_3_   Student competently met the stated criteria without assistance.

_2_   Student required assistance in order to meet the stated criteria.

_1_   Student showed uncertainty when performing the stated criteria.

_0_   Student was not prepared and needs to repeat the step.

_N/A_   No evaluation of this step.

Instructor shall define grades for each point range earned on completion of each performance-evaluated task.

Performance Standards

The minimum number of satisfactory performances required before final evaluation is _____.

Instructor shall identify by * those steps considered critical. If a step is missed or minimum competency is not met, the evaluated procedure fails and must be repeated.

PERFORMANCE CRITERIA	*	SELF	PEER	INSTRUCTOR	COMMENT
1. Assembled the appropriate setup.					
2. Placed personal protective equipment according to the procedure.					
3. Cleaned and disinfected the partial or denture for repair.					
4. Aligned the fractured denture parts and applied sticky wax over the fracture line on the external surface of the denture.					
5. Examined the denture and, using a slurry mix or block-out wax, blocked out all undercuts on the internal surface that would be exposed to the plaster.					
6. Prepared a plaster mix using a rubber bowl and spatula.					
7. Slowly poured the plaster into the internal surface of the denture so that the plaster covered the fracture line, but not the entire denture.					
8. Placed the denture in an upright position and allowed the plaster to set.					
9. Once the plaster had set, gently removed it from the cast.					

Continued

501

10. Removed the sticky wax and pumice.				
11. With an acrylic bur, widened the fracture lines on the denture and placed retentive grooves along the fracture line.				
12. Applied a thin coat of the acrylic monomer to the fracture lines and then placed a small amount of the acrylic powder. Alternated the liquid and powder until the fracture line was filled.				
13. Once the material had cured, smoothed and polished the area on the dental lathe.				
14. Cleaned and disinfected the denture before trying it for fit on the patient.				
15. Documented the procedure in the patient record.				

ADDITIONAL COMMENTS

Total number of points earned _____

Grade _____ Instructor's initials _____

53 Dental Implants

SHORT-ANSWER QUESTIONS

1. List the indications and contraindications to receiving a dental implant.

2. Discuss how a patient is screened to receive a dental implant.

3. Give the types of dental implants.

4. Give an overview of the surgical procedure for implantation.

5. Describe postoperative home care and follow-up visits required after placement of a dental implant.

FILL-IN-THE-BLANK STATEMENTS

Select the best term from the list below and complete the following statements.

circumoral   stent
endosteal   subperiosteal
implants   titanium
osseointegration   transosteal

1. A type of implant that a metal framework is surgically inserted in the inferior border of the mandible is a(n) _____ implant.

2. The _____ implant is surgically placed into the maxilla or mandible.

3. _____ is the process of introducing certain metals into a living bone to form a biocombatiable bond.

4. _____ means surrounding the mouth.

5. A(n) _____ implant has a metal frame that is surgically placed under the periosteum of the maxilla or mandible.

6. A _____ is a clear acrylic template placed over the alveolar ridge to aid the dentist in placement of a dental implant.

7. Artificial teeth attached to anchors that have been surgically embedded into the bone or surrounding structures are termed _____.

8. _____ is a type of metal used for implants.

Complete each question by circling the best answer.

1. Which dental specialist can be skilled in the placement of dental implants?
   a. Oral and maxillofacial surgeon
   b. Periodontist
   c. Prosthodontist
   d. All the above

2. The success rate for dental implants have shown to be
   _____.
   a. 50%
   b. 70%
   c. 90%
   d. 100%

3. Which of the following is the minimum number of years a dental implant is expected to last?
   a. 5 years
   b. 10 years
   c. 20 years
   d. 30 years

4. Compared with fixed prosthodontics, what is the financial investment for an implant?
   a. An implant is a larger investment than fixed prosthodontics.
   b. Fixed prosthodontics is a larger investment than an implant.
   c. Both procedures average about the same cost.
   d. Insurance will not cover this procedure.

5. What is the time commitment for an implant procedure?
   a. Approximately 2 to 4 weeks
   b. Approximately 6 to 8 weeks
   c. Approximately 3 to 9 months
   d. Approximately 1 year

6. Which extraoral radiographic image will the dentist use to evaluate a patient for implants?
   a. Panoramic radiograph
   b. Cephalometric radiograph
   c. Tomogram
   d. All the above

7. How is a surgical stent utilized for implant surgery?
   a. To hold the tissue in place
   b. To guide placement for the dentist in the initial placement
   c. To maintain the teeth in an upright position
   d. To assist in the healing process

8. What material is the dental implant generally fabricated from?
   a. Bone graft
   b. Stainless steel
   c. Titanium
   d. Enamel

9. *Osseo* means _____.
   a. implant
   b. tissue
   c. stent
   d. bone

10. What *component of the* endosteal implant attaches to the artificial tooth or teeth?
    a. Abutment post
    b. Cylinder
    c. Stent
    d. a and b

11. A subperiosteal implant is commonly recommended for a _____.
    a. maxillary anterior bridge
    b. mandibular full denture
    c. mandibular posterior crown
    d. maxillary full denture

12. Plaque and calculus are easier to remove from implants than from natural teeth because _____.
    a. implants have a rough surface
    b. implants have a natural cleansing cover
    c. implants have a smooth surface
    d. implants have fluoride embedded in the teeth

13. An example of a cleaning accessory used for implants is a _____.
    a. toothbrush
    b. clasp brush
    c. interproximal brush
    d. All of the above

14. What type of environment should be maintained during a surgical implant procedure?
    a. Aseptic
    b. Sterile
    c. Clean
    d. Cold

15. What type of assessment will a prospective implant patient undergo?
    a. Medical history evaluation
    b. Dental examination
    c. Psychological evaluation
    d. All of the above

CASE STUDY

Your patient is considering implants. There are two drawbacks associated with this procedure. One is cost, and the other is that it will take longer for the procedure to be completed.

1. Are there any contraindications that should be reviewed with a patient before an implant is placed?

2. Explain why the process of implants takes so long and the importance of not rushing this type of procedure.

3. What role does infection control play in the procedure of implants?

4. What financial assistance options could the patient be informed of regarding implants?

5. Describe the most important home care advice that this patient should receive regarding implants.

INTERACTIVE DENTAL OFFICE PATIENT CASE EXERCISE

Access the *Interactive Dental Office* on the *Evolve* website and click on the patient case file for Gregory Brooks.
- Review Mr. Brooks's record.
- Complete all exercises on the website for Mr. Brooks's case.
- Answer the following questions.

1. Are there any other types of fixed prosthodontics in Mr. Brooks's mouth?

2. Which type of implant did Mr. Brooks decide to have?

3. If Mr. Brooks decided not to proceed with the placement of an implant because of cost, what would be the second choice for treatment?

4. What type of home care is recommended for implants?

5. After the implant procedure is completed, what will Mr. Brooks be scheduled for next?

COMPETENCY 53.1: ASSISTING IN ENDOSTEAL IMPLANT SURGERY

Performance Objective

By following a routine procedure that meets stated protocols, the student will demonstrate the proper techniques to be used when assisting during the stages of implant surgery.

Evaluation and Grading Criteria

 3   Student competently met the stated criteria without assistance.

 2   Student required assistance in order to meet the stated criteria.

 1   Student showed uncertainty when performing the stated criteria.

 0   Student was not prepared and needs to repeat the step.

 N/A   No evaluation of this step.

Instructor shall define grades for each point range earned on completion of each performance-evaluated task.

Performance Standards

The minimum number of satisfactory performances required before final evaluation is _____.

Instructor shall identify by * those steps considered critical. If a step is missed or minimum competency is not met, the evaluated procedure fails and must be repeated.

PERFORMANCE CRITERIA	*	SELF	PEER	INSTRUCTOR	COMMENT
1. Gathered the appropriate setup.					
2. Placed personal protective equipment according to the procedure.					
3. Assisted in stage I surgery: implant placement.					
4. Maintained patient comfort and followed appropriate infection control measures throughout the procedure.					
5. Assisted in stage II surgery: implant exposure.					
6. Maintained patient comfort and followed appropriate infection control measures throughout the procedure.					
7. Documented the procedure in the patient record.					
ADDITIONAL COMMENTS					

Total number of points earned _____

Grade _____ Instructor's initials _____

54 Endodontics

SHORT-ANSWER QUESTIONS

1. List the types of tests used to determine pulp vitality.

2. Describe diagnostic conclusions for endodontic therapy.

3. Discuss the medicaments and materials used in endodontics.

4. Give an overview of a root canal therapy.

5. Describe surgical endodontics and explain why it is performed.

FILL-IN-THE-BLANK STATEMENTS

Select the best term from the list below and complete the following statements.

apicoectomy
debridement
direct pulp cap
endodontist
gutta-percha
control tooth
indirect pulp cap
non-vital
palpation

percussion
perforation
periradicular
abscess
pulpitis
pulpotomy
retrograde restoration
reversible pulpitis
root canal therapy

1. _____ is the surgical removal of infectious material surrounding the apex of a root.

2. A(n) _____ is a healthy tooth used as a standard to compare questionable teeth of a similar size and structure during pulp vitality testing.

3. A(n) _____ is a localized area of pus that originates from an infection.

4. _____ is an examination technique that involves tapping on the incisal or occlusal surface of a tooth to determine vitality.

5. _____ is a plastic type of filling material used in root canal therapy.

6. A(n) _____ is the placement of calcium hydroxide over a not completely exposed pulp.

7. _____ means not living.

8. _____ is a term used to remove or clean out the pulpal canal.

9. _____ is a technique to touch or feel for abnormalities of the soft tissue.

10. _____ is the procedure whereby the dental pulp is removed, and the canal is filled with a permanent dental material.

11. A(n) _____ is the application of calcium hydroxide to a cavity preparation in which the dental pulp is fully or partially exposed.

12. To break through and extend beyond the apex of the root is _____.

13. Nerves, blood vessels, and tissue that surround the root of a tooth are called _____.

14. A(n) _____ is the removal of a vital pulp from the coronal portion of a tooth.

15. _____ is inflammation of the dental pulp.

16. A small restoration placed at the apex of a root is _____.

17. A dentist who specializes in the prevention, diagnosis, and treatment of the dental pulp and periradicular tissues is a(n) _____.

18. _____ occurs when there is pulpal inflammation, but the pulp may be salvageable.

MULTIPLE-CHOICE QUESTIONS

Complete each question by circling the best answer.

1. Periradicular tissues are _____.
   a. pulp tissues
   b. tissues that surround the root of a tooth
   c. tissues that surround the crown of a tooth
   d. buccal mucosa

2. What specialist performs root canal therapy?
   a. Prosthodontist
   b. Implantologist
   c. Endodontist
   d. Periodontist

3. What dental emergency can result if bacteria reach the nerves and blood vessels of a tooth?
   a. Abscess
   b. Decay
   c. Tumor
   d. Calculus

4. Is pain a subjective or objective component of a diagnosis?
   a. Subjective
   b. Objective
   c. Neither
   d. Both

5. Tooth #5 is being considered for possible root canal therapy. Which tooth would be used as a control tooth?
   a. #6
   b. #9
   c. #12
   d. #15

6. When the dentist taps on a tooth, what diagnostic test is being performed?
   a. Mobility
   b. Heat
   c. Palpation
   d. Percussion

7. What type of radiograph would be exposed throughout root canal therapy?
   a. Cephalometric
   b. Bitewing
   c. Periapical
   d. Panorex

8. The diagnosis of inflamed pulp tissues is _____.
   a. pulpitis
   b. pulpotomy
   c. pulpectomy
   d. abscess

9. Another term for necrotic is _____.
   a. living
   b. vital
   c. nonvital
   d. a and b

10. The dental material selected for a pulp cap is _____.
    a. amalgam
    b. zinc phosphate
    c. calcium hydroxide
    d. glass ionomer

11. What portion of the pulp would the dentist remove in a pulpotomy?
    a. Coronal portion
    b. Root portion
    c. Complete pulp
    d. Only the infected portion

12. What instrument has tiny projections and is used to remove pulp tissue?
    a. File
    b. Broach
    c. Reamer
    d. Pesso file

13. What type of file would be selected for the final enlargement of a pulpal canal
    a. Broach
    b. Reamer
    c. Pesso
    d. Hedstrom

14. A rubber stop is placed on a file to _____.
    a. prevent perforation
    b. maintain the correct measurement of the canal
    c. identify the file
    d. a and b

15. To *obturate* means to _____.
    a. open a pulpal canal
    b. examine a pulpal canal
    c. fill a pulpal canal
    d. surgically remove a pulpal canal

16. The irrigation solution recommended during root canal therapy is _____.
    a. a combination of air and water from the air-water syringe
    b. diluted sodium hypochlorite
    c. concentrated sodium hypochlorite
    d. diluted phosphoric acid

17. The dental material commonly selected for obturation of a canal is _____.
    a. amalgam
    b. composite
    c. gutta-percha
    d. IRM

18. The type of moisture control recommended by the ADA for root canal therapy is _____.
    a. cotton pellets
    b. cotton rolls
    c. dry angles
    d. dental dam

19. What surface of a posterior tooth would the dentist enter with a rotary bur when opening a canal for root canal therapy?
    a. Occlusal
    b. Facial
    c. Mesial
    d. Incisal

20. _____ is a surgical procedure that involves the removal of the apex of a root.
    a. Hemisection
    b. Apicoectomy
    c. Forceps extraction
    d. Pulpotomy

CASE STUDY

John Allen is scheduled for a diagnosis on tooth #20. This is Mr. Allen's first time to the endodontist, and his subjective comments describe pain when chewing on the affected side and a constant dull pain lasting for approximately a week.

1. How did Mr. Allen know to see an endodontist for dental treatment?

2. What type of tooth is #20 and how many canals could be affected?

3. What type of diagnostic testing will the dentist perform to determine the type of endodontic treatment required?

4. Which tooth is used as the control tooth during diagnostic evaluation and why is a control tooth used?

5. It was determined that the tooth would need a pulpectomy. Describe what this procedure entails.

6. What type of pain control would the endodontist use during the procedure to help alleviate unwarranted stress as well as discomfort?

7. How would tooth #20 be completely restored and what dentist would complete this procedure?

INTERACTIVE DENTAL OFFICE PATIENT CASE EXERCISE

Access the *Interactive Dental Office* on the *Evolve* website and click on the patient case file for Antonio DeAngelis.
- Review Mr. DeAngelis's record.
- Complete all exercises on the website for Mr. DeAngelis's case.
- Answer the following questions.

1. Does the chart indicate that Mr. DeAngelis has any existing root canals?

2. What tooth was used as a control tooth for electric pulp testing?

3. How would tooth #10 be charted after completion of the root canal?

4. What specialist will Mr. DeAngelis be referred to for the porcelain-fused-to-metal crown?

5. Now that the existing work is completed, should Mr. DeAngelis be rescheduled for anything?

COMPETENCY 54.1: ASSISTING IN ELECTRIC PULP VITALITY TEST

Performance Objective

By following a routine procedure that meets stated protocols, in states where it is legal, the student will demonstrate the proper procedure for performing an electric pulp vitality test.

Evaluation and Grading Criteria

 3 Student competently met the stated criteria without assistance.

 2 Student required assistance in order to meet the stated criteria.

 1 Student showed uncertainty when performing the stated criteria.

 0 Student was not prepared and needs to repeat the step.

 N/A No evaluation of this step.

Instructor shall define grades for each point range earned on completion of each performance-evaluated task.

Performance Standards

The minimum number of satisfactory performances required before final evaluation is _____.

Instructor shall identify by * those steps considered critical. If a step is missed or minimum competency is not met, the evaluated procedure fails and must be repeated.

PERFORMANCE CRITERIA	*	SELF	PEER	INSTRUCTOR	COMMENT
1. Gathered the appropriate setup.					
2. Placed personal protective equipment according to the procedure.					
3. Described the procedure to the patient.					
4. Identified the tooth to be tested and the appropriate control tooth.					
5. Isolated the teeth to be tested and dried them thoroughly.					
6. Set the control dial at zero.					
7. Placed a thin layer of toothpaste on the tip of the pulp tester electrode.					
8. Tested the control tooth first; placed the tip of the electrode on the facial surface of the tooth at the cervical third.					
9. Gradually increased the level of current until the patient felt a response; recorded the response on the patient's record.					

Continued

10. Repeated the procedure on the suspect tooth and recorded the response on the patient's record.				
11. Maintained patient comfort and followed appropriate infection control measures throughout the procedure.				
12. Documented the procedure in the patient record.				

ADDITIONAL COMMENTS

Total number of points earned _____

Grade _____ Instructor's initials _____

COMPETENCY 54.2: ASSISTING IN ROOT CANAL THERAPY

Performance Objective

By following a routine procedure that meets stated protocols, the student will demonstrate the proper procedure for making pretreatment preparations and assisting in root canal therapy.

Evaluation and Grading Criteria

3	Student competently met the stated criteria without assistance.
2	Student required assistance in order to meet the stated criteria.
1	Student showed uncertainty when performing the stated criteria.
0	Student was not prepared and needs to repeat the step.
N/A	No evaluation of this step.

Instructor shall define grades for each point range earned on completion of each performance-evaluated task.

Performance Standards

The minimum number of satisfactory performances required before final evaluation is _____.

Instructor shall identify by * those steps considered critical. If a step is missed or minimum competency is not met, the evaluated procedure fails and must be repeated.

PERFORMANCE CRITERIA	*	SELF	PEER	INSTRUCTOR	COMMENT
1. Prepared the appropriate setup.					
2. Placed personal protective equipment according to the procedure.					
3. Assisted with the administration of a local anesthetic and with placing and disinfecting the dental dam.					
4. Anticipated the dentist's needs.					
5. Maintained moisture control and a clear operating field throughout the procedure.					
6. Exchanged instruments as necessary.					
7. On request, irrigated the canals gently with a solution of sodium hypochlorite and used the HVE tip to remove excess solution.					
8. On request, placed a rubber stop at the desired working length for that canal.					
9. Assisted in preparation of the trial-point radiograph.					
10. Exposed and processed the trial-point radiograph.					
11. At a signal from the endodontist, prepared the endodontic sealer.					

Continued

#					
12. Dipped a file or Lentulo spiral into the material, and transferred it to the endodontist.					
13. Dipped the tip of the gutta-percha point into the sealer and transferred it to the endodontist.					
14. Transferred the hand instruments and additional gutta-percha points to the endodontist.					
15. Continued the instrument exchange until the procedure was complete and the tooth was sealed with temporary cement.					
16. Exposed and processed a post-treatment radiograph.					
17. Gave the patient posttreatment instructions.					
18. Maintained patient comfort and followed appropriate infection control measures throughout the procedure.					
19. Documented the procedure in the patient record.					

ADDITIONAL COMMENTS

Total number of points earned _____

Grade _____ Instructor's initials _____

55 Periodontics

SHORT-ANSWER QUESTIONS

1. What role does the dental assistant assume in a periodontal practice?

2. What is included in a comprehensive periodontal exam?

3. Give the types of instruments that are used in periodontal therapy.

4. When would a periodontal surgical dressing be indicated?

5. What type of systemic conditions can have a negative influence on periodontal treatment?

6. Explain the purpose of radiographs in periodontal treatment.

7. Give the indications and contraindications of the ultrasonic scaler.

8. Describe the various types of non-surgical periodontal therapy.

9. Describe the various types of surgical periodontal therapy.

FILL-IN-THE-BLANK STATEMENTS

Select the best term from the list below and complete the following statements.

gingivoplasty
mobility
osseous surgery
ostectomy
laser beam
osteoplasty
periodontal dressing
bleeding index

periodontal explorer
periodontal pocket
furcation probe
periodontics
gingivectomy
periodontist
periotomes
ultrasonic scaler

519

1. The dental specialty that includes the diagnosis and treatment of diseases of the supporting tissues for the teeth is _____.

2. A(n) _____ is a dentist with advanced education in the specialty of periodontics.

3. A(n) _____ is a deepening of the gingival sulcus beyond normal, resulting from periodontal disease.

4. A covering that is applied to the surgical site for protection, like a bandage, is a(n) _____.

5. _____ is the movement of the tooth within its socket.

6. The _____ is a method used to measure the amount of hemorrhage present.

7. A(n) _____ is a thin, fine, instrument easily adapted around root surfaces to locate calculus.

8. A(n) _____ is a insturment that operates on a high-frequency sound wave for the removal of calculus.

9. _____ is indicated when there is loss of connective tissue and alveolar bone.

10. A(n) _____ is the surgical removal of diseased gingival tissues.

11. A type of surgery in which gingival tissues are reshaped and contoured is _____.

12. _____ is a type of surgery in which bone is added, contoured, and reshaped.

13. _____ is a type of surgery that involves the removal of bone.

14. A highly concentrated beam of light is a(n) _____.

15. _____ is an intrument used to cut periodontal ligaments for atraumatic tooth extraction.

16. A(n) _____ is used to measure horizontal and vertical pocket depths for multirooted teeth.

MULTIPLE-CHOICE QUESTIONS

Complete each question by circling the best answer.

1. How do patients most often seek periodontal care?
   a. Prescription from their general dentist
   b. Referral by their general dentist
   c. Referral by another specialist
   d. Referral by their insurance company

2. What information is included in periodontal charting?
   a. Pocket readings
   b. Furcations
   c. Tooth mobility
   d. All of the above

3. Should teeth have any mobility?
   a. No
   b. Depends on the teeth
   c. A slight amount
   d. Yes

4. What is the depth of a normal sulcus?
   a. 1 to 3 mm
   b. 2 to 4 mm
   c. 3 to 5 mm
   d. 4 to 6 mm

5. What units of measurement are used on the periodontal probe?
   a. Centimeters
   b. Millimeters
   c. Inches
   d. Milligrams

6. What type of radiograph is especially useful in periodontics?
   a. Panoramic
   b. Occlusal
   c. Vertical bitewing
   d. Periapical

7. Which instrument is used to remove calculus from supragingival surfaces?
   a. Spoon excavator
   b. Scaler
   c. Explorer
   d. Curette

8. Which type of instrument is used to remove calculus from subgingival surfaces?
   a. Spoon excavator
   b. Scaler
   c. Explorer
   d. Curette

9. What is the purpose of explorers in periodontal treatment?
   a. To detect pathology
   b. To provide tactile information
   c. To locate calculus
   d. b and c

10. A type of curette with two cutting edges is a _____.
    a. universal
    b. Kirkland
    c. Gracey
    d. sickle

11. What is the purpose of a periodontal pocket marker?
    a. To carry items to and from the mouth
    b. To mark bleeding points in the gingival tissue
    c. To measure the sulcus
    d. To remove calculus from the sulcus

12. How does an ultrasonic scaler work?
    a. Water pressure
    b. Air pressure
    c. Sound waves
    d. RPM

13. What oral conditions contraindicate the use of an ultrasonic scaler?
    a. Patients with demineralization
    b. Narrow periodontal pockets
    c. Exposed dentin
    d. All of the above

14. Is an ultrasonic scaler indicated for a patient with a communicable disease?
    a. Yes
    b. No
    c. It does not matter.

15. What is the common term for a dental prophylaxis?
    a. Prophy
    b. Sealants
    c. Scaling
    d. Treatment

16. Who can perform a dental prophylaxis?
    a. Dentist
    b. Dental assistant
    c. Dental hygienist
    d. a and c

17. _____ is considered a surgical periodontal procedure.
    a. Scaling
    b. Root planing
    c. Gingivectomy
    d. Gingival curettage

18. What drug is often used for the treatment of periodontitis, juvenile periodontitis, and rapidly destructive periodontitis?
    a. Fluoride
    b. Tetracycline
    c. Ibuprofen
    d. Acetaminophen

CASE STUDY

You will be assisting Dr. Lanier with an incisional periodontal surgical procedure. Dr. Lanier has noted in the patient record that teeth #23 through #26 do not have adequate tissue coverage and will need to move the flap of tissue into position to cover more tooth structure.

1. What type of dental specialist would complete this procedure?

2. What is another name for incisional periodontal surgery?

3. To close the flap, what would the surgeon most commonly use?

4. To protect the surgical site and promote healing, what would you prepare for placement? Where would it be placed?

MULTIMEDIA PROCEDURES RECOMMENDED REVIEW

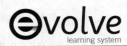

- Noneugenol Periodontal Dressings
- Removing a Periodontal Dressing

INTERACTIVE PATIENT CASE EXERCISE

Access the *Interactive Dental Office* on the *Evolve* website and click on the patient case file for Mrs. Louisa Van Doren.
- Review Mrs. Van Doren's record.
- Complete all exercises for Mrs. Van Doren's case.
- Answer the following questions.

1. Are there contraindications to the use of an ultrasonic scaler on Mrs. Van Doren's teeth?

2. A gingivectomy is scheduled for which area in Mrs. Van Doren's mouth?

3. Will Dr. Bowman need to place a periodontal dressing?

Access the *Interactive Dental Office* on the *Evolve* website and click on the patient case file for Mrs. Janet Folkner.
- Review Mrs. Folkner's record.
- Complete all exercises for Mrs. Folkner's case.
- Answer the following questions.

4. Are there any special precautions that should be taken before an ultrasonic scaler is used on Mrs. Folkner's teeth?

5. What do you notice about the level of bone on Mrs. Folkner's radiographs?

6. What types of instruments would be used to remove the subgingival calculus?

COMPETENCY 55.1: ASSISTING WITH A DENTAL PROPHYLAXIS

Performance Objective

By following a routine procedure that meets stated protocols, the student will demonstrate the proper procedure for assisting with a dental prophylaxis.

Evaluation and Grading Criteria

3	Student competently met the stated criteria without assistance.
2	Student required assistance in order to meet the stated criteria.
1	Student showed uncertainty when performing the stated criteria.
0	Student was not prepared and needs to repeat the step.
N/A	No evaluation of this step.

Instructor shall define grades for each point range earned on completion of each performance-evaluated task.

Performance Standards

The minimum number of satisfactory performances required before final evaluation is _____.

Instructor shall identify by * those steps considered critical. If a step is missed or minimum competency is not met, the evaluated procedure fails and must be repeated.

PERFORMANCE CRITERIA	*	SELF	PEER	INSTRUCTOR	COMMENT
1. Placed personal protective equipment according to the procedure.					
2. Adjusted the light as necessary and was prepared to dry the teeth with air when requested to do so.					
3. Provided retraction of the lips, tongue, and cheeks.					
4. Rinsed and evacuated the fluid from the patient's mouth.					
5. Exchanged instruments with the operator.					
6. Passed the dental floss and/or tape.					
7. Reinforced oral hygiene instructions when requested to do so.					
8. Maintained patient comfort and followed appropriate infection control measures throughout the procedure.					
9. Documented the procedure in the patient record.					

ADDITIONAL COMMENTS

Total number of points earned _____

Grade _____ Instructor's initials _____

COMPETENCY 36-1: ASSISTING WITH A DENTAL PROPHYLAXIS

Performance Objective

By following a routine procedure that aided by others, the student will demonstrate the proper procedure for assisting with a dental prophylaxis.

Evaluation and Grading Criteria

3   Student competently met the highest standards without assistance.

2   Student required assistance in order to meet the stated criteria.

1   Student needed more training when performing the listed criteria.

0   Student was not prepared and needs to repeat the step.

N/A   No evaluation of this step.

Instructor shall define grade for each point range earned at completion of each performance-evaluated task.

Performance Standards

The minimum number of satisfactory performances required before final evaluation is _____

Instructor shall indicate by * those steps considered critical. If a step is missed or minimum competency is not met, the evaluated procedure fails and must be repeated.

PERFORMANCE CRITERIA	SELF	PEER	INSTRUCTOR	COMMENT
1. Placed personal protective equipment according to the treat date.				
2. Adjusted the light as necessary and was prepared to dry the teeth with the air-water syringe and evacuator.				
3. Provided retraction of the tongue, cheek and lips.				
4. Rinsed and evacuated the mouth from the patient's mouth.				
5. Exchanged instruments with the operator.				
6. Rinsed the dental floss and air tips.				
7. Rinsed and dried ... when necessary ... returned to dry.				
8. Maintained ... the suction and record ... throughout the procedure.				
9. Documented the procedure in the patient record.				

ADDITIONAL COMMENTS

Total number of points earned _____

Grade _____   Instructor initials _____

COMPETENCY 55.2: ASSISTING WITH GINGIVECTOMY AND GINGIVOPLASTY

Performance Objective

By following a routine procedure that meets stated protocols, the student will demonstrate the proper procedure for assisting with a gingivectomy and gingivoplasty.

Evaluation and Grading Criteria

 3   Student competently met the stated criteria without assistance.

 2   Student required assistance in order to meet the stated criteria.

 1   Student showed uncertainty when performing the stated criteria.

 0   Student was not prepared and needs to repeat the step.

 N/A   No evaluation of this step.

Instructor shall define grades for each point range earned on completion of each performance-evaluated task.

Performance Standards

The minimum number of satisfactory performances required before final evaluation is _____.

Instructor shall identify by * those steps considered critical. If a step is missed or minimum competency is not met, the evaluated procedure fails and must be repeated.

PERFORMANCE CRITERIA	*	SELF	PEER	INSTRUCTOR	COMMENT
1. Set out the patient's health history, radiographs, and periodontal chart.					
2. Placed personal protective equipment according to the procedure.					
3. Anticipated the operator's needs and was prepared to pass and retrieve the surgical instruments.					
4. Had gauze ready to remove tissue from the instruments.					
5. Provided oral evacuation and retraction.					
6. Irrigated with sterile saline.					
7. Assisted with suture placement.					
8. Placed or assisted with placement of the periodontal dressing.					
9. Provided postoperative instructions.					

Continued

10. Maintained patient comfort and followed appropriate infection control measures throughout the procedure.					
11. Documented the procedure in the patient record.					

ADDITIONAL COMMENTS

Total number of points earned _____

Grade _____ Instructor's initials _____

COMPETENCY 55.3: PREPARING AND PLACING A NONEUGENOL PERIODONTAL DRESSING (EXPANDED FUNCTION*)

Performance Objective

By following a routine procedure that meets stated protocols, the student will demonstrate the proper procedure for preparing and placing a non-eugenol periodontal dressing.

Evaluation and Grading Criteria

3 Student competently met the stated criteria without assistance.

2 Student required assistance in order to meet the stated criteria.

1 Student showed uncertainty when performing the stated criteria.

0 Student was not prepared and needs to repeat the step.

N/A No evaluation of this step.

Instructor shall define grades for each point range earned on completion of each performance-evaluated task.

Performance Standards

The minimum number of satisfactory performances required before final evaluation is _____.

Instructor shall identify by * those steps considered critical. If a step is missed or minimum competency is not met, the evaluated procedure fails and must be repeated.

PERFORMANCE CRITERIA	*	SELF	PEER	INSTRUCTOR	COMMENT
1. Placed personal protective equipment according to the procedure.					
Mixing					
1. Extruded equal lengths of the two pastes on a paper pad.					
2. Mixed the pastes until a uniform color was obtained (2 to 3 minutes).					
3. Placed the material in the paper cup.					
4. Lubricated the gloved fingers with vaseline					
5. Rolled the paste into strips.					
Placement					
1. Pressed small triangular pieces of dressing into the interproximal spaces.					
2. Adapted one end of the strip around the distal surface of the last tooth in the surgical site.					
3. Gently pressed the remainder of the strip along the incised gingival margin.					

Continued

4. Gently pressed the strip into the interproximal areas.					
5. Applied the second strip from the lingual surface.					
6. Joined the facial and lingual strips.					
7. Applied gentle pressure on the facial and lingual surfaces.					
8. Checked the dressing for over-extension and interference.					
9. Removed any excess dressing and adjusted the new margins.					
10. Maintained patient comfort and followed appropriate infection control measures throughout the procedure.					
11. Documented the procedure in the patient record.					

ADDITIONAL COMMENTS

Total number of points earned _____

Grade _____ Instructor's initials _____

*This procedure may not be considered an expanded function in your area. Check your local regulations.

COMPETENCY 55.4: REMOVING A PERIODONTAL DRESSING

Performance Objective

By following a routine procedure that meets stated protocols, the student will demonstrate the proper procedure for removing a periodontal dressing.

Evaluation and Grading Criteria

_3_   Student competently met the stated criteria without assistance.

_2_   Student required assistance in order to meet the stated criteria.

_1_   Student showed uncertainty when performing the stated criteria.

_0_   Student was not prepared and needs to repeat the step.

_N/A_   No evaluation of this step.

Instructor shall define grades for each point range earned on completion of each performance-evaluated task.

Performance Standards

The minimum number of satisfactory performances required before final evaluation is _____.

Instructor shall identify by * those steps considered critical. If a step is missed or minimum competency is not met, the evaluated procedure fails and must be repeated.

PERFORMANCE CRITERIA	*	SELF	PEER	INSTRUCTOR	COMMENTS
1. Placed personal protective equipment according to the procedure.					
2. Gently inserted the spoon excavator under the margin.					
3. Used lateral pressure to gently pry the dressing away from the tissue.					
4. Checked for sutures and removed any present.					
5. Gently used dental floss to remove all fragments of the dressing material.					
6. Irrigated the entire area gently with a warm saline solution.					
7. Used the HVE tip or saliva ejector to remove the fluid from the patient's mouth.					
8. Maintained patient comfort and followed appropriate infection control measures throughout the procedure.					
9. Documented the procedure in the patient record.					

ADDITIONAL COMMENTS

Total number of points earned _____

Grade _____ Instructor's initials _____

56 Oral and Maxillofacial Surgery

SHORT-ANSWER QUESTIONS

1. Define the specialty of oral and maxillofacial surgery.

2. Describe the role of an oral surgery assistant.

3. State the importance of the chain of asepsis for this specialized area of dentistry.

4. List the instruments used for a forceps extraction.

5. Describe the surgical procedures that are commonly performed in a general and oral and maxillofacial surgery practice.

6. Describe the type of postoperative instructions provided to a patient after a surgical procedure.

7. Discuss the possible complications of surgery.

FILL-IN-THE-BLANK STATEMENTS

Select the best term from the list below and complete the following statements.

impacted	oral and maxillofacial surgeon
bone file	oral and maxillofacial surgery
chisel	oral brush biopsy
rongeur	outpatient
elevator	donning
forceps	retractor
hemostat	scalpel
incisional biopsy	soft tissue impaction
alveoplasty	surgical curette
mallet	hard tissue impaction

1. The _____ is a surgical instrument used for cutting or severing the tooth and bone structure.

2. The surgical instrument used to reflect and retract the periodontal ligament and periosteum is the _____.

3. In a(n) _____, a tooth is partially to fully covered by bone and gingival tissue.

4. An instrument used to hold or grasp an item is a(n) _____.

5. A surgical instrument used to remove tissue and debris from the tooth socket is the _____.

6. _____ is the procedure of surgical reduction and reshaping of the alveolar ridge.

7. A surgical instrument used to smooth the rough edges of a bone structure is the _____.

8. In a(n) _____, a tooth is partially to fully covered by gingival tissue.

9. A(n) _____ is rotated on the oral mucosa to remove tissue from a suspicious oral lesion.

10. A surgical instrument used to grasp a tooth, hold it, and remove it from its socket is a(n) _____.

11. _____ is the act of placing your protective eyewear, mask and gloves on.

12. A tooth that has not erupted is termed _____.

13. The removal of a portion of a questionable lesion for evaluation is an _____.

14. A(n) _____ is a hammer-like instrument used with a chisel to section teeth or bone.

15. A(n) _____ is a surgical knife.

16. A(n) _____ is a dentist who specializes in surgery of the head and neck region.

17. _____ is the dental specialty that focuses on treatment of the head and neck.

18. A patient who is seen and treated by a doctor and then is sent home for recovery is considered a(n) _____.

19. A(n) _____ is an instrument used to hold back soft tissue.

20. A surgical instrument used to cut and trim the alveolar bone is the _____.

MULTIPLE-CHOICE QUESTIONS

Complete each question by circling the best answer.

1. What type of surgical procedure would a general dentist most commonly perform?
   a. Single extraction
   b. Removal of impacted teeth
   c. Reconstructive surgery
   d. Biopsy

2. How can a dental assistant further their career as a surgical assistant?
   a. Obtain a dental hygiene degree
   b. Obtain a nursing degree
   c. Obtain continuing credentials in oral and maxillo-facial surgery
   d. Obtain a dental degree

3. In what type of setting are oral surgery procedures completed?
   a. Dental office
   b. Outpatient surgical center
   c. Hospital
   d. All the above

4. Most surgical procedures completed in the dental office are considered _____.
   a. major surgery
   b. minor surgery
   c. dental procedures
   d. medical procedures

5. The periosteal elevator is used to reflect and retract
   _____.
   a. calculus
   b. teeth
   c. periosteum
   d. lips

6. Universal forceps are designed to be used for
   _____.
   a. right side only
   b. left side only
   c. left or right of the opposite arch
   d. left or right of the same arch

7. What surgical instrument resembles a spoon
   excavator?
   a. Rongeur
   b. Surgical curette
   c. Elevator
   d. Scalpel

8. What surgical instrument is used to trim and shape
   bone?
   a. Rongeur
   b. Surgical curette
   c. Elevator
   d. Scalpel

9. If a chisel is placed on the tray setup, what additional
   surgical instrument must be set out?
   a. Elevator
   b. Scalpel
   c. Mallet
   d. Hemostat

10. What equipment is used to perform a surgical scrub?
    a. Orange stick
    b. Antimicrobial soap
    c. Scrub brush
    d. All the above

11. The term *donning* means _____.
    a. taking off
    b. putting on
    c. procedure
    d. prior to

12. What procedure is generally completed by the sur-
    geon following the removal of multiple adjacent
    teeth?
    a. Implants
    b. Sutures
    c. Alveoplasty
    d. b or c

13. When a impacted tooth is directly under gingival
    tissue, it is said to be _____.
    a. ankylosed
    b. soft tissue impacted
    c. exposed
    d. hard tissue impacted

14. _____ is completed when cells are scraped
    from a surface lesion.
    a. Incisional biopsy
    b. Excisional biopsy
    c. Oral brush biopsy
    d. Surgical biopsy

15. The term *suture* refers to _____.
    a. impaction
    b. stitching
    c. control of bleeding
    d. expose

16. Which is an absorbable suture material?
    a. Silk
    b. Polyester
    c. Nylon
    d. Catgut

17. What is the approximate time frame for the removal
    of non-absorbable sutures?
    a. 1 to 3 days
    b. 4 to 6 days
    c. 5 to 7 days
    d. 12 to 14 days

18. How long should the patient be instructed to keep
    sterile gauze on the surgical site to control bleeding?
    a. 30 minutes
    b. 2 to 3 hours
    c. 12 hours
    d. 24 hours

19. What analgesic may be prescribed for mild pain?
    a. Antibiotic
    b. Ibuprofen
    c. Aspirin
    d. Codeine

20. What is advised to control swelling during the first 24
    hours?
    a. Gauze pack
    b. Tea bag
    c. Cold pack
    d. Heat pack

Katie Samuels's mother has called the surgeon about extreme pain in Katie's lower right jaw. The business assistant reviews her record and sees that Katie underwent surgical extraction of teeth #17 and #32 three days ago. The teeth were impacted, but the surgeon's progress notes indicate that there were no complications and the patient tolerated the procedure well. Katie is scheduled to return in a week for follow-up and for suture removal.

1. Why would this patient be referred to a specialist for this procedure?

2. What does the term *impacted* describe about the teeth that were removed?

3. What type of material would the surgeon have used for sutures that would require the patient to return for their removal?

4. Give a possible analysis for Katie's pain.

5. What type of questions would you ask Katie's mom to help the surgeon determine the diagnosis.

6. If the diagnosis is correct, what should be performed to alleviate the patient's pain?

7. Can the patient wait until her scheduled checkup to be seen? If not, when should she be seen?

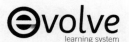
- Suture Removal

 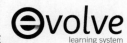
Access the *Interactive Dental Office* on the *Evolve* website and click on the patient case file for Mr. Lee Wong.
- Review Mr. Wong's record.
- Complete all exercises on the website for Mr. Wong's case.
- Answer the following questions.

1. What does the charting indicate for tooth #30?

2. Could any additional methods of pain control be used to calm Mr. Wong?

3. What type of PPE was worn during the procedure?

4. Were sutures placed after the extraction?

5. How is the medicated dressing placed in the tooth socket for the treatment of alveolitis?

COMPETENCY 56.1: PREPARING A STERILE FIELD FOR INSTRUMENTS AND SUPPLIES

Performance Objective

By following a routine procedure that meets stated protocols, the student will demonstrate the proper procedure for preparing a sterile field for instruments and supplies.

Evaluation and Grading Criteria

<u>3</u>   Student competently met the stated criteria without assistance.

<u>2</u>   Student required assistance in order to meet the stated criteria.

<u>1</u>   Student showed uncertainty when performing the stated criteria.

<u>0</u>   Student was not prepared and needs to repeat the step.

<u>N/A</u>   No evaluation of this step.

Instructor shall define grades for each point range earned on completion of each performance-evaluated task.

Performance Standards

The minimum number of satisfactory performances required before final evaluation is _____.

Instructor shall identify by * those steps considered critical. If a step is missed or minimum competency is not met, the evaluated procedure fails and must be repeated.

PERFORMANCE CRITERIA	*	SELF	PEER	INSTRUCTOR	COMMENT
1. Washed and dried hands.					
2. Positioned the surgical tray and placed the sterile pack.					
3. Opened the outer wrapping in a direction away from the assistant.					
4. Held the outside flaps open and allowed the sterile contents to fall on the tray.					
5. Added items to the field.					
ADDITIONAL COMMENTS					

Total number of points earned _____

Grade _____ Instructor's initials _____

COMPETENCY 56.2: PERFORMING A SURGICAL SCRUB

Performance Objective

By following a routine procedure that meets stated protocols, the student will demonstrate the proper procedure for performing a surgical scrub for a sterile surgical procedure.

Evaluation and Grading Criteria

3	Student competently met the stated criteria without assistance.
2	Student required assistance in order to meet the stated criteria.
1	Student showed uncertainty when performing the stated criteria.
0	Student was not prepared and needs to repeat the step.
N/A	No evaluation of this step.

Instructor shall define grades for each point range earned on completion of each performance-evaluated task.

Performance Standards

The minimum number of satisfactory performances required before final evaluation is _____.

Instructor shall identify by * those steps considered critical. If a step is missed or minimum competency is not met, the evaluated procedure fails and must be repeated.

PERFORMANCE CRITERIA	*	SELF	PEER	INSTRUCTOR	COMMENT
1. Wet the hands and forearms with warm water.					
2. Placed antimicrobial soap on hands.					
3. Scrubbed each side of each finger, between the fingers, and the back and front of both hands.					
4. Proceeded to scrub the arms, keeping the hands higher than the arms at all times.					
5. Washed each side of each arm to 3 inches above the elbow.					
6. Rinsed the hands and arms by passing them through the water in one direction only, from the fingertips to elbow.					
7. Accomplished washing in 7 minutes.					
8. Dried the hands using a sterile disposable towel.					
9. Placed personal protective equipment according to the procedure.					

ADDITIONAL COMMENTS

Total number of points earned _____

Grade _____ Instructor's initials _____

COMPETENCY 56.3: PERFORMING STERILE GLOVING

Performance Objective

By following a routine procedure that meets stated protocols, the student will demonstrate the proper procedure for gloving with the use of a sterile technique.

Evaluation and Grading Criteria

 3   Student competently met the stated criteria without assistance.

 2   Student required assistance in order to meet the stated criteria.

 1   Student showed uncertainty when performing the stated criteria.

 0   Student was not prepared and needs to repeat the step.

 N/A   No evaluation of this step.

Instructor shall define grades for each point range earned on completion of each performance-evaluated task.

Performance Standards

The minimum number of satisfactory performances required before final evaluation is _____.

Instructor shall identify by * those steps considered critical. If a step is missed or minimum competency is not met, the evaluated procedure fails and must be repeated.

PERFORMANCE CRITERIA	*	SELF	PEER	INSTRUCTOR	COMMENT
1. Opened the glove package before the surgical scrub.					
2. Touched only the inside of the package after the surgical scrub.					
3. Gloved the dominant hand first, touching only the folded cuff.					
4. Placed the other glove on, touching only the sterile portion of the glove with the dominant hand.					
5. Unrolled the cuff from the gloves.					

ADDITIONAL COMMENTS

Total number of points earned _____

Grade _____ Instructor's initials _____

COMPETENCIES 56.4 TO 56.6: ASSISTING IN SURGICAL EXTRACTION

Performance Objective

By following a routine procedure that meets stated protocols, when provided with information concerning the type of surgery, the tooth, and the anesthetics to be used, the student will prepare the setup, prepare the patient, and assist in a surgical procedure.

Evaluation and Grading Criteria

_3_	Student competently met the stated criteria without assistance.
_2_	Student required assistance in order to meet the stated criteria.
_1_	Student showed uncertainty when performing the stated criteria.
_0_	Student was not prepared and needs to repeat the step.
_N/A_	No evaluation of this step.

Instructor shall define grades for each point range earned on completion of each performance-evaluated task.

Performance Standards

The minimum number of satisfactory performances required before final evaluation is _____.

Instructor shall identify by * those steps considered critical. If a step is missed or minimum competency is not met, the evaluated procedure fails and must be repeated.

PERFORMANCE CRITERIA	*	SELF	PEER	INSTRUCTOR	COMMENT
Preparing the Treatment Room					
1. Prepared the treatment room.					
2. Kept instruments in their sterile wraps until ready for use; if a surgical tray was preset, opened the tray and placed a sterile towel over the instruments.					
3. Placed the appropriate local anesthetic on the tray.					
4. Placed the appropriate forceps on the tray.					
Preparing the Patient					
1. Seated the patient and positioned a sterile patient drape or towel.					
2. Took the patient's vital signs and recorded them in the patient record.					
3. Adjusted the dental chair to the proper position.					
4. Stayed with the patient until the dentist entered the treatment room.					

Continued

During the Surgical Procedure					
1. Placed personal protective equipment according to the procedure.					
2. Maintained the chain of asepsis.					
3. Monitored vital signs.					
4. Aspirated and retracted as needed.					
5. Transferred and received instruments as needed.					
6. Assisted in suture placement as needed.					
7. Maintained a clear operating field with adequate light and irrigation.					
8. Steadied the patient's head and mandible if necessary.					
9. Observed the patient's condition and anticipated the dentist's needs.					
10. Provided postoperative instructions for the patient.					
11. Maintained patient comfort and followed appropriate infection control measures throughout the procedure.					
12. Documented the procedure in the patient record.					

ADDITIONAL COMMENTS

Total number of points earned _____

Grade _____ Instructor's initials _____

COMPETENCY 56.7: ASSISTING IN SUTURE PLACEMENT

Performance Objective

By following a routine procedure that meets stated protocols, the student will demonstrate the proper procedure for assisting the surgeon in suture placement.

Evaluation and Grading Criteria

 3   Student competently met the stated criteria without assistance.

 2   Student required assistance in order to meet the stated criteria.

 1   Student showed uncertainty when performing the stated criteria.

 0   Student was not prepared and needs to repeat the step.

 N/A   No evaluation of this step.

Instructor shall define grades for each point range earned on completion of each performance-evaluated task.

Performance Standards

The minimum number of satisfactory performances required before final evaluation is _____.

Instructor shall identify by * those steps considered critical. If a step is missed or minimum competency is not met, the evaluated procedure fails and must be repeated.

PERFORMANCE CRITERIA	*	SELF	PEER	INSTRUCTOR	COMMENT
1. Placed personal protective equipment according to the procedure.					
2. Removed the suture material from the sterile package.					
3. Clamped the suture needle at the upper third.					
4. Transferred the needle holder to the surgeon.					
5. Retracted during suture placement.					
6. Cut the suture where indicated by the surgeon.					
7. Placed the suture material on the tray.					
8. Recorded the numbers and types of sutures placed in the patient record.					
ADDITIONAL COMMENTS					

Total number of points earned _____

Grade _____ Instructor's initials _____

COMPETENCY 56.8: PERFORMING SUTURE REMOVAL (EXPANDED FUNCTION)

Performance Objective

By following a routine procedure that meets stated protocols, the student will demonstrate the proper procedure for removing sutures.

Evaluation and Grading Criteria

 3   Student competently met the stated criteria without assistance.

 2   Student required assistance in order to meet the stated criteria.

 1   Student showed uncertainty when performing the stated criteria.

 0   Student was not prepared and needs to repeat the step.

 N/A No evaluation of this step.

Instructor shall define grades for each point range earned on completion of each performance-evaluated task.

Performance Standards

The minimum number of satisfactory performances required before final evaluation is _____.

Instructor shall identify by * those steps considered critical. If a step is missed or minimum competency is not met, the evaluated procedure fails and must be repeated.

PERFORMANCE CRITERIA	*	SELF	PEER	INSTRUCTOR	COMMENT
1. Confirmed with surgeon the removal of sutures placed at the extraction site.					
2. Set out the instruments correctly.					
3. Placed personal protective equipment according to the procedure.					
4. Wiped the area with an antiseptic agent.					
5. Held the suture away from the tissue with cotton pliers.					
6. Cut the suture with suture scissors, ensuring that the scissors were lying flat near the tissue.					
7. Grasped the knot with cotton pliers and removed it, keeping it away from the tissue.					
8. Counted the number of sutures removed and recorded the total in the patient record.					

Continued

9. Maintained patient comfort and followed appropriate infection control measures throughout the procedure.				
10. Documented the procedure in the patient record.				
ADDITIONAL COMMENTS				

Total number of points earned _____

Grade _____ Instructor's initials _____

COMPETENCY 56.9: ASSISTING IN THE TREATMENT OF ALVEOLAR OSTEITIS

Performance Objective

By following a routine procedure that meets stated protocols, the student will assist the surgeon in the treatment of alveolitis.

Evaluation and Grading Criteria

__3__   Student competently met the stated criteria without assistance.

__2__   Student required assistance in order to meet the stated criteria.

__1__   Student showed uncertainty when performing the stated criteria.

__0__   Student was not prepared and needs to repeat the step.

__N/A__   No evaluation of this step.

Note: In some states, it is legal for the dental assistant to perform this procedure.

Instructor shall define grades for each point range earned on completion of each performance-evaluated task.

Performance Standards

The minimum number of satisfactory performances required before final evaluation is _____.

Instructor shall identify by * those steps considered critical. If a step is missed or minimum competency is not met, the evaluated procedure fails and must be repeated.

PERFORMANCE CRITERIA	*	SELF	PEER	INSTRUCTOR	COMMENT
1. Gathered the appropriate setup.					
2. Placed personal protective equipment according to the procedure.					
3. Assisted the dentist in irrigating the site with a saline solution.					
4. Prepared a strip of iodoform gauze in the appropriate length.					
5. Transferred the gauze with medication to the site to be packed.					
6. Retrieved the prescription pad and pen for surgeon to prescribe analgesics and antibiotics.					
7. Provided postoperative instructions to the patient.					
8. Documented the procedure in the patient record.					

ADDITIONAL COMMENTS

Total number of points earned _____

Grade _____ Instructor's initials _____

57 Pediatric Dentistry

SHORT-ANSWER QUESTIONS

1. Describe the appearance and layout of a pediatric dental office.

2. List the stages of development according to Erikson from birth through adolescence.

3. Discuss the specific behavioral techniques that work as a positive reinforcement in the treatment of children.

4. Describe why children and adults with certain special needs would be seen in a pediatric practice.

5. List what would be included in the clinical examination of a pediatric patient.

6. Discuss the importance of preventive dentistry in pediatrics.

7. Compare the clinical procedures for treating pediatric patients to adults.

FILL-IN-THE-BLANK STATEMENTS

Select the best term from the list below and complete the following statements.

autonomy	mouth guard
cerebral palsy	chronologic age
Down's syndrome	neural
athetosis	open bay
extrusion	protective stabilization
Frankl scale	pediatric dentistry
intellectual disability	postnatal
intrusion	prenatal
avulsed	pulpotomy
mental age	T-band

1. _____ is a neural disorder or loss of motor function caused by brain damage.

2. A child's actual age is the _____.

3. _____ is the process of being independent.

4. A tooth that has been torn away or dislodged by force is said to be _____.

5. _____ is a disorder caused by a chromosomal defect.

6. _____ is a term used to describe involuntary movement of the body, face, arms, and legs.

7. _____ occurs when teeth are displaced from their position in the mouth.

8. When a tooth has been pushed into the socket as a result of injury, it is _____.

9. The _____ is a type of matrix used for primary teeth.

10. Wearing a(n) _____ is recommended to a child playing certain sports to protect the dentition.

11. The child's _____ is his or her level of intellectual capacity and development.

12. The _____ is a measurement designed to evaluate behavior.

13. The specialty of dentistry concerned with infants through adolescent and special needs patients is _____.

14. _____ means after birth.

15. _____ is a disorder in which an individual's intelligence is underdeveloped.

16. Another term for referring to the brain, nervous system, and nerve pathways is _____.

17. _____ is a concept of layout used in pediatric dental practices.

18. A(n) _____ is a type of confining device used to hold the hands, arms, and legs still.

19. A(n) _____ is a dental procedure in which the coronal portion of the dental pulp is removed.

20. _____ means before birth.

MULTIPLE-CHOICE QUESTIONS

Complete each question by circling the best answer.

1. How long will a pediatric dentist continue his or her education after dental school?
   a. 1-2 years
   b. 2-3 years
   c. 3-4 years
   d. 4-5 years

2. What is unique about the treatment areas of a pediatric practice?
   a. The dental chairs are close together.
   b. More than one dentist can use a treatment area.
   c. Many are designed with the open-bay concept.
   d. There are chairs for parents.

3. Describe the types of patients seen in a pediatric practice.
   a. Healthy adolescents
   b. Special needs children
   c. Special needs adults
   d. All the above

4. You are describing a child's _____ when a 10-year-old is behaving like a 6-year-old.
   a. chronologic age
   b. emotional age
   c. physical age
   d. size

5. At what stage of life does a child first want control and structure in his or her environment?
   a. 1 to 3 years of age
   b. 3 to 5 years of age
   c. 6 to 9 years of age
   d. 9 to 12 years of age

6. How would Dr. Frankl describe a positive child?
   a. Accepts treatment
   b. Is willing to comply
   c. Follows directions
   d. All the above

7. Which of the following is a device that can be used to gently restrain pediatric patients?
   a. T-band
   b. Protective stabilization
   c. Frankl scale
   d. Open bay

8. Which of the following is a limitation in children who are mentally challenged?
   a. Physical ability
   b. Speech
   c. IQ
   d. b and c

9. Another name for Down's syndrome is _____.
   a. trisomy 21
   b. mentally challenged
   c. cerebral palsy
   d. learning disorder

10. Cerebral palsy is a non-progressive neural disorder caused by _____.
    a. a chromosomal defect
    b. a stroke
    c. brain damage
    d. an overdose

11. When should children first see a dentist for regular examinations?
    a. When they first start solid foods
    b. When they say their first words
    c. When their first tooth erupts
    d. When they have teeth visible in both their maxilla and mandible

12. How often are radiographs recommended to be taken in a child with a high risk of decay?
    a. Monthly
    b. Every six months
    c. Once a year
    d. Before each tooth is restored

13. Fluoride varnish is applied as _____.
    a. direct gel
    b. a rinse
    c. an application in trays
    d. an application in toothpaste

14. What procedure is recommended to protect the pits and fissures of posterior teeth?
    a. Pulpotomy
    b. Fluoride rinse
    c. Coronal polishing
    d. Sealants

15. At what phase of orthodontics would a pediatric dentist intercede in getting a patient to stop sucking his or her thumb?
    a. Interceptive
    b. Preventive
    c. Corrective
    d. Elective

16. If your patient plays soccer, would you recommend that he or she wears a mouth guard?
    a. No
    b. Yes

17. What type of matrix is used on primary teeth?
    a. Metal contoured
    b. T-band
    c. Tofflemire
    d. b and c

18. What endodontic procedure is performed on a primary molar
    a. Apicoectomy
    b. Pulpectomy
    c. Pulpotomy
    d. Retrograde

19. Would a child be referred to a prosthodontist for the placement of a stainless steel crown?
    a. Yes
    b. No

20. In children, which teeth are most commonly injured?
    a. Mandibular anterior
    b. Mandibular posterior
    c. Maxillary anterior
    d. Maxillary posterior

21. When a tooth is avulsed, it has _____.
    a. been fractured
    b. come out
    c. been pushed back into the socket
    d. become loose

555

22. How would the dentist stabilize a tooth after an avulsion?
    a. With a temporary splint
    b. With a thermoplastic resin tray
    c. With wax
    d. With sutures

23. Who in the dental office is legally required to report child abuse?
    a. Dental assistant
    b. Business assistant
    c. Dental hygienist
    d. Dentist

24. What could be a possible sign of child abuse?
    a. Chipped or fractured teeth
    b. Bruises
    c. Scars on the lips or tongue
    d. All the above

25. What organization should be contacted if someone suspects child abuse?
    a. American Dental Association
    b. Child Protective Services of the Public Health Department
    c. Local hospital
    d. Pediatric Dental Association

CASE STUDY

Ashley is a 12-year-old patient of the practice who is being seen as an emergency patient. Ashley was hit in the face while playing intramural basketball. Her maxillary central incisors were knocked back into the sockets.

1. Your schedule is filled for the day, when would you instruct Ashley to come in for an emergency visit?

2. What type of examination techniques is to be used to enable the dentist to make a correct diagnosis of the complexity of the damage to the teeth and surrounding area?

3. What is the diagnosis when a person's teeth are knocked inward?

4. Would Ashley's maxillary central incisors be her primary or permanent central incisors?

5. What letter or number would those teeth be noted on a charting form?

6. What form of treatment would be provided for Ashley?

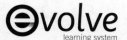

Access the *Interactive Dental Office* on the *Evolve* website and click on the patient case file for Raul Ortega, Jr.
- Review Raul's record.
- Complete all exercises on the website for Raul's case.
- Answer the following questions.

1. What teeth are visible on Raul's maxillary occlusal film?

2. Could the absence of fluoridated water be the reason for Raul's having baby bottle mouth syndrome?

3. What is the normal age range for the eruption of permanent first molars?

4. Would the placement of a stainless steel crown in Raul be considered an expanded function for the dental assistant?

5. Is the cement used for cementation of the stainless steel crown permanent or temporary?

COMPETENCY 57.1: ASSISTING IN PULPOTOMY OF A PRIMARY TOOTH

Performance Objective

By following a routine procedure that meets stated protocols, the student will demonstrate the proper technique when assisting in the pulpotomy of a primary tooth.

Evaluation and Grading Criteria

 3   Student competently met the stated criteria without assistance.

 2   Student required assistance in order to meet the stated criteria.

 1   Student showed uncertainty when performing the stated criteria.

 0   Student was not prepared and needs to repeat the step.

 N/A   No evaluation of this step.

Instructor shall define grades for each point range earned on completion of each performance-evaluated task.

Performance Standards

The minimum number of satisfactory performances required before final evaluation is _____.

Instructor shall identify by * those steps considered critical. If a step is missed or minimum competency is not met, the evaluated procedure fails and must be repeated.

PERFORMANCE CRITERIA	*	SELF	PEER	INSTRUCTOR	COMMENT
1. Gathered the appropriate setup.					
2. Placed personal protective equipment according to the procedure.					
3. Assisted in the administration of the local anesthetic.					
4. Assisted in placement of, or placed dental dam.					
5. Assisted in removal of dental caries; used an HVE and air-water syringe during removal.					
6. Transferred instruments throughout the procedure.					
7. Prepared formocresol and cotton pellet, and transferred when needed.					
8. Mixed ZOE for a base and transferred it to be placed.					

Continued

9. Maintained patient comfort and followed appropriate infection control measures throughout the procedure.					
10. Documented the procedure in the patient record.					
ADDITIONAL COMMENTS					

Total number of points earned _____

Grade _____ Instructor's initials _____

COMPETENCY 57.2: ASSISTING IN PLACEMENT OF A STAINLESS STEEL CROWN

Performance Objective

By following a routine procedure that meets stated protocols, the student will demonstrate the proper technique when assisting in the preparation and placement of a stainless steel crown.

Evaluation and Grading Criteria

3   Student competently met the stated criteria without assistance.

2   Student required assistance in order to meet the stated criteria.

1   Student showed uncertainty when performing the stated criteria.

0   Student was not prepared and needs to repeat the step.

N/A   No evaluation of this step.

Instructor shall define grades for each point range earned on completion of each performance-evaluated task.

Performance Standards

The minimum number of satisfactory performances required before final evaluation is _____.

Instructor shall identify by * those steps considered critical. If a step is missed or minimum competency is not met, the evaluated procedure fails and must be repeated.

PERFORMANCE CRITERIA	*	SELF	PEER	INSTRUCTOR	COMMENT
1. Gathered the appropriate setup.					
2. Placed personal protective equipment according to the procedure.					
3. Assisted in the administration of the local anesthetic.					
4. Assisted in the sizing of the stainless steel crown.					
5. Transferred instruments as requested in the transfer zone.					
6. Assisted in trimming and contouring of the stainless steel crown.					
7. Prepared cement and assisted in the cementation of the stainless steel crown.					
8. Maintained patient comfort and followed appropriate infection control measures throughout the procedure.					
9. Documented the procedure in the patient record.					

ADDITIONAL COMMENTS

Total number of points earned _____

Grade _____ Instructor's initials _____

COMPETENCY 5.2 ASSISTING IN PLACEMENT OF A STAINLESS STEEL CROWN

Performance Objective

By following a routine procedure that includes stated protocols, the student will demonstrate the proper techniques when assisting in the preparation and placement of a stainless steel crown.

Evaluation and Grading Criteria

3   Student consistently met the stated criteria without assistance.

2   Student required assistance in order to meet the stated criteria.

1   Student was unable to demonstrate when performing the stated criteria.

0   Student was not prepared and needs to repeat the skill.

N/A   Not applicable for this step.

In the space provided, for each point earned, rate the completion of each performance criterion task.

Performance Standards

A minimum number of satisfactory performances required is one (1) unassisted.

Instructor shall identify by * those steps considered critical. If a step is missed or performed incorrectly, competency is not met and the procedure must be stopped and then repeated.

PERFORMANCE CRITERIA	SELF	PEER	INSTRUCTOR	COMMENT
1. Gathered the appropriate setup.				
2. Placed patient in a protective napkin according to the procedure.				
3. Assisted in the administration of the local anesthetic.				
4. Assisted in the selection of the stainless steel crown.				
5. Transferred instruments as required in the procedure.				
6. Assisted in trimming and contouring if necessary, step by step.				
7. Prepared, mixed, and assisted in the placement of the stainless steel crown.				
8. Mixed the cement, loaded the crown, and assisted in the placement during the cementation process.				
9. Dismissed the patient according to the procedure.				

ADDITIONAL COMMENTS

Instructor's signature _____

Date _____

58 Coronal Polishing

SHORT-ANSWER QUESTIONS

1. Explain the difference between a prophylaxis and coronal polishing.

2. Give the indications and contraindications to coronal polishing.

3. Name and describe the types of extrinsic stains.

4. Name and describe the two categories of intrinsic stains.

5. Describe the types of abrasives used for polishing teeth.

6. Discuss considerations when polishing esthetic-type restorations.

FILL-IN-THE-BLANK STATEMENTS

Select the best term from the list below and complete the following statements.
extrinsic stains

fulcrum
calculus
intrinsic stains

oral prophylaxis
rubber cup polishing
clinical crown

1. _____ is a hard, mineralized deposit attached to the teeth.

2. A(n) _____ is the complete removal of calculus, debris, stain, and plaque from the teeth.

3. The portion of the tooth that is visible in the oral cavity is the _____.

4. _____ occurs within the tooth structure and can not be removed by polishing.

5. _____ occurs on the external surfaces of the teeth and can be removed by polishing.

6. The _____ is a position that provides stability for the operator.

7. _____ is a technique used to remove plaque and stains from the coronal surfaces of teeth.

MULTIPLE-CHOICE QUESTIONS

Complete each question by circling the best answer.

1. The purpose of coronal polishing is to
   _____.
   a. Remove calculus
   b. Remove stains and plaque
   c. Prepare teeth for a restoration
   d. Remove inflamed gingiva

2. An oral prophylaxis includes which of the following.
   a. fluoride treatment
   b. removal of calculus and debris
   c. examination
   d. removal of decay

3. The purpose of selective polishing is to
   _____.
   a. polish only teeth that are visible
   b. polish the occlusal surfaces of teeth
   c. polish only teeth with stain
   d. polish the facial surfaces of teeth

4. Stains that may be removed from the surfaces of the
   teeth are _____.
   a. extrinsic
   b. natural
   c. intrinsic
   d. infected

5. Stains that cannot be removed from the teeth are
   _____.
   a. extrinsic
   b. natural
   c. intrinsic
   d. infected

6. Which is the most recommended technique for stain removal?
   a. Using a scaler
   b. Using a toothbrush
   c. Using floss
   d. Rubber cup polishing

7. The recommended grasp for the low-speed handpiece
   is the _____.
   a. reverse-palm grasp
   b. pen grasp
   c. thumb-to-nose grasp
   d. palm grasp

8. The purpose of a fulcrum is to _____.
   a. provide pressure to the fingers
   b. provide better retraction
   c. provide stability to the hand
   d. provide movement for the arm

9. What precaution is taken when using a bristle brush?
   a. Not to allow the brush to get dry
   b. Not to traumatize the tissue
   c. Not to wear away enamel
   d. Not to use on occlusal surfaces

10. Which tooth surface should coronal polishing begin on?
    a. Occlusal surface of most anterior
    b. Distal surface of most anterior
    c. Occlusal surface of most posterior
    d. Distal surface of most posterior

11. What can result from using the prophy angle at a high speed?
    a. It can cause frictional heat.
    b. It can remove dentin.
    c. It can cool the tooth.
    d. It can etch enamel.

12. The patient's head is positioned _____ for access to the maxillary anterior teeth.
    a. chin downward
    b. head turned to the right
    c. chin upward
    d. head turned to the left

CASE STUDY

As a practicing dental assistant in a busy pediatric office, your daily schedule can include performing coronal polish on 8 to 10 children. You see a variety of conditions in their mouths.

1. Describe what specific procedures you would be responsible for while performing a coronal polish.

2. Is it possible for a pediatric practice to have a dental hygienist? If so, why?

3. Because you work with children, what contraindications would prevent you from completing a coronal polish in a patient?

4. During the evaluation of a recall patient, you notice calculus on the lingual surfaces of the lower anteriors. What should you do?

5. Would calculus be removed before the coronal polishing or after?

MULTIMEDIA PROCEDURES RECOMMENDED REVIEW

Ɵvolve
learning system

- Coronal Polishing

COMPETENCY 58.1: RUBBER CUP CORONAL POLISHING (EXPANDED FUNCTION)

Performance Objective

By following a routine procedure that meets stated protocols, in states where coronal polishing by a dental assistant is legal, the student will demonstrate the proper procedure for a complete mouth coronal polish.

Evaluation and Grading Criteria

3	Student competently met the stated criteria without assistance.
2	Student required assistance in order to meet the stated criteria.
1	Student showed uncertainty when performing the stated criteria.
0	Student was not prepared and needs to repeat the step.
N/A	No evaluation of this step.

Instructor shall define grades for each point range earned on completion of each performance-evaluated task.

Performance Standards

The minimum number of satisfactory performances required before final evaluation is_____.

Instructor shall identify by * those steps considered critical. If a step is missed or minimum competency is not met, the evaluated procedure fails and must be repeated.

PERFORMANCE CRITERIA	*	SELF	PEER	INSTRUCTOR	COMMENT
1. Gathered appropriate supplies.					
2. Placed personal protective equipment according to the procedure.					
3. Prepared the patient and explained the procedure.					
4. Maintained the correct operator position and posture for each quadrant.					
5. Maintained adequate retraction and an appropriate fulcrum for each quadrant.					
6. Used the rubber polishing cup and abrasive with the proper polishing movements in all quadrants.					
7. Used the bristle brush and abrasive properly in all quadrants.					
8. Controlled the handpiece speed and pressure throughout the procedure while maintaining patient safety and comfort.					
9. Flossed between the patient's teeth.					

Continued

10. Rinsed the patient's mouth.				
11. Evaluated the coronal polish; repeated steps as necessary.				
12. Maintained patient comfort and followed appropriate infection control measures throughout the procedure.				
13. Documented the procedure in the patient record.				

ADDITIONAL COMMENTS

Total number of points earned _____

Grade _____ Instructor's initials _____

59 Dental Sealants

SHORT-ANSWER QUESTIONS

1. Describe the objective of dental sealants.

2. List the clinical indications for dental sealants?

3. List the clinical contraindications to dental sealants?

4. Discuss the differences between filled and unfilled sealant materials.

5. Give the two types of polymerization for sealant material.

6. List the steps in the application of dental sealants.

7. Describe the safety steps necessary for the patient and the operator during sealant placement.

8. What is the most important factor in sealant retention?

FILL-IN-THE-BLANK STATEMENTS

Select the best term from the list below and complete the following statements.

light-cured
dental sealant
microleakage
polymerization
acrylate

retention
self-cured
unfilled resin
microabrasion

1. Resin material applied to the pits and fissures of teeth is a(n) _____.

2. _____ is a chemical reaction that changes a fluid substance to a hard substance

3. A type of resin material that is polymerized by a chemical reaction is _____.

4. A type of resin material that is polymerized by a curing light is _____.

5. A technique that prepares the enamel surface prior to the placement of sealant material is _____.

6. _____ is a sealant material that does not contain filler particles.

7. _____ is a movement of bacteria and oral fluids at the border of tooth structure or margin of the sealant or restoration.

8. _____ is a component of acid etchant material.

9. The sealant firmly adheres to the tooth surface because of _____.

MULTIPLE-CHOICE QUESTIONS

Complete each question by circling the best answer.

1. The purpose of dental sealants is to _____.
   a. prevent decay from spreading
   b. prevent decay in pits and fissures of teeth
   c. promote good oral health
   d. prevent decay in interproximal spaces

2. Why are pits and fissures susceptible to caries?
   a. Saliva pools in these areas.
   b. Fluoride is less effective in these areas.
   c. These areas are difficult to clean.
   d. b and c

3. Are sealants the main preventive measure prescribed by the dentist?
   a. Yes
   b. No

4. What are the ways for sealant materials to harden?
   a. Polymerization
   b. Light curing
   c. Self-curing
   d. All of the above

5. Why is clear sealant material less desirable?
   a. It is less attractive.
   b. It is more difficult to evaluate.
   c. It does not match tooth color.
   d. It is contraindicated with dental restorations.

6. What is the difference between filled and unfilled sealants regarding retention rates?
   a. There is no difference.
   b. Filled sealants are much stronger.
   c. Unfilled sealants will last longer.
   d. The filler is weaker.

7. Sealants are placed _____.
   a. in pits and fissures
   b. on cingula
   c. in grooves
   d. on marginal ridges

8. What is the range of shelf life for a sealant material?
   a. 3 to 6 months
   b. 6 to 12 months
   c. 18 to 36 months
   d. Indefinite

9. What patient safety precautions should be considered when placing the etchant?
   a. Keep the etchant off the soft tissue.
   b. Use only after the patient has been anesthetized.
   c. Have the patient wear eyewear.
   d. a and c

10. What is the main cause of sealant failures?
    a. Polymerization
    b. Moisture contamination
    c. Deep pits and fissures
    d. Occlusion interference

Cindy Evans is an 8-year-old patient who is scheduled for placement of sealants on all of her molars. Dr. Allen is running behind and has told you to go ahead with the placement and to call her if you have any questions.

1. What must Dr. Allen complete before you can begin the procedure?

2. How many teeth will receive sealants today?

3. What type of moisture control will you use?

4. Describe your plan for preparation and placement of sealants.

5. After placement, Cindy says when she closes her teeth they "feel funny". What is wrong and how is this corrected?

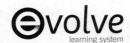
- Applying Dental Sealants

Access the *Interactive Dental Office* on the *Evolve* website and click on the patient case file for Todd Ledbetter.
- Review Todd's record.
- Complete all exercises on the website for Todd's case.
- Answer the following questions.

1. Which of Todd's teeth are going to have dental sealants?

2. Why did Dr. Roberts not recommend sealants for Todd's anterior teeth?

3. Identify the materials in the sealant setup.

Access the *Interactive Dental Office* on the *Evolve* website and click on the patient case file for Christopher Brooks.
- Review Christopher's record.
- Complete all exercises on the website for Christopher's case.
- Answer the following questions.

4. Which of Christopher's teeth are going to have dental sealants?

5. What type of moisture control is used during sealant placement?

6. Before the sealants are placed, how should the teeth be cleaned?

7. What should be done if Christopher accidentally contaminates the conditioned surface of a tooth with his saliva?

COMPETENCY 59.1: APPLICATION OF DENTAL SEALANTS (EXPANDED FUNCTION)

Performance Objective

By following a routine procedure that meets stated protocols, in states where application of dental sealants by a dental assistant is legal, the student will demonstrate the proper procedure for applying pit-and-fissure sealants.

Evaluation and Grading Criteria

<u>3</u>   Student competently met the stated criteria without assistance.

<u>2</u>   Student required assistance in order to meet the stated criteria.

<u>1</u>   Student showed uncertainty when performing the stated criteria.

<u>0</u>   Student was not prepared and needs to repeat the step.

<u>N/A</u>   No evaluation of this step.

Instructor shall define grades for each point range earned on completion of each performance-evaluated task.

Performance Standards

The minimum number of satisfactory performances required before final evaluation is _____.

Instructor shall identify by * those steps considered critical. If a step is missed or minimum competency is not met, the evaluated procedure fails and must be repeated.

PERFORMANCE CRITERIA	*	SELF	PEER	INSTRUCTOR	COMMENT
1. Gathered appropriate supplies.					
2. Placed personal protective equipment according to the procedure.					
3. Seated the patient and explained the procedure.					
4. Polished the teeth to be treated.					
5. Used appropriate steps to prevent contamination by moisture or saliva.					
6. Placed the etching agent on the appropriate surfaces for the time specified by the manufacturer.					
7. Rinsed and dried the teeth and then verified the appearance of the etched surfaces. If the appearance was not satisfactory, etched the surfaces again.					
8. Placed the sealant on the etched surfaces.					
9. Light-cured the material according to the manufacturer's instructions.					
10. Examined the application with an explorer for discrepancy in the material.					

Continued

11. Wiped the sealant with a cotton applicator to remove the thin film on the surface. Checked occlusion using articulation paper and instructed the dentist to make adjustments as necessary.				
12. Asked the dentist to evaluate the result before the patient was dismissed.				
13. Maintained patient comfort and followed appropriate infection control measures throughout the procedure.				
14. Documented the procedure in the patient record.				
ADDITIONAL COMMENTS				

Total number of points earned _____

Grade _____ Instructor's initials _____

60 Orthodontics

SHORT-ANSWER QUESTIONS

1. Describe the environment of an orthodontic practice.

2. List the three types of malocclusion.

3. Discuss corrective orthodontics and what types of treatment are involved.

4. List the types of diagnostic records used to assess orthodontic problems.

5. Describe the components of the fixed appliance.

6. Describe the use and function of headgear.

7. Describe how you would convey to the patient and/or parent(s) the importance of dietary and good oral hygiene habits to orthodontic treatment.

FILL-IN-THE-BLANK STATEMENTS

Select the best term from the list below and complete the following statements.

open bite	separator
band	distoclusion
ligature tie	auxiliary
positioner	fetal molding
braces	headgear
bracket	mesioclusion
cephalometric	orthodontics
arch wire	overbite
cross-bite	retainer
dentofacial	
overjet	

1. A(n) _____ is a stainless steel ring cemented to molars to hold the arch wire for orthodontics.

2. A common term used for fixed orthodontics is _____.

3. A(n) _____ is a small device bonded to teeth to hold the arch wire in place.

4. A(n) _____ is used to secure the arch wire within a bracket.

5. A(n) _____ attachment is located on either a bracket or a band to hold an arch wire or elastic in place.

6. A preformed metal wire that provides the force to guide teeth into position for orthodontics is a(n) _____.

7. A(n) _____ is a device used to wedge molars open before fitting and placement of orthodontic bands.

8. A(n) _____ is a condition that occurs when the maxillary teeth are not properly aligned with the mandibular teeth.

9. _____ is another term for class III malocclusion.

10. An extraoral radiograph of the bones and tissues of the head is a(n) _____ radiographic image.

11. _____ is another term used for class II malocclusion.

12. An extraoral orthodontic appliance used to control growth and tooth movement is _____.

13. An appliance used to maintain the set position of teeth and jaws after orthodontic treatment is a(n) _____.

14. The excessive protrusion of the maxillary incisors is diagnosed as _____.

15. A _____ is the lack of vertical overlap of the maxillary incisors that creates an opening between the anterior teeth.

16. The specialty of dentistry designed to prevent, intercept, and correct skeletal and dental problems is _____.

17. _____ is a term that describes the structures of the teeth, jaws, and surrounding facial bones.

18. A(n) _____ is a removable appliance used during the final stage of orthodontic treatment to retain teeth in their desired position.

19. An increased vertical overlap of the maxillary incisors is a(n) _____.

20. _____ can occur when pressure is applied to the jaw in vitro, which could cause a distortion.

Complete each question by circling the best answer.

1. Individuals in what age group seek orthodontic care?
   a. Adolescents
   b. Teenagers
   c. Adults
   d. All the above

2. What could be a genetic cause for malocclusion?
   a. Parent with a small jaw
   b. Ectopic eruption
   c. Fetal molding
   d. Thumb sucking

3. What is the term used for abnormal occlusion?
   a. Distoclusion
   b. Mesioclusion
   c. Malocclusion
   d. Facial occlusion

4. What tooth is used to determine a person's occlusion?
   a. Maxillary central incisor
   b. Mandibular first premolar
   c. Mandibular first molar
   d. Maxillary first molar

5. If a person's tooth is not properly aligned with its opposing tooth, the malalignment is referred to as
   _____.
   a. overjet
   b. cross-bite
   c. open bite
   d. overbite

6. If a person occludes his or her teeth and the mandibular anterior teeth are not visible, the diagnosis is
   _____.
   a. overjet
   b. cross-bite
   c. open bite
   d. overbite

7. What views will the orthodontist use to evaluate facial symmetry?
   a. Frontal view
   b. Distal view
   c. Profile view
   d. a and c

8. What type of radiograph is most commonly exposed in orthodontics?
   a. Periapical
   b. Cephalometric
   c. Occlusal
   d. Bitewing

9. What is the minimum number of photographs taken in the diagnostic records appointment?
   a. Two
   b. Four
   c. Five
   d. Six

10. What gypsum material is most commonly used for fabricating orthodontic diagnostic models?
    a. Plaster
    b. Stone
    c. Alginate
    d. Polyether

11. The instrument used for seating a mandibular molar band is the _____.
    a. Howe pliers
    b. bite stick
    c. explorer
    d. hemostat

12. The orthodontic scaler is used for _____.
    a. removing excess material from around bands and brackets
    b. placing separators
    c. tying in arch wires
    d. a and b

13. Another name for #110 pliers is _____.
    a. contouring pliers
    b. Howe pliers
    c. Weingart pliers
    d. band-removing pliers

14. To ease the placement of orthodontic bands, what procedure is completed to open the contact between specific teeth?
    a. Wearing of a positioner
    b. Placement of a ligature tie
    c. Bonding of a bracket
    d. Placement of a separator

15. During cementation of bands, what can be used to keep cement from getting into the buccal tubes or attachments?
    a. String
    b. Lip balm
    c. Utility wax
    d. b and c

16. How is a bracket adhered to a tooth?
    a. Cement
    b. Sealant
    c. Bonding agent
    d. Wax

577

17. Where are auxiliary attachments found on braces?
    a. Brackets
    b. Arch wire
    c. Bands
    d. a and c

18. What shape of arch wire is indicated for correcting the initial stages of malalignment of teeth?
    a. Round wire
    b. Rectangular wire
    c. Braided wire
    d. Twisted wire

19. What would be used to size an arch wire for a patient that does not involve placing the wire in the patient's mouth?
    a. Cephalometric radiograph
    b. Study model
    c. Used arch wire
    d. b and c

20. Besides ligature ties, what can be used to hold an arch wire in place?
    a. Cement
    b. Elastomeric ties
    c. Wax
    d. Positioner

21. What appliance might the orthodontist use to maintain growth and/or tooth movement?
    a. Space maintainer
    b. Retainer
    c. Headgear
    d. All of the above

22. How can a hard piece of candy possibly harm a person's braces?
    a. It can bend a wire.
    b. It can loosen a bracket.
    c. It can pull off a band.
    d. All of the above

23. _____ can make flossing easier for someone wearing braces.
    a. A floss threader
    b. Waxed floss
    c. Unwaxed floss
    d. A toothpick

24. When braces are removed, is orthodontic treatment over?
    a. Yes
    b. No

25. An example of a retention appliance is the _____.
    a. Hawley retainer
    b. positioner
    c. lingual retainer
    d. all of the above

CASE STUDY

Matt is 14 years old and has completed the diagnostic phase for corrective orthodontics. After discussion with his parents and the orthodontist, Matt is anxious to get his braces on to correct crowding in the anterior area and a cross-bite on his left side. He is scheduled today for his first appointment.

1. What diagnostic tools were used to evaluate Matt's case?

2. Discuss the importance of having Matt, his parents, and the orthodontist together when the final decision about having braces is made.

3. What procedure will be completed on Matt today?

4. He should be scheduled for which procedure next time? How long should the appointment last?

5. What is your role in the fitting and cementation of orthodontic bands?

6. After banding, what would be the next procedure to be scheduled?

7. What is the common response to a patient when they ask how long will they have braces?

8. Once the braces are removed, what will Matt wear to make sure everything remains aligned?

MULTIMEDIA PROCEDURES RECOMMENDED REVIEW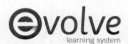

- Placing and Removing Ligature Ties
- Placing and Removing Elastomeric Ties

INTERACTIVE DENTAL OFFICE PATIENT CASE EXERCISE

Access the *Interactive Dental Office* on the *Evolve* website and click on the patient case file for Kevin McClelland.
- Review Kevin's record.
- Complete all exercises on the website for Kevin's case.
- Answer the following questions.

1. On Kevin's panoramic radiograph, which teeth are banded?

2. What types of ligatures are being used for Kevin's orthodontic treatment?

3. The bands have labial hooks. What are they used for?

4. What type of oral hygiene instructions should be provided to Kevin while orthodontic treatment is in progress?

5. Kevin is scheduled to have a sealant placed on tooth #19. Can a sealant be placed while Kevin is receiving orthodontic treatment?

COMPETENCIES 60.1 AND 60.2: PLACING AND REMOVING SEPARATORS (EXPANDED FUNCTION)

Performance Objective

By following a routine procedure that meets stated protocols, the student will demonstrate the proper technique when placing separators.

Evaluation and Grading Criteria

_3_   Student competently met the stated criteria without assistance.

_2_   Student required assistance in order to meet the stated criteria.

_1_   Student showed uncertainty when performing the stated criteria.

_0_   Student was not prepared and needs to repeat the step.

_N/A_   No evaluation of this step.

Instructor shall define grades for each point range earned on completion of each performance-evaluated task.

Performance Standards

The minimum number of satisfactory performances required before final evaluation is _____.

Instructor shall identify by * those steps considered critical. If a step is missed or minimum competency is not met, the evaluated procedure fails and must be repeated.

PERFORMANCE CRITERIA	*	SELF	PEER	INSTRUCTOR	COMMENT
1. Gathered the appropriate setup.					
2. Explained the procedure to the patient.					
3. Placed personal protective equipment according to the procedure.					
4. Carried the separator with the appropriate instrument for placement.					
5. Inserted the separator below the proximal contact.					
6. Recorded in the patient record the number of separators used.					
7. Provided postoperative instructions to the patient.					
8. Maintained patient comfort and followed appropriate infection control measures throughout the procedure.					
9. Documented the procedure in the patient record.					

Continued

Removal of Separators				
1. Used an orthodontic scaler to remove the separator.				
2. Slid the instrument under and continued to remove the separator from the bracket wings.				
3. Documented the procedure in the patient record.				
ADDITIONAL COMMENTS				

Total number of points earned _____

Grade _____ Instructor's initials _____

COMPETENCY 60.3: ASSISTING IN THE FITTING AND CEMENTATION OF ORTHODONTIC BANDS (EXPANDED FUNCTION)

Performance Objective

By following a routine procedure that meets stated protocols, the student will prepare the appropriate setup and will assist in the cementation of orthodontic bands.

Evaluation and Grading Criteria

3	Student competently met the stated criteria without assistance.
2	Student required assistance in order to meet the stated criteria.
1	Student showed uncertainty when performing the stated criteria.
0	Student was not prepared and needs to repeat the step.
N/A	No evaluation of this step.

Instructor shall define grades for each point range earned on completion of each performance-evaluated task.

Performance Standards

The minimum number of satisfactory performances required before final evaluation is _____.

Instructor shall identify by * those steps considered critical. If a step is missed or minimum competency is not met, the evaluated procedure fails and must be repeated.

PERFORMANCE CRITERIA	*	SELF	PEER	INSTRUCTOR	COMMENT
1. Gathered the appropriate setup.					
2. Placed personal protective equipment according to the procedure.					
3. Placed each preselected orthodontic band on a small square of masking tape with the occlusal surface on the tape.					
4. Wiped any buccal tubes or attachments with the lip balm.					
5. Mixed the cement according to the manufacturer's instructions.					
6. Loaded the bands with cement correctly by flowing cement into the band.					
7. Transferred the band correctly.					
8. For a maxillary band, transferred the band pusher.					
9. For a mandibular band, transferred the band seater.					
10. Repeated the process until all bands were cemented.					

Continued

11. Cleaned the cement spatula and slab.				
12. Used a scaler or explorer to remove excess cement on the enamel surfaces and then rinsed the patient's mouth.				
13. Maintained patient comfort and followed appropriate infection control measures throughout the procedure.				
14. Documented the procedure in the patient record.				

ADDITIONAL COMMENTS

Total number of points earned _____

Grade _____ Instructor's initials _____

COMPETENCY 60.4: ASSISTING IN THE DIRECT BONDING OF ORTHODONTIC BRACKETS

Performance Objective

By following a routine procedure that meets stated protocols, the student will prepare the appropriate setup and will assist in the bonding of orthodontic brackets.

Evaluation and Grading Criteria

3   Student competently met the stated criteria without assistance.

2   Student required assistance in order to meet the stated criteria.

1   Student showed uncertainty when performing the stated criteria.

0   Student was not prepared and needs to repeat the step.

N/A   No evaluation of this step.

Instructor shall define grades for each point range earned on completion of each performance-evaluated task.

Performance Standards

The minimum number of satisfactory performances required before final evaluation is _____.

Instructor shall identify by * those steps considered critical. If a step is missed or minimum competency is not met, the evaluated procedure fails and must be repeated.

PERFORMANCE CRITERIA	*	SELF	PEER	INSTRUCTOR	COMMENT
1. Gathered the appropriate setup.					
2. Placed personal protective equipment according to the procedure.					
3. If stain or plaque was present, prepared tooth surfaces using a rubber cup and a pumice slurry.					
4. Isolated the teeth.					
5. Assisted throughout the etching of the teeth.					
6. Applied a small quantity of bonding material on the back of the bracket.					
7. Used bracket placement tweezers to transfer the brackets to the orthodontist.					
8. Transferred an orthodontic scaler for final placement and removal of the excess bonding material.					

Continued

9. Maintained patient comfort and followed appropriate infection control measures throughout the procedure.					
10. Documented the procedure in the patient record.					
ADDITIONAL COMMENTS					

Total number of points earned _____

Grade _____ Instructor's initials _____

COMPETENCIES 60.5 TO 60.7: PLACING AND REMOVING ARCH WIRES AND TIES (EXPANDED FUNCTION)

Performance Objective

By following a routine procedure that meets stated protocols, the student will demonstrate the proper technique for placing and removing ligature wires and elastomeric ties.

Evaluation and Grading Criteria

_3_   Student competently met the stated criteria without assistance.

_2_   Student required assistance in order to meet the stated criteria.

_1_   Student showed uncertainty when performing the stated criteria.

_0_   Student was not prepared and needs to repeat the step.

_N/A_   No evaluation of this step.

Instructor shall define grades for each point range earned on completion of each performance-evaluated task.

Performance Standards

The minimum number of satisfactory performances required before final evaluation is _____.

Instructor shall identify by * those steps considered critical. If a step is missed or minimum competency is not met, the evaluated procedure fails and must be repeated.

PERFORMANCE CRITERIA	*	SELF	PEER	INSTRUCTOR	COMMENT
Placing the Arch Wires					
1. Gathered the appropriate setup.					
2. Placed personal protective equipment according to the procedure.					
3. Premeasured the wire before placing it in patient's mouth.					
4. If additional bends were needed, transferred appropriate pliers to the orthodontist.					
5. Centered the arch wire.					
6. Placed the distal ends of the wire in a buccal tube with correct length.					
Placing the Ligature Wires					
1. Placed the ligature wire around the bracket and used the ligature director to push the wire against the tie wing.					
2. Used the hemostat to twist the wire snugly against the bracket; repeated the procedure until all brackets were ligated.					
3. Used a ligature cutter to cut the excess wire, leaving a 4- to 5-mm pigtail.					

Continued

4. Tucked the pigtails under the arch wire using the correct instruments.				
5. The wire was not protruding to injure the patient.				
Removing the Ligature Wire				
1. Held the ligature cutter properly and used the beaks of the pliers to cut the wire at the easiest access.				
2. Carefully unwrapped the ligature and removed it.				
3. Did not twist or pull as the ligatures were cut and removed.				
4. Continued cutting and removing until all brackets were untied.				
5. Maintained patient comfort and followed appropriate infection control measures throughout the procedure.				
Placing the Elastomeric Tie				
1. Gathered the appropriate setup.				
2. Used a hemostat and placed the beaks of the pliers on a tie; then locked the pliers.				
3. Placed the tie on the gingival portion of one tie wing and slipped the tie around the edges of the bracket.				
4. Released the pliers.				
Removing the Elastomeric Tie				
1. Used the orthodontic scaler held in a pen grasp and supported the teeth and tissue with the other hand.				
2. Placed the scaler tie between the bracket and tie wings and pulled the tie at the gingival position with a rolling motion.				
3. Removed the tie in an occlusal direction.				

4. Maintained patient comfort and followed appropriate infection control measures throughout the procedure.					
5. Documented the procedure in the patient record.					

ADDITIONAL COMMENTS

Total number of points earned _____

Grade _____ Instructor's initials _____

61 Communication in the Dental Office

SHORT-ANSWER QUESTIONS

1. Describe the type of relationship the dental team and their patients should have.

2. Discuss the differences between verbal and non-verbal communications.

3. What is professional phone courtesy?

4. Describe how to handle a difficult patient on the phone.

5. Explain the difference between external marketing and internal marketing.

6. Discuss the types of stress that exist in a dental practice.

7. Discuss what "team" concept can do to improve communication.

FILL-IN-THE-BLANK STATEMENTS

Select the best term from the list below and complete the following statements.

objective fears	subjective fears
salutation	non-verbal communication
letterhead	verbal communication
marketing	word processing software

1. The part of the letter that contains the introductory greeting is the _____.

2. _____ is the type of communication by which we use words to express ourselves.

3. _____ is utilized to create most types of business documents.

4. _____ are learned from a person's memory or experience

5. Feelings, attitudes and concerns developed by the suggestion of others are _____.

6. _____ is the type of communication that uses body language for expression.

7. The _____ is the part of a letter that contains the name and address of the person sending the letter.

8. _____ is a way of advertising or recruiting people to your business.

MULTIPLE-CHOICE QUESTIONS

Complete each question by circling the best answer.

1. What type of communication describes our body language?
   a. Verbal
   b. Written
   c. Nonverbal
   d. Speech

2. What percentage of verbal communication is never heard?
   a. 50%
   b. 75%
   c. 90%
   d. 100%

3. What non-verbal behavior could signify tension and uneasiness in a dental patient?
   a. Body language
   b. Grasping the chair arms
   c. Rapid shallow breathing
   d. All of the above

4. Select a less intimidating term for the word "drill."
   a. Anesthetic
   b. Remove decay
   c. Prepare tooth
   d. b and c

5. How could a patient be psychologically influenced by the attitudes of others?
   a. By subjective fears
   b. By negative fears
   c. By objective fears
   d. all of the above

6. How are objective fears attained?
   a. By hearing others express their experiences
   b. By learning fears from past experiences
   c. By dreaming up fears
   d. By reading about fears

7. The best way to calm an irate patient is to _____ _____.
   a. listen
   b. maintain eye contact
   c. nod your head when the patient is talking
   d. all the above

8. The _____ is the most important item in a dental office used for public relations.
   a. professional letter
   b. fax machine
   c. telephone
   d. newsletter

9. The business telephone should be answered after _____ ring.
   a. the first
   b. the second
   c. the third
   d. any

10. How should telephone messages be obtained when the dental office is closed?
    a. Answering service
    b. Answering machine
    c. Email
    d. a and b

11. Which component is included in the salutation of a letter?
    a. Date
    b. Inside address
    c. Greeting
    d. Closing

12. Besides patients of the practice, who else would the business assistant correspond with?
    a. Other dental professionals
    b. Physicians
    c. Dental insurance companies
    d. All of the above

13. Which dental professional is key in the marketing of a practice because they have first contact with the patient?
    a. Dentist
    b. Business assistant
    c. Dental laboratory technician
    d. Dental assistant

14. What percentage of gross revenue should a dental practice invest in marketing?
    a. 1% to 2%
    b. 3% to 5%
    c. 8% to 10%
    d. 15% to 20%

15. An example of an external marketing activity is _____.
    a. home visits
    b. website
    c. sending flowers
    d. all of the above

16. What is the key to a successful work environment?
    a. High salaries
    b. Teamwork
    c. Good benefits
    d. Job flexibility

17. Which would *not* be a stress factor for someone working in a dental office?
    a. Job flexibility
    b. Overbooking of patients
    c. Performing multiple tasks
    d. No job advancement

18. Which is a valuable communication tool for a dental practice?
    a. Business letter
    b. Practice newsletter
    c. Email
    d. Greeting card

ACTIVITY

Create a professional letter using the following directions:

1. Create a dental practice heading.

2. Compose an introduction in the letter of a new dentist to the practice, how it will affect scheduling, and any changes in staff that will occur.

3. How would you address the letter, and close a letter to your patients.

COMPETENCY 61.1: ANSWERING THE PHONE

Performance Objective

By following a routine procedure that meets stated protocols, the student will demonstrate the proper technique when answering the phone in a place of business.

Evaluation and Grading Criteria

3	Student competently met the stated criteria without assistance.
2	Student required assistance in order to meet the stated criteria.
1	Student showed uncertainty when performing the stated criteria.
0	Student was not prepared and needs to repeat the step.
N/A	No evaluation of this step.

Instructor shall define grades for each point range earned on completion of each performance-evaluated task.

Performance Standards

The minimum number of satisfactory performances required before final evaluation is _____.

Instructor shall identify by * those steps considered critical. If a step is missed or minimum competency is not met, the evaluated procedure fails and must be repeated.

PERFORMANCE CRITERIA	*	SELF	PEER	INSTRUCTOR	COMMENT
1. Answered the phone after the first ring.					
2. Spoke directly into the receiver.					
3. Identified the office and self.					
4. Acknowledged the caller by name.					
5. Followed through on the caller's specific inquiry.					
6. Took a message if appropriate.					
7. Completed the call in a professional manner.					
8. Replaced the receiver after the caller hung up.					
ADDITIONAL COMMENTS					

Total number of points earned _____

Grade _____ Instructor's initials _____

COMPETENCY 61.2: COMPOSING A BUSINESS LETTER

Performance Objective

By following a routine procedure that meets stated protocols, the student will demonstrate the proper technique when composing and typing a professional letter.

Evaluation and Grading Criteria

3	Student competently met the stated criteria without assistance.
2	Student required assistance in order to meet the stated criteria.
1	Student showed uncertainty when performing the stated criteria.
0	Student was not prepared and needs to repeat the step.
N/A	No evaluation of this step.

Instructor shall define grades for each point range earned on completion of each performance-evaluated task.

Performance Standards

The minimum number of satisfactory performances required before final evaluation is _____.

Instructor shall identify by * those steps considered critical. If a step is missed or minimum competency is not met, the evaluated procedure fails and must be repeated.

PERFORMANCE CRITERIA	*	SELF	PEER	INSTRUCTOR	COMMENT
1. Prepared the first draft for review.					
2. Checked for correct information, grammar, spelling, and punctuation.					
3. Ensured that the letter had correct margins, font, spacing, and order of text.					
4. Signed name to close the letter.					

ADDITIONAL COMMENTS

Total number of points earned _____

Grade _____ Instructor's initials _____

62 Business Operating Systems

SHORT-ANSWER QUESTIONS

1. Describe the roles of the office manager and business assistant in a dental office.

2. List three types of practice records or files commonly used in a dental practice.

3. Describe each of the following filing systems: alphabetic, numeric, chronologic, and electronic.

4. Describe the importance of appointment scheduling for maximum productivity.

5. Identify three types of preventive recall systems and give the benefits of each.

6. Compare the functions of computerized practice management systems with manual bookkeeping systems.

7. Describe the importance of managing an inventory system.

FILL-IN-THE-BLANK STATEMENTS

Select the best term from the list below and complete the following statements.

patient of record	filing
warranty	inactive
buffer time	lead time
chronologic file	ledger
units	purchase order
cross-reference file	call list
active	rate of use
outguide	reorder tags
requisition	shelf life
daily schedule	want list

1. The _____ is the estimated period to allow for items shipped and arrival.

2. A(n) _____ patient is one who has been seen within the past 2 to 3 years.

3. A filing system that divides materials into months and days of the month is a(n) _____.

4. The specific time reserved on the schedule for emergency patients is the _____.

5. A patient who has not been seen in the office for the past 5 years is considered _____.

6. A filing system that uses an alphabetic order by name and an assigned number is the _____.

7. A(n) _____ is a list of patients who can come in for an appointment on short notice.

8. A printed schedule of that day's procedures placed throughout the office for viewing by staff is a(n) _____.

9. _____ is the means of classifying and arranging records so that they can be easily retrieved when needed.

10. A(n) _____ is a type of file or statement that contains the patient's financial records.

11. A bookmark for a filing system is called a _____.

12. A written statement that outlines the manufacturer's responsibility for replacement and repair of a product is a(n) _____.

13. A(n) _____ is a form that authorizes the buying of supplies from the supplier.

14. A(n) _____ is one that has been seen by the dentist and has a plan of care.

15. The _____ of an item is the period before it begins to deteriorate and is no longer usable.

16. Time increments used in scheduling appointments are the _____.

17. A(n) _____ is a list of supplies to be ordered.

18. The _____ is the amount of a product used within a given time.

19. A formal request for supplies is a(n) _____.

20. _____ are placed on items when the supplies are close to being low and the items need to be replaced.

MULTIPLE-CHOICE QUESTIONS

Complete each question by circling the best answer.

1. Who oversees the daily financial activities of a dental practice?
   a. Dentist
   b. Clinical assistant
   c. Accountant
   d. Business assistant

2. How would a new employee be introduced to the office protocol?
   a. Instructed to contact the American Dental Association
   b. Through an office procedure and policy manual
   c. By attending a continuing education course
   d. By watching a video

3. What continues to replace the manual work in a dental practice?
   a. A temporary service
   b. A typewriter
   c. A fax machine
   d. A computer

4. Another term used for a "patient statement" is the
   _____.
   a. patient record
   b. ledger
   c. file
   d. document

5. How much free space should remain in a filing cabinet to allow for easier access to documents?
   a. 2 inches
   b. 4 inches
   c. 6 inches
   d. 1 foot

6. What is used to mark a space where a paper file has been removed?
   a. Bookmark
   b. Empty file
   c. Ledger
   d. Outguide

7. What is considered to be the easiest filing system used?
   a. Chronologic
   b. Alphabetic
   c. Numeric
   d. Color-coded

8. If a patient has not been seen within the past 4 years, what is his or her status as a patient of the practice?
   a. Active
   b. On recall
   c. Backorder
   d. Inactive

9. How many minutes commonly make up 1 unit of time for scheduling?
   a. 5 to 7 minutes
   b. 10 to 15 minutes
   c. 20 to 40 minutes
   d. 60 minutes

10. What elements should be outlined in an appointment book?
    a. Office hours
    b. Buffer times
    c. Meetings
    d. All the above

11. If a patient does not keep his or her appointment, where should this event be recorded?
    a. On the ledger
    b. In the patient record
    c. On the daily schedule
    d. b and c

12. What is the normal time frame for scheduling recall appointments?
    a. 3 months
    b. 6 months
    c. 9 months
    d. 1 year

13. If a patient is seen in September, what would be the recall month for a 6-month appointment?
    a. August
    b. September
    c. February
    d. March

14. Which factors are determined when a product must be reordered?
    a. Rate of use
    b. Shelf life
    c. Lead time
    d. All the above

15. How is an item marked for reorder?
    a. Reorder tag
    b. Blue slip
    c. Outguide
    d. Inguide

16. Supplies are ordered _____.
    a. through a sales representative
    b. by telephone/email
    c. online
    d. all of the above

17. What might happen if an item is not available at the time from your regular supply company?
    a. You could be referred to another company.
    b. You call another dental office to see if you could borrow the item.
    c. It goes on backorder.
    d. You are instructed to wait until a new shipment is received.

18. Which is not considered an expendable item?
    a. Handpiece
    b. Plastic suction tip
    c. Patient napkin
    d. Gloves

601

19. If a dental unit is not operational, what is the effect on a dental practice?
    a. Loss of income
    b. Inconvenience to the dental team
    c. Time management
    d. All the above

20. A written statement received from the manufacturer that describes the responsibility of equipment replacement and repair is a _____.
    a. requisition
    b. warranty
    c. contract
    d. a and c

TOPICS FOR DISCUSSION

As the business assistant in the office, your job is to organize and maintain the operating systems of the dental practice. During your weekly team meeting, the dentist has expressed concern about the decline in number of patients being scheduled. Because of this decrease, the revenue of the practice has also fallen.

1. Does the scheduling issue concern the clinical or business staff of the practice?

2. How could the decrease in revenue affect the staff?

3. Describe how the following could increase the number of daily patients who are active patients of the practice.
    a. Scheduling
    b. Recall
    c. Broken appointments
    d. Quality assurance

4. Describe different methods that may be used to increase the number of new patients in the practice.

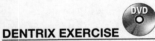

DENTRIX EXERCISE

The Dentrix Appointment Book is an electronic scheduler that allows you to manage your patient appointments without paper. Convenient toolbars and exclusive Flip Tabs help you navigate through appointments, search for available time slots, organize appointments and notes, and handle all the common tasks needed to run the dental office schedule. Please refer to the Dentrix *User's Guide,* Chapter 7, to review how to complete scheduling.

Exercise: Scheduling Appointments

Please refer to the information on the *Evolve* website on **Scheduling Appointments** and **Moving Appointments.** Then complete scheduling for the Brooks family. They would all like to schedule appointments in the third week of February. Listed below are the preferences for each family member, along with the procedures that are to be completed on the day of the appointment.

1. Gregory Brooks (prefers afternoon appointment).
   - Complete examination
   - Four bitewing radiographs
   - Prophylaxis

2. Jessica Brooks (prefers morning appointment).
   - MOD composite resin: Tooth #5
   - DO composite resin: Tooth #7

3. Christopher Brooks (prefers to be scheduled with his mother).
   - Periodic oral examination
   - Two bitewing radiographs
   - Prophylaxis
   - Fluoride treatment

63 Financial Management in the Dental Office

1. Explain why a computerized financial management system is significant for the operation of a dental practice.

2. Describe how financial arrangements of services would be incorporated into a dental practice.

3. Describe the importance and management of collections in the dental office.

4. What is the reason for providing a business summary.

5. Describe payroll withholding taxes and discuss the financial responsibility of the employer regarding these.

6. Discuss the importance of having dental insurance.

7. Identify all parties involved with dental insurance.

8. Identify the various types of prepaid dental programs.

9. Define managed care.

10. Explain dual coverage.

11. Explain the reasons for dental procedures and coding.

12. Give the breakdown of the CDT procedure codes.

FILL-IN-THE-BLANK STATEMENTS

Select the best term from the list below and complete the following statements.

net income
accounts payable
carrier
provider
check
statement
customary
deposit slip
expenses
gross income

invoice
ledger
accounting
petty cash
posting
reasonable
CDT
responsible party
transaction
walkout statement

1. Expenses and disbursements paid out from a business are _____.

2. A(n) _____ is a draft or an order on a bank for payment of a specific amount of money.

3. _____ constitute the overhead that a business needs in order to keep operating.

4. _____ is a system designed to maintain the financial records of a business.

5. A fee that is within the range of the usual fee charged for a service is the _____ fee.

6. A(n) _____ is an itemized list of the funds to be deposited into the bank.

7. A(n) _____ is the insurance company that pays the claims and collects premiums.

8. _____ are procedure codes that are assigned to dental services in the process of dental insurance.

9. _____ is the total of all professional income received.

10. A(n) _____ is an itemized list of goods that specifies the prices and terms of sale.

11. A financial statement that maintains all account transactions of a patient is a(n) _____.

12. _____ is the result of the income minus the expenses.

13. The term used for documenting money transactions within a business is _____.

14. The _____ is the dentist who offers treatment to a patient.

15. The _____ is like a receipt that the patient receives to show account balance.

16. A fee that is considered fair for an extensive or complex treatment is called _____.

17. The person who agrees to pay for an account is the _____.

18. A small amount of money kept on hand for small daily expenses is _____.

19. The _____ is a summary of all charges, payments, credits, and debits for the month.

20. The _____ is a change in payment or an adjustment made to a financial account.

MULTIPLE-CHOICE QUESTIONS

Complete each question by circling the best answer.

1. What type of bookkeeping systems are utilized in a dental practice?
   a. Accounts receivable
   b. Accounts payable
   c. Accounts taxable
   d. a and b

2. What form is used to gather financial information from a patient?
   a. Treatment plan
   b. Consent form
   c. Registration form
   d. Ledger

3. The business assistant should discuss financial arrangements with a patient _____.
   a. in front of the dentist
   b. in the reception area
   c. during the dental exam
   d. in a private area

4. Money that is owed to the practice is considered _____.
   a. accounts payable
   b. revenue
   c. accounts receivable
   d. gross income

5. If a dental office does not have a computerized accounts receivable system, what manual system would be used?
   a. Check register
   b. Posting slip
   c. Pegboard system
   d. Ledger

6. What form is used to transmit a patient's fee for service from the treatment area to the business office?
   a. Receipt
   b. Patient record
   c. Ledger
   d. Charge slip

7. What means of payment could a patient use for his or her account?
   a. Cash
   b. Credit card
   c. Insurance
   d. All the above

8. How often should bank deposits be made?
   a. Daily
   b. Weekly
   c. Monthly
   d. Quarterly

9. A dental office should begin collection efforts on a past due account?
   a. After 15 days
   b. After 30 days
   c. After 60 days
   d. After 90 days

10. How would a business follow through with the collection of fees?
    a. Letters
    b. Phone call
    c. Collection agency
    d. All of the above

11. An example of fixed overhead is _____.
    a. dental supplies
    b. continuing education
    c. salaries
    d. business supplies

12. A paycheck is a person's _____.
    a. gross income
    b. net income
    c. reimbursement
    d. accounts receivable

13. Which document arrives with the shipment of supplies?
    a. Packing slip
    b. Invoice
    c. Statement
    d. All of the above

14. COD means _____.
    a. cancel order delivered
    b. cost of dental service
    c. cash on delivery
    d. cash order delinquent

15. Where would you record check deposits made on an account?
    a. Daily schedule
    b. Check register
    c. Recall system
    d. Patient registration

16. What term indicates that an account does not have enough money to cover a check?
    a. Non-sufficient funds
    b. Bounced
    c. Inadequate funds
    d. Delinquent

17. The method of calculating fee-for-service benefits is
    _____.
    a. UCR
    b. schedule of benefits
    c. fixed fee
    d. all of the above

18. The specified amount of money that an insured person must pay before his or her insurance goes into
    effect is the _____.
    a. overhead
    b. deductible
    c. customary fee
    d. reimbursement fee

19. A child or spouse of an insurance subscriber is considered a(n) _____.
    a. uninsured
    b. copayer
    c. dependent
    d. deductible

20. A patient's insurance information is submitted by means of _____.
    a. a fax
    b. registered mail
    c. a claim form
    d. a table of allowances

ACTIVITY

Complete the insurance form on the next page. Use the information listed on the back of the insurance form on the following page.

Chapter **63** **Financial Management in the Dental Office**

American Dental Association Dental Claim Form

HEADER INFORMATION

1. Type of Transaction (Mark all applicable boxes)

☐ Statement of Actual Services　　☐ Request for Predetermination / Preauthorization

☐ EPSDT / Title XIX

2. Predetermination / Preauthorization Number

INSURANCE COMPANY/DENTAL BENEFIT PLAN INFORMATION

3. Company/Plan Name, Address, City, State, Zip Code

Insurance Company Name
Address 1
Address 2
City　　　　　　　ST　　ZIP

OTHER COVERAGE

4. Other Dental or Medical Coverage?　☐ No (Skip 5-11)　☐ Yes (Complete 5-11)

5. Name of Policyholder/Subscriber in #4 (Last, First, Middle Initial, Suffix)

6. Date of Birth (MM/DD/CCYY)　7. Gender ☐ M ☐ F　8. Policyholder/Subscriber ID (SSN or ID#)

9. Plan/Group Number　10. Patient' s Relationship to Person Named in #5 ☐ Self ☐ Spouse ☐ Dependent ☐ Other

11. Other Insurance Company/Dental Benefit Plan Name, Address, City, State, Zip Code

Other Insurance Company Name
Address
City　　　　　ST　　ZIP

POLICYHOLDER/SUBSCRIBER INFORMATION (For Insurance Company Named in #3)

12. Policyholder/Subscriber Name (Last, First, Middle Initial, Suffix), Address, City, State, Zip Code

Policyholder Name
Address 1
Address 2
City　　　　　　　ST　　　ZIP

13. Date of Birth (MM/DD/CCYY)　14. Gender ☐ M ☐ F　15. Policyholder/Subscriber ID (SSN or ID#)

16. Plan/Group Number　17. Employer Name

PATIENT INFORMATION

18. Relationship to Policyholder/Subscriber in #12 Above ☐ Self ☐ Spouse ☐ Dependent Child ☐ Other　19. Student Status ☐ FTS ☐ PTS

20. Name (Last, First, Middle Initial, Suffix), Address, City, State, Zip Code

Patient Name
Address 1
Address 2
City　　　　　　　ST　　　ZIP

21. Date of Birth (MM/DD/CCYY)　22. Gender ☐ M ☐ F　23. Patient ID/Account # (Assigned by Dentist)

RECORD OF SERVICES PROVIDED

	24. Procedure Date (MM/DD/CCYY)	25. Area of Oral Cavity	26. Tooth System	27. Tooth Number(s) or Letter(s)	28. Tooth Surface	29. Procedure Code	30. Description	31. Fee
1								
2								
3								
4								
5								
6								
7								
8								
9								
10								

MISSING TEETH INFORMATION

34. (Place an 'X' on each missing tooth)

			Permanent														Primary						
1	2	3	4	5	6	7	8	9	10	11	12	13	14	15	16	A	B	C	D	E	F	G	H	I	J
32	31	30	29	28	27	26	25	24	23	22	21	20	19	18	17	T	S	R	Q	P	O	N	M	L	K

32. Other Fee(s)

33. Total Fee　0

35. Remarks

AUTHORIZATIONS

36. I have been informed of the treatment plan and associated fees. I agree to be responsible for all charges for dental services and materials not paid by my dental benefit plan, unless prohibited by law, or the treating dentist or dental practice has a contractual agreement with my plan prohibiting all or a portion of such charges. To the extent permitted by law, I consent to your use and disclosure of my protected health information to carry out payment activities in connection with this claim.

X _____
Patient/Guardian signature　　　　　　　Date

37. I hereby authorize and direct payment of the dental benefits otherwise payable to me, directly to the below named dentist or dental entity.

X _____
Subscriber signature　　　　　　　Date

BILLING DENTIST OR DENTAL ENTITY (Leave blank if dentist or dental entity is not submitting claim on behalf of the patient or insured/subscriber)

48. Name, Address, City, State, Zip Code

Dentist Name
Address 1
Address 2
City　　　　　ST　　ZIP

49. NPI　50. License Number　51. SSN or TIN

52. Phone Number ( ) –　52A. Additional Provider ID

ANCILLARY CLAIM/TREATMENT INFORMATION

38. Place of Treatment ☐ Provider's Office ☐ Hospital ☐ ECF ☐ Other

39. Number of Enclosures (00 to 99) Radiograph(s) Oral Image(s) Model(s)

40. Is Treatment for Orthodontics? ☐ No (Skip 41-42) ☐ Yes (Complete 41-42)

41. Date Appliance Placed (MM/DD/CCYY)

42. Months of Treatment Remaining　43. Replacement of Prosthesis? ☐ No ☐ Yes (Complete 44)　44. Date Prior Placement (MM/DD/CCYY)

45. Treatment Resulting from ☐ Occupational illness/injury ☐ Auto accident ☐ Other accident

46. Date of Accident (MM/DD/CCYY)　47. Auto Accident State

TREATING DENTIST AND TREATMENT LOCATION INFORMATION

53. I hereby certify that the procedures as indicated by date are in progress (for procedures that require multiple visits) or have been completed.

X _____
Signed (Treating Dentist)　　　　　　　Date

54. NPI　55. License Number

56. Address, City, State, Zip Code　56A. Provider Specialty Code

Address
City　　　　　　ST　　　ZIP

57. Phone Number ( ) –　58. Additional Provider ID

Personal Information

Birth Date:	5-22-79
Social Security Number:	402-38-2853
Name:	Jason F. Scott
Address:	8402 Alexander Drive Colorado Springs, CO 39720
Home Phone:	486-555-1847
Employer:	U.S. Olympic Association
Work Phone:	486-555-4910
Responsible Party:	Same as above

Dental Insurance Information

Name of Insured:	Jason F. Scott
Insurance Company:	Dental Support
Group Number:	48204
Employee Certificate Number:	40238285-20
Address:	P.O. Box 313 Denver, CO 13750
Annual Benefits:	1800.00

Treatment to Be Recorded

Date	Tooth and Surface	Treatment	Fee
3/12/20		Periodic Oral Evaluation	75.00
3/12/20		Full Mouth Series	65.00
3/12/20		Oral Prophylaxis	80.00
4/10/20	3 MOD	Amalgam	90.00
4/10/20	4 DO	Amalgam	60.00
5/03/20	10 F	Composite	32.00
5/03/20	11 DI	Composite	64.00
6/10/20	20	Root Canal	700.00
6/20/20	20	PFM Crown	800.00

DENTRIX EXERCISE

The Dentrix Ledger component works just like a paper ledger, only it's faster, easier, and more powerful. The main Ledger screen packs a wealth of information in an easy-to-read format, making it possible to find necessary information without toggling among endless screens and menus. The Ledger facilitates entry of payments, claim filing, statement printouts, and much more—all from a single location.

Exercise: Patient Checkout Procedures

Please refer to the information on the *Evolve* website on **Creating a Pretreatment Estimate, Generating a Payment Agreement, Posting Scheduled Work,** and **Completing a Patient Checkout.** Then complete the following procedures for the Brooks family.

1. Pretreatment Estimate
   - Create a pretreatment estimate for Gregory Brooks.
   - Create a pretreatment estimate for Jessica Brooks.
   - Create a pretreatment estimate for Christopher Brooks.

   a. What is the total estimated charge for each patient?

   b. What is the estimated insurance payment for each patient?

   c. What is the total out-of-pocket payment for the Brooks family?

2. Payment Agreement
   - Complete a Payment Agreement for Gregory Brooks.
   - Print a Truth in Lending Disclosure Statement for Gregory Brooks.
   - Print a Coupon Book for Scheduled Payments.

3. Patient Checkout
   - The Brooks family has completed their treatment.

   a. Post the procedures attached to Gregory Brooks' appointment to show that they have been completed.
   b. Print the Insurance Claim for Gregory Brooks.
   c. Print a Walkout Statement for Gregory Brooks.

64 Marketing Your Skills

SHORT-ANSWER QUESTIONS

1. What are your career goals?

2. Identify potential career opportunities.

3. Describe how to prepare for a job interview.

4. Discuss factors to consider when negotiating salary.

5. List the elements of an employment agreement.

6. Describe the steps taken to achieve career objectives.

7. Describe the steps that lead to job termination.

FILL-IN-THE-BLANK STATEMENTS

Select the best term from the list below and complete the following statements.

termination   **career**
employment   **professional**
interview   **resume**

1. A(n) _____ is a formal meeting held in person to assess the qualifications of an applicant.

2. _____ is the end of an employee's contract.

3. A profession or occupation is one's _____.

4. A(n) _____ is the term used to describe a person who conforms to the standards of his or her job.

5. A(n) _____ is a written description of one's professional or work experience and qualifications.

6. A day-to-day job or service performed on a routine basis is one's _____.

MULTIPLE-CHOICE QUESTIONS

Complete each question by circling the best answer.

1. Which employment opportunity could a dental assistant not apply for?
   a. Teaching
   b. Sales
   c. Dental hygiene
   d. Insurance

2. Where might you find a dental assisting job position advertised?
   a. Online Advertisment
   b. Dental assisting program
   c. Dental society newsletter
   d. All of the above

3. A cover letter _____.
   a. provides your educational background
   b. describes your past work experience
   c. gives a list of references
   d. introduces you

4. What should not be included in a resume?
   a. Marital status
   b. Race
   c. Religion
   d. All of the above

5. How long should a resume be?
   a. One paragraph
   b. One page
   c. Two pages
   d. It does not matter.

6. The most critical part of an interview is the _____.
   a. closing remarks
   b. salary discussion
   c. first 10 minutes
   d. follow-up

7. Termination without notice should be handled in accordance with _____.
   a. your job description
   b. ADA
   c. your employment agreement
   d. application form

8. What is the most important factor in achieving professional success?
   a. The amount of money you make
   b. Liking the people you work with
   c. Having a positive attitude
   d. Your professional title

9. What time frame is routinely considered interim employment?
   a. 1 week
   b. 1 month
   c. 3 months
   d. 1 year

ACTIVITIES

1. Prepare a cover letter to be used for seeking employment.

2. Prepare a resume to be used for seeking employment.

3. Prepare a follow-up letter to be used after an interview.

COMPETENCY 64.1: PREPARING A PROFESSIONAL RÉSUMÉ

Performance Objective

By following a routine procedure that meets stated protocols, and given a computer, printer, and paper, the student will prepare a one-page resume.

Evaluation and Grading Criteria

3   Student competently met the stated criteria without assistance.

2   Student required assistance in order to meet the stated criteria.

1   Student showed uncertainty when performing the stated criteria.

0   Student was not prepared and needs to repeat the step.

N/A   No evaluation of this step.

Instructor shall define grades for each point range earned on completion of each performance-evaluated task.

Performance Standards

The minimum number of satisfactory performances required before final evaluation is _____.

Instructor shall identify by * those steps considered critical. If a step is missed or minimum competency is not met, the evaluated procedure fails and must be repeated.

PERFORMANCE CRITERIA	*	SELF	PEER	INSTRUCTOR	COMMENT
1. Used common typefaces.					
2. Used a 10-, 12-, or 14-point font size.					
3. Used 1-inch margins on all sides.					
4. Resume was one page in length.					
5. Resume was neat and error-free.					
6. Resume was concise and easy to read.					
ADDITIONAL COMMENTS					

Total number of points earned _____

Grade _____ Instructor's initials _____

Dental Assisting Clinical Externship Guide

I. The clinical externship for the dental assisting student is an integral part of the dental assisting program. Your externship is designed to allow you to gain proficiency in the general, specialty, and expanded dental assisting functions from the knowledge and skills acquired in the classroom, preclinical, and laboratory settings. The specific guidelines you as a dental assisting student must adhere to are as follows: You will be assigned to _____ (#) clinical rotations. A rotation can take place within a general dental practice, group dental practice, specialty practice, public health facility, or dental school clinic.
- A dental assisting faculty member, along with an identified staff member within the setting, will supervise and evaluate your clinical experience.
- A formal agreement between the dental assisting program and the facility providing the experience has been reviewed and accepted.

II. The major portion of your time in your clinical assignment is chairside assisting in patient care.

III. You must maintain the following records of the activities in rotations; forms of these records are included later in the section:
- Attendance logs about assigned clinical rotations.
- Time-sheets: You must complete a minimum of _____ hours of clinical experience.
- List of clinical activities to be completed.
- Student journal.

IV. A dental assisting faculty member will be assigned to your externship and will visit to assess your progress.

V. A seminar class is a component of your externship and will be held weekly for discussion of your clinical experience.

VI. Competency evaluation forms are utilized by the faculty and office/clinical personnel to evaluate your performance in the following areas (refer to specific competencies in the MDA workbook):
   A. Patient information and assessment
   B. Infection control
   C. Radiology
   D. General dental procedures
   E. Specialty dental procedures
   F. Expanded function procedures
   G. Business procedures

Externship Site: _____

Date of Externship: _____

Address: _____

_____

Phone: _____

Contact Person: _____

Externship Site: _____

Date of Externship: _____

Address: _____

Phone: _____

Contact Person: _____

Externship Site: _____

Date of Externship: _____

Address: _____

Phone: _____

Contact Person: _____

TIME SHEET FOR CLINICAL EXTERNSHIP

Student Name: _____

Externship Site: _____

A completed and signed form is to be maintained in the externship folder and submitted.

Week 1	Date	Total Hours Present	Comments	Evaluator Initials
Monday				
Tuesday				
Wednesday				
Thursday				
Friday				
Week 2	**Date**	**Total Hours Present**	**Comments**	**Evaluator Initials**
Monday				
Tuesday				
Wednesday				
Thursday				
Friday				
Week 3	**Date**	**Total Hours Present**	**Comments**	**Evaluator Initials**
Monday				
Tuesday				
Wednesday				
Thursday				
Friday				
Week 4	**Date**	**Total Hours Present**	**Comments**	**Evaluator Initials**
Monday				
Tuesday				
Wednesday				
Thursday				
Friday				

TIME SHEET FOR CLINICAL EXTERNSHIP

Student Name: _____

Externship Site: _____

A completed and signed form is to be maintained in the externship folder and submitted.

Week 1	Date	Total Hours Present	Comments	Evaluator Initials
Monday				
Tuesday				
Wednesday				
Thursday				
Friday				
Week 2	Date	Total Hours Present	Comments	Evaluator Initials
Monday				
Tuesday				
Wednesday				
Thursday				
Friday				
Week 3	Date	Total Hours Present	Comments	Evaluator Initials
Monday				
Tuesday				
Wednesday				
Thursday				
Friday				
Week 4	Date	Total Hours Present	Comments	Evaluator Initials
Monday				
Tuesday				
Wednesday				
Thursday				
Friday				

TIME SHEET FOR CLINICAL EXTERNSHIP

Student Name: _____

Externship Site: _____

A completed and signed form is to be maintained in the externship folder and submitted.

Week 1	Date	Total Hours Present	Comments	Evaluator Initials
Monday				
Tuesday				
Wednesday				
Thursday				
Friday				
Week 2	Date	Total Hours Present	Comments	Evaluator Initials
Monday				
Tuesday				
Wednesday				
Thursday				
Friday				
Week 3	Date	Total Hours Present	Comments	Evaluator Initials
Monday				
Tuesday				
Wednesday				
Thursday				
Friday				
Week 4	Date	Total Hours Present	Comments	Evaluator Initials
Monday				
Tuesday				
Wednesday				
Thursday				
Friday				

DENTAL ASSISTING STUDENT RECORD OF CLINICAL ACTIVITIES

Below is a list of advanced functions that you will either assist in or perform. Use this form as a record of your experiences. When you are to be evaluated, use the evaluation form provided by your program. Enter the date and any additional notes or comments in this record, which will provide an organized log of your clinical activities.

Clinical Procedure	Date	Notes/Comments
Patient Information and Assessment		
Register a New Patient		
Obtain Medical/Dental Health History		
Take Vital Signs		
Chart Teeth		
Assist in Periodontal Screening Exam		
Infection Control		
Place PPE		
Perform a Surgical Scrub		
Perform Sterile Gloving		
Disinfect an Impression		
Place/Remove Surface Barriers		
Clean/Disinfect a Treatment Room		
Operate the Ultrasonic		
Use an Autoclave		
Use Chemical Vapor		
Use a Dry Heat Sterilizer		
Use Liquid Sterilant		
Perform Biologic Monitoring		
Sterilize a Handpiece		
Create a Label for a Secondary Container		
Test a Dental Unit		
Radiology		
Process Dental Films Manually		
Process Dental Films in an Automatic Film Processor		
Perform a Full-Mouth Survey Using the Paralleling Technique		
Perform a Full-Mouth Survey Using the Bisecting Technique		
Perform Bitewing Survey		
Perform Occlusal Survey		
Take a Panoramic Image		
Take a Cephalometric Image		

Continued

Dental Assisting Clinical Externship Guide

Clinical Procedure	Date	Notes/Comments
General Dental Procedures		
Assist with Class I Restoration		
Assist with Class II Restoration		
Assist with Class III/IV Restoration		
Assist with Class V Restoration		
Assist with Placement of a Veneer		
Specialty Dental Procedures		
Assist with Crown and Bridge		
Assist with Partial Denture		
Assist with Full Denture		
Assist with Endosteal Implant Surgery		
Assist in Pulp Vitality Test		
Assist with Root Canal Therapy		
Assist with Gingivectomy/Gingivoplasty		
Assist with an Extraction		
Assist with an Impaction		
Assist with Alveolitis		
Assist in Cementation of Orthodontic Bands		
Assist in Bonding of Orthodontic Brackets		
Expanded Functions		
Take Pulse Oximetry		
Take ECG		
Take Extraoral/Intraoral Photographs		
Perform Soft Tissue Exam		
Perform Caries Detection		
Perform Caries Risk Assessment		
Perform Coronal Polishing		
Place Sealants		
Apply Calcium Hydroxide		
Apply Liners		
Apply Base		
Apply Etchant		
Apply a Bonding System		
Place a Matrix Band		
Place Intermediate Restoration		
Take Preliminary Impression		
Take Final Impressions		
Take Bite Registration		
Take Face Bow Registration		

Clinical Procedure	Date	Notes/Comments
Place a Gingival Retraction Cord		
Construct and Cement a Provisional		
Remove Cement		
Repair Fractured Prosthesis		
Place Periodontal Dressing		
Remove Sutures		
Place Separators		
Place Arch Wires		
Place Ligature Ties		
Business Procedures		
Answer the Phone		
Prepare a Business Letter		
Prepare a Resume		

Student Signature: _____

Dental Assisting Supervisor Signature: _____

Dental Assisting Program: _____

To optimize your personal clinical experiences, you will keep a journal to record your personal objectives (specific goals) and learning experiences throughout the externship. Your journal is to be maintained in a small notepad and carried to the externship daily.

Description

1. Daily/weekly, write down a personal objective that you would like to meet.
2. At the end of that time, record your experiences in your journal.
3. Explain whether you were able to meet your personal learning objective.
4. Discuss whether you would do the same thing or something different to ensure you met your objective if you could repeat the experience.
5. At the end of the externship, write a reflection on the total experience as a final entry in your journal.

Examples of personal goals can include, but are not limited to the following:

- Expectations of your role
- Organization of the office
- Prioritization of the workday
- Communication and interaction with patients
- Communication and interaction with staff
- Delegation of duties

Dental Assisting Program: _____

Student Name: _____